KAPLAN & SADOCK'S POCKET HANDBOOK OF **PSYCHIATRIC DRUG TREATMENT**

Seventh Edition

CONSULTING EDITOR

SAMOON AHMAD, M.D.

Associate Professor and Attending Physician
Department of Psychiatry
NYU School of Medicine
New York, New York

KAPLAN & SADOCK'S POCKET HANDBOOK OF PSYCHIATRIC DRUG TREATMENT

Seventh Edition

BENJAMIN J. SADOCK, M.D.

Menas S. Gregory Professor of Psychiatry
Department of Psychiatry, New York University School of Medicine
Attending Psychiatrist, Tisch Hospital
Attending Psychiatrist, Bellevue Hospital Center
New York, New York

NORMAN SUSSMAN, M.D.

Professor of Psychiatry, Department of Psychiatry
New York University School of Medicine
New York, New York

VIRGINIA A. SADOCK, M.D.

Professor of Psychiatry, Department of Psychiatry
New York University School of Medicine
Attending Psychiatrist, Tisch Hospital
Attending Psychiatrist, Bellevue Hospital Center
New York, New York

🌐. Wolters Kluwer

Philadelphia • Baltimore • New York • London
Buenos Aires • Hong Kong • Sydney • Tokyo

Acquisitions Editor: Chris Teja
Development Editor: Ashley Fischer
Editorial Coordinator: Alexis Pozonsky
Marketing Manager: Rachel Mante-Leung
Production Project Manager: Bridgett Dougherty
Design Coordinator: Teresa Mallon
Manufacturing Coordinator: Beth Welsh
Prepress Vendor: Aptara, Inc.

7th edition

Library of Congress Cataloging-in-Publication Data

Names: Sadock, Benjamin J., 1933- author. | Sussman, Norman, author. |
  Sadock, Virginia A., author.
Title: Kaplan & Sadock's pocket handbook of psychiatric drug treatment /
  Benjamin J. Sadock, Norman Sussman, Virginia A. Sadock.
Other titles: Kaplan and Sadock's pocket handbook of psychiatric drug
  treatment | Pocket handbook of psychiatric drug treatment
Description: Seventh edition. | Philadelphia : Wolters Kluwer, [2019] |
  Includes bibliographical references and index.
Identifiers: LCCN 2017055311 | ISBN 9781496389589 (alk. paper)
Subjects: | MESH: Mental Disorders–drug therapy | Psychotropic
  Drugs–therapeutic use | Handbooks
Classification: LCC RC483 | NLM WM 34 | DDC 616.89/18—dc23
  LC record available at https://lccn.loc.gov/2017055311

LWW.com

Dedicated
to our children
James and Victoria
and to our grandchildren
Celia, Emily, Oliver, and Joel
B.J.S.
V.A.S.

Dedicated
to my wife Susan
and my children
Rebecca and Zachary
N.S.

Preface

This is the seventh edition of *Kaplan & Sadock's Pocket Handbook of Psychiatric Drug Treatment*, the first of which was published almost 25 years ago. During that time, a revolution in the treatment of mental illness occurred, sparked by the introduction of psychotropic drugs. This book has kept up with that revolution and contains information about every drug used in the treatment of mental illness. It has served the needs of many professionals who provide care for the mentally ill—psychiatrists and nonpsychiatric physicians, psychiatric residents, medical students, clinical psychologists, psychiatric nurses, and others.

GOALS OF THIS BOOK

This book covers the entire spectrum of psychiatric drug therapy used in the clinical practice of psychiatry. As with each new edition, every section has been updated and revised and new sections added. Many drugs approved by the FDA as treatments for psychiatric disorders have been found to have benefits beyond those recognized at the time of their initial marketing, thus expanding the range of disorders that can be treated. Some have also been found to have unanticipated risks. These developments serve to emphasize the importance of having updated information about drug selection and use that reflects both research data and clinical experience. The goals of this book are to present this information clearly and concisely.

ORGANIZATION OF THIS BOOK

Following the format of previous editions, whenever possible, we classify drugs according to their pharmacological activity and mechanism of action rather than using such categories as antidepressants, antipsychotics, anxiolytics, and mood stabilizers which are overly broad. For example, many antidepressant drugs are used to treat anxiety disorders; some anxiolytics are used to treat depression and bipolar disorders; and drugs from all categories are used to treat other conditions such as eating disorders and impulse control disorders to name but two. This organization is used in textbooks of pharmacology and we believe psychopharmacology should follow that organization as much as possible, given the current state of our knowledge.

HOW TO USE THIS BOOK

At the beginning of the book, the reader will find a chart (Table A) that lists each and every drug and the chapter in which it is found. In addition, the index lists each drug separately under its generic and brand name and the page number on which it can be found. Each section provides a wealth of data that includes (1) the drug's chemical name; (2) preparation and dosages; (3) pharmacologic actions including its pharmacokinetics and pharmacodynamics; (4) the indications for use and clinical applications; (5) use in children, elderly persons, and pregnant and nursing women; (6) side effects and adverse and allergic reactions; and (7) drug–drug interactions.

NUTRITIONAL SUPPLEMENTS

We continue to include an updated chapter covering nutritional supplements as well as herb and plant preparations with psychoactive properties because their use is increasing. Many persons medicate themselves with these compounds and while some may be beneficial, no standards of use have been developed; however, many are being evaluated under the auspices of the National Center for Complementary and Alternative Medicine (NCCAM). Clinicians must be alert to the possibility of adverse effects of these agents in addition to their interactions with prescribed psychotropic medications.

DRUGS USED IN THE TREATMENT OF OBESITY

We include a chapter on drugs used to treat obesity for two reasons: Many psychotropic drugs influence metabolism in such a way that significant weight gain occurs as a side effect; and obesity, now classified as a disease by the American Medical Association, occurs in conjunction with many psychiatric disorders and psychiatrists have a role to play in its management.

MEDICATION-INDUCED MOVEMENT DISORDERS

Movement disorders are commonly associated with the use of potent psychotropic medications and for that reason a special chapter has been devoted to this topic. Some movement disorders, such as neuroleptic-induced tardive dyskinesia can be potentially disabling and others such as neuroleptic malignant syndrome can be life threatening. Psychiatrists must know which drugs are associated with these effects and must remain vigilant when these drugs are prescribed. This new section will be very helpful to clinicians in this regard.

Acknowledgments

We want to thank our assistants, especially Heidiann Grech, who worked on this and other books of ours. We also wish to thank James Sadock, M.D. and Victoria Sadock Gregg, M.D., both emergency physicians, for their help. Rebecca Sussman, M.D. and Zachary Sussman were also of great help and deserve thanks. We also extend our deepest thanks to Samoon Ahmad, M.D., whose expertise in psychopharmacology was of invaluable help to the authors.

Finally, we extend our thanks to Charles Marmar, M.D., Chairman of the Department of Psychiatry at New York School of Medicine, whose support and encouragement of all our academic accomplishments are highly appreciated.

Contents

Table A
Index to Book by Generic Name of Drug

(continued)

Table A—*continued*
Index to Book by Generic Name of Drug

Table A—*continued*
Index to Book by Generic Name of Drug

(continued)

Table A—*continued*
Index to Book by Generic Name of Drug

Table A—*continued*
Index to Book by Generic Name of Drug

[a]No longer manufactured.

General Principles of Psychopharmacology

INTRODUCTION

There are three general terms, used interchangeably, that describe drugs that treat psychiatric disorders—psychotropic drugs, psychoactive drugs, and psychotherapeutic drugs. Traditionally, these agents have been divided into the following four categories: (1) antipsychotic drugs or neuroleptics used to treat psychosis, (2) antidepressant drugs used to treat depression, (3) antimanic drugs or mood stabilizers used to treat bipolar disorder, and (4) antianxiety drugs or anxiolytics used to treat anxious states (which are also effective as hypnotics in high dosages). Such categoric distinctions, however, have become less valid for the following reasons:

1. Many drugs of one class are used to treat disorders previously assigned to another class. For example, most antidepressant drugs are now also used to treat a broad range of anxiety disorders.
2. Drugs introduced as treatments for schizophrenia, agents such as the second-generation antipsychotics (SGAs), are also indicated for the management of bipolar disorder and appear to have some antidepressant activity.
3. Drugs from all four categories are used to treat symptoms and disorders such as insomnia, eating disorders, behavioral disturbances associated with dementia, and impulse-control disorders.
4. Drugs such as clonidine (Catapres), propranolol (Inderal), verapamil (Isoptin), modafinil (Provigil), and gabapentin (Neurontin) can effectively treat a variety of psychiatric disorders and do not fit easily into the traditional classification of drugs.
5. Some descriptive psychopharmacologic terms are arbitrary and overlap in meaning. For example, anxiolytics decrease anxiety, sedatives produce a calming or relaxing effect, and hypnotics produce sleep. However, most anxiolytics function as sedatives and at high doses can be used as hypnotics, and all hypnotics at low doses can be used for daytime sedation.

CLASSIFICATION

This book uses a classification in which each drug is discussed according to its pharmacologic category. Each drug is described in terms of its pharmacologic actions, including pharmacodynamics and pharmacokinetics. Indications, contraindications, drug–drug interactions, and adverse side effects are also discussed.

Table A (see p. xi) lists each psychotherapeutic drug according to its generic name, trade name, and chapter title and number in which it is discussed.

PHARMACOLOGIC ACTIONS

The main determinants of the clinical effects of a drug on an individual are determined by its pharmacokinetic and pharmacodynamic properties. In simple terms, pharmacokinetics describes *what the body does to the drug,* and pharmacodynamics describes *what the drug does to the body.* Pharmacokinetic data trace the *absorption, distribution, metabolism,* and *excretion* of the drug in the body. Pharmacodynamic data measure the *effects* of the drug on cells in the brain and other tissues of the body.

Pharmacokinetics

Absorption.   Drugs reach the brain through the bloodstream. Orally administered drugs dissolve in the fluid of the gastrointestinal (GI) tract—depending on their lipid solubility and the GI tract's local pH, motility, and surface area—and are then absorbed into the blood.

Stomach acidity may be reduced by proton pump inhibitors, such as omeprazole (Prilosec), esomeprazole (Nexium), and lansoprazole (Prevacid); by histamine H_2 receptor blockers, such as cimetidine (Tagamet), famotidine (Pepcid), nizatidine (Axid), and ranitidine (Zantac); or by antacids. Gastric and intestinal motility may be either slowed by anticholinergic drugs or increased by dopamine receptor antagonists (DRAs), such as metoclopramide (Reglan). Food can also increase or decrease the rate and degree of drug absorption.

As a rule, parenteral administration can achieve therapeutic plasma concentrations more rapidly than can oral administration. However, some drugs are deliberately emulsified in an insoluble carrier matrix for intramuscular (IM) administration, which results in the drug's gradual release over several weeks. These formulations are called *depot* preparations. Intravenous (IV) administration is the quickest route for achieving therapeutic blood concentrations, but it also carries the highest risk of sudden and life-threatening adverse effects.

Distribution and Bioavailability.   Drugs that circulate bound to plasma proteins are called *protein bound,* and those that circulate unbound are called *free.* Only the free fraction can pass through the blood–brain barrier.

The *distribution* of a drug to the brain is governed by the brain's regional blood flow, the blood–brain barrier, and the drug's affinity with its receptors in the brain. High cerebral blood flow, high lipid solubility, and high receptor affinity promote the therapeutic actions of the drug.

A drug's *volume of distribution* is a measure of the apparent space in the body available to contain the drug, which can vary with age, sex, adipose tissue content, and disease state. A drug that is very lipid soluble, such as diazepam (Valium), and thus is extensively distributed in adipose tissue, may have a short duration of clinical activity despite a very long elimination half-life.

Bioavailability refers to the fraction of the total amount of administered drug that can subsequently be recovered from the bloodstream. Bioavailability is an important variable because the U.S. Food and Drug Administration (FDA) regulations specify that the bioavailability of a generic formulation can differ from that of the brand-name formulation by no more than 30%.

Metabolism and Excretion

Metabolic Routes.   The four major metabolic routes for drugs are *oxidation, reduction, hydrolysis,* and *conjugation.* Metabolism usually yields inactive metabolites that are readily excreted. However, metabolism also transforms many inactive prodrugs into therapeutically active metabolites.

The liver is the principal site of *metabolism,* and bile, feces, and urine are the major routes of *excretion.* Psychotherapeutic drugs can also be excreted in sweat, saliva, tears, and breast milk.

Quantification of Metabolism and Excretion. Four important parameters regarding metabolism and excretion are time of *peak plasma concentration, half-life, first-pass effect,* and *clearance.*

The time between the administration of a drug and the appearance of *peak plasma concentrations* varies according to the route of administration and rate of absorption.

A drug's *half-life* is the amount of time it takes for metabolism and excretion to reduce a particular plasma concentration by half. This is not the same as duration of action. The clinical effects of a drug may persist long after a drug has been cleared from the body. A drug administered steadily at time intervals shorter than its half-life will reach 97% of its steady-state plasma concentration after five half-lives.

The *first-pass effect* refers to the initial metabolism of orally administered drugs within the portal circulation of the liver, and is described as the fraction of absorbed drug reaching the systemic circulation unmetabolized.

Clearance is a measure of the amount of the drug excreted from the body in a specific period of time.

Pharmacogenomic Testing

Pharmacogenetics research is attempting to identify the role of genetics in drug response.

Several companies now offer pharmacogenetic testing, though psychiatrists have not yet incorporated this into daily practice. This is due to questionable clinical relevance; absence of recommendation by the FDA and lack of endorsement by any expert panels. Insurance also may not cover the cost of testing.

In theory pharmacodynamics gene testing of the serotonin transporter (SLC6A4) may help predict response and adverse effects of selective serotonin reuptake inhibitor (SSRI) and serotonin–norepinephrine reuptake inhibitor (SNRI) antidepressants. Another serotonin receptor 2C ($5-HT_{2C}$) mutation may predict weight gain with atypical antipsychotics. The pharmacokinetic genes, discussed below, CYP450 (CYP1A2, CYP2B6, CYP2C9, CYP2C19, CYP2D6, CYP3A4/5), may predict rate of metabolism of medications and predict dose adjustment. Despite the limitations and clinical utility of pharmacogenomic testing, psychiatrists should familiarize themselves with genetic terminology, genes and alleles affecting various psychotropic medications as well as understanding metabolizing factors that may impact the use of psychotropic medicines and inform the patients about potential issues and individualizing treatment choices.

Drug Selection

Although all FDA-approved psychotropics are similar in overall effectiveness for their indicated disorder, they differ considerably in their pharmacology and in their efficacy and adverse effects on individual patients. The ability of a drug to prove effective, thus, is only partially predictable and is dependent on poorly understood patient variables. Nevertheless, it is possible that some drugs have a niche in which they can be uniquely helpful for a subgroup of patients, without demonstrating any overall superiority in efficacy. No drug is universally effective, and no evidence indicates the unambiguous superiority of any single agent as a treatment for any major psychiatric disorders. The only exception, clozapine (Clozaril), has been approved by the FDA as a treatment for cases of treatment-refractory schizophrenia.

Cytochrome P450 Enzymes.   The cytochrome P450 (CYP) enzyme system is responsible for the inactivation of most psychotherapeutic drugs. It is so named because the heme-containing enzymes strongly absorb light at a wavelength of 450 nm. Although present throughout the body, these enzymes act primarily in the endoplasmic reticulum of the hepatocytes and the cells of the intestine. Therefore, cellular pathophysiology, such as that caused by viral hepatitis or cirrhosis, may affect the efficiency of drug metabolism by the CYP enzymes.

The human CYP enzymes comprise several distinct families and subfamilies. In the CYP nomenclature, the family is denoted by a numeral, the subfamily by a capital letter, and the individual member of the subfamily by a second numeral (e.g., 2D6). Persons with genetic polymorphisms in the CYP genes that encode inefficient versions of CYP enzymes are considered *poor metabolizers.*

There are two mechanistic processes involving the CYP system: induction and inhibition (Table 1–1).

Induction.   Expression of the CYP genes may be induced by alcohol, certain drugs (barbiturates, anticonvulsants), or smoking. For example, an inducer of CYP3A4, such as cimetidine, may increase the metabolism and decrease the plasma concentrations of a substrate of 3A4, such as alprazolam (Xanax).

Inhibition.   Certain drugs are not substrates for a particular enzyme but may nonetheless indirectly inhibit the enzyme and slow its metabolism of other drug substrates. For example, concurrent administration of a CYP2D6 inhibitor, such as fluoxetine (Prozac), may inhibit the metabolism and thus raise the plasma concentrations of CYP2D6 substrates, including amitriptyline (Elavil). If one CYP enzyme is inhibited, then its substrate accumulates until it is metabolized by an alternate CYP enzyme. Table 1–2 lists representative psychotropic drug substrates of human CYPs along with representative inhibitors.

Table 1–1
Comparison of Metabolic Inhibition and Metabolic Induction

	Inhibition	Induction
Mechanism	Direct chemical effect on existing enzyme	Increased synthesis of metabolizing enzyme
Immediate exposure needed	Yes	No
Prior exposure needed	No	Yes
Rate of onset	Rapid	Slow
Rate of offset	Rapid	Slow
In vitro study	Straightforward (cell homogenates)	Difficult (requires intact cells in culture)

Table 1-2
Representative Psychotropic Drug Substrates of Human Cytochrome P450's Along with Representative Inhibitors

CYP3A	CYP2D6	CYP2C19
Substrates	Substrates	Substrates
Triazolam (Halcion)	Desipramine (Norpramin)	Diazepam^a
Alprazolam (Xanax)	Nortriptyline (Aventyl)	Amitriptyline^a
Midazolam (Versed)	Paroxetine (Paxil)	Citalopram^a
Quetiapine (Seroquel)	Venlafaxine (Effexor)	Inhibitors
Nefazodone (Serzone)	Tramadol (Ultram)	Fluvoxamine
Buspirone (BuSpar)	Fluoxetine^a (Prozac)	Omeprazole (Prilosec)
Trazodone (Desyrel)	Citalopram^a	
Ramelteon (Rozerem)	Inhibitors	
Zolpidem^a (Ambien)	Quinidine (Cardioquin)	
Amitriptyline^a (Endep)	Fluoxetine	
Imipramine^a (Tofranil)	Paroxetine	
Haloperidol^a (Haldol)	Bupropion (Wellbutrin, Zyban)	
Citalopram^a (Celexa)	Terbinafine (Lamisil)	
Clozapine^a (Clozaril)	Diphenhydramine (Benadryl)	
Diazepam^a (Valium)		
Inhibitors		
Ritonavir (Norvir)		
Ketoconazole (Nizoral)		
Itraconazole (Sporanox)		
Nefazodone		
Fluvoxamine (Luvox)		
Erythromycin (E-Mycin)		
Clarithromycin (Biaxin)		

^{a}Partial substrate.

Pharmacodynamics

The major pharmacodynamic considerations include *molecular site of action*; the *dose–response curve*; the therapeutic index; and the development of tolerance, dependence, and withdrawal symptoms.

Molecular Site of Action. Psychotropic drugs may act at any of several molecular sites in brain cells. Some activate (agonists) or inactivate (antagonists) receptors for a specific neurotransmitter. Other drugs, particularly antidepressant drugs, bind to and block transporters that normally take up serotonin or norepinephrine from the synaptic cleft into the presynaptic nerve ending (reuptake inhibitors).

Some drugs block the passage of cations or anions through ion channels embedded in cellular membranes (channel inhibitors or blockers). Other drugs bind to and inhibit catabolic enzymes that normally inactivate neurotransmitters, thereby prolonging the life span of the active neurotransmitters (e.g., monoamine oxidase inhibitors [MAOIs]). Finally, several drugs have numerous molecular sites of action, although the sites that are therapeutically relevant may remain unknown.

Dose–Response Curves. The dosage–response curve plots the clinical response to the drug as a function of drug concentration (Fig. 1–1). *Potency* refers to comparisons of the dosages of different drugs required to achieve a certain effect. For example, haloperidol (Haldol) is more potent than chlorpromazine (Thorazine) because about 2 mg of haloperidol is required to achieve the same therapeutic effect as

Examples of Dose–Response Curves

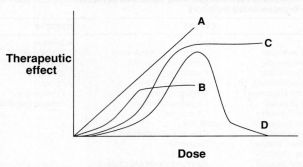

Figure 1-1. The dosage–response curves plot the therapeutic effect as a function of increasing dose, often calculated as the log of the dose. Drug A has a linear dosage response, drugs B and C have sigmoidal curves, and drug D has a curvilinear dosage–response curve. Although smaller doses of drug B are more potent than are equal doses of drug C, drug C has a higher maximum efficacy than does drug B. Drug D has a therapeutic window such that both low and high doses are less effective than midrange doses.

100 mg of chlorpromazine. However, haloperidol and chlorpromazine are equal in their *clinical efficacy*—that is, the maximum achievable clinical response.

Therapeutic Index.   The *therapeutic index* is a relative measure of a drug's toxicity or safety. It is defined as the ratio of the median toxic dosage (TD_{50})—the dosage at which 50% of persons experience toxic effects—to the median effective dosage (ED_{50})—the dosage at which 50% of persons experience therapeutic effects. For example, haloperidol has a high therapeutic index, as evidenced by the wide range of dosages in which it is prescribed without monitoring of plasma concentrations. Conversely, lithium (Eskalith, Lithobid, and Lithonate) has a low therapeutic index, thereby requiring the close monitoring of plasma concentrations to avoid toxicity.

Persons exhibit both interindividual and intraindividual variation in their responses to a specific drug. An individual may be hyporeactive, normally reactive, or hyperreactive to a particular drug. For example, whereas some persons require 50 mg a day of sertraline, other persons require 200 mg a day for control of their symptoms. An unpredictable, non–dosage-related drug response is called *idiosyncratic*. For example, diazepam administered as a sedative paradoxically causes agitation in some persons.

Tolerance, Dependence, and Withdrawal Symptoms.   A person who becomes less responsive to a particular drug over time is said to develop *tolerance* to the effects of the drug. The development of tolerance can be associated with the appearance of physical *dependence*, which is the necessity to continue administering the drug to prevent the appearance of *withdrawal symptoms* (also called discontinuation syndrome).

DRUG INTERACTIONS

Drug interactions may be either pharmacokinetic or pharmacodynamic, and they vary greatly in their potential to cause serious problems. Pharmacokinetic drug interactions concern the effects of drugs on their respective plasma concentrations, and pharmacodynamic drug interactions concern the effects of drugs on their respective receptor activities.

Pharmacodynamic drug–drug interactions causing additive biochemical changes may trigger toxic adverse effects. For example, MAOIs when coadministered with either tricyclic antidepressants or SSRIs, may precipitate a serotonin syndrome in which serotonin is metabolized slowly and thus accumulates in excessive concentrations. The interaction of disulfiram (Antabuse) and alcohol is another example of toxicity caused by pharmacodynamic drug interactions.

Some clinically important drug interactions are well studied and well proven; other interactions are well documented but have only modest effects; and still other interactions are true but unproven, although reasonably plausible. Clinicians must remember that (1) animal pharmacokinetic data are not always readily generalizable to humans; (2) in vitro data do not necessarily replicate the results obtained under in vivo conditions; (3) single-case reports can contain misleading information; and (4) studies of acute conditions should not be uncritically regarded as relevant to chronic, steady-state conditions.

An additional consideration is one of phantom drug interactions. The person may be taking only drug A and then later receive both drug A and drug B. The clinician may then notice some effect and attribute it to the induction of metabolism. In fact, what may have occurred is that the person was more compliant at one point in the observation period than in another or there may have been some other effect of which the clinician was unaware. The clinical literature may contain reports of phantom drug interactions that are rare or nonexistent.

Informed clinicians need to keep these considerations in mind and to focus on the clinically important interactions, not on the ones that may be mild, unproven, or entirely phantom. At the same time, clinicians should maintain an open and receptive attitude toward the possibility of pharmacokinetic and pharmacodynamic drug interactions.

DRUG SELECTION

There is no psychotropic drug that is effective in all patients with a given diagnosis. The ability of a drug to prove effective is only partially predictable and depends on the properties of the drug and the biology of the patient. Decisions about drug selection and use are made on a case-by-case basis, relying on the individual judgment of the physician. There are three factors in drug selection: (1) the drug, (2) the patient, and (3) the expertise and judgment of the prescribing physician. Each of these components affects the probability of a successful outcome.

An often-overlooked consideration in drug selection involves possible long-term consequences of being on a particular drug. For example, when starting antidepressant treatment in a young woman, thought needs to be given to which drug would be less problematic should she become pregnant and need to remain on medication. Paroxetine (Paxil), as an example, carries a higher risk of birth defects and would not be the best choice of medication in this instance. Another reason that paroxetine would not be the most appropriate agent for this patient group is its more severe withdrawal syndrome, which would make it more difficult for a woman who wants to discontinue medication in order to become pregnant. Similarly, drugs such as quetiapine (Seroquel) or citalopram (Celexa) that can prolong the QT interval may be reasonable choices for a healthy adult with no congenital long QT interval, but may be problematic if that patient needs to be treated for a medical problem with other medications that prolong the QT interval. Thinking long term is important because many psychiatric disorders are chronic and involve treatment over extended periods.

THERAPEUTIC INDICATIONS

A therapeutic indication is a psychiatric diagnosis, as defined in the 10th revision of the *International Statistical Classification of Diseases and Related Health Problems* (ICD-10) or the fifth edition of the *Diagnostic and Statistical Manual of Mental Disorders* (DSM-5), for which a specific drug ameliorates signs or symptoms. Drugs are approved on the basis of carefully designed large-scale clinical trials that prove the drug is safe and that clinical improvement is attributable to the drug and not to the placebo. The FDA then grants a manufacturer the official right to advertise the drug as safe and effective for that therapeutic indication.

Clinicians must distinguish between official and unofficial therapeutic indications. This is necessary because many drugs are in fact safe and effective for treating not only those indications proven in FDA-scale trials but also for a much broader range of indications described in smaller trials.

Drug Approval Process in the United States

Under the Federal Food, Drug, and Cosmetic (FD&C) Act, initially passed in 1938 and subsequently heavily amended, the FDA has the authority to (1) control the initial availability of a drug by approving only those new drugs that demonstrate both safety and effectiveness and (2) ensure that the drug's proposed labeling is truthful and contains all pertinent information for the safe and effective use of that drug. An additional concentration of government regulation is directed by the Drug Enforcement Administration (DEA), which classifies drugs according to their abuse potential (Table 1–3). Clinicians are advised to exercise increased caution when prescribing controlled substances.

In general, the FDA not only ensures that a new medication is safe and effective but also that a new medication compares favorably with existing agents used for the same indications. The new agent is usually not approvable unless it is at least equivalent in safety and efficacy to existing agents, if not superior. Table 1–4 summarizes the phases of research that lead to approval of a new drug.

Off-Label Uses

After a drug has been approved for commercial use, the clinician may, as part of the practice of medicine, lawfully prescribe a different dosage for a person or otherwise vary the conditions of use from what is approved in the package labeling without

Table 1–3
Characteristics of Drugs at Each DEA Level

Schedule (Control Level)	Characteristics of Drug at Each Schedule	Examples of Drugs at Each Schedule
I	High abuse potential No accepted use in medical treatment in the United States at the present time; therefore, not for prescription use Can be used for research	LSD, heroin, marijuana, peyote, PCP, mescaline, psilocybin, nicocodeine, nicomorphine
II	High abuse potential Severe physical dependence liability Severe psychological dependence liability No refills; no telephone prescriptions	Amphetamine, opium, morphine, codeine, hydromorphone, phenmetrazine, amobarbital, secobarbital, pentobarbital, ketamine, methylphenidate
III	Abuse potential lower than levels I and II Moderate or low physical dependence liability High psychological liability Prescriptions must be rewritten after 6 months or five refills	Glutethimide; methyprylon; nalorphine; sulfonmethane; benzphetamine; phendimetrazine; chlorphentermine; compounds containing codeine, morphine, opium, hydrocodone, dihydrocodeine; diethylpropion; dronabinol
IV	Low abuse potential Limited physical dependence liability Limited psychological dependence liability Prescriptions must be rewritten after 6 months or five refills	Phenobarbital, benzodiazepines,[a] chloral hydrate, ethchlorvynol, ethinamate, meprobamate, paraldehyde
V	Lowest abuse potential of all controlled substances	Narcotic preparations containing limited amounts of nonnarcotic active medicinal ingredients

[a]In New York State, benzodiazepines are treated as schedule II substances, which require a triplicate prescription for a maximum of 3 months' supply.
DEA, Drug Enforcement Administration; LSD, lysergic acid diethylamide; PCP, phencyclidine.

Table 1–4
Phases of Drug Development

Nonclinical (Preclinical) Studies. Nonclinical studies that are sufficient to establish a tolerable dose and to identify the target organs of toxicity for a new drug must be conducted before first use of a new chemical entity in humans. A standard battery of animal studies and in vitro studies is required.

Phase I. Phase I studies represent the initial introduction of the new drug into humans. These studies, usually conducted in healthy volunteers, typically in closely monitored (often inpatient) settings, serve to characterize the absorption, distribution, metabolism, and excretion of the compound; to identify overt toxicities associated with drug administration; and to establish a tolerable dose for use in further studies.

Phase II. Phase II includes the initial controlled clinical efficacy studies. These studies typically include carefully selected patients with the disease or condition under study and are usually well controlled, closely monitored, and optimized for the collection of efficacy data. In phase II, exploratory work is undertaken to help determine the optimal doses of the drug.

Phase III. After preliminary evidence suggesting the effectiveness of the drug has been established in phase II trials, additional information about effectiveness and safety is needed to evaluate the overall risk–benefit relationship of the drug and to provide an adequate basis for product labeling. Phase III studies, expanded controlled and uncontrolled trials, provide this information.

Phase IV. After the drug has been approved, subsequent postmarketing activities may be conducted in phase IV. Studies to elucidate new indications or adverse effects and risks occur in this phase.

notifying the FDA or obtaining its approval. In other words, the FD&C Act does not limit the manner in which a clinician may use an approved drug.

However, although clinicians may treat persons with an approved drug for unapproved purposes—that is, for indications not included on the drug's official labeling—without violating the FD&C Act, this practice exposes the clinician to increased risk for medical malpractice liability. This is a significant concern because the failure to follow the FDA-approved label may create an inference that the clinician is varying from the prevailing standard of care. Clinicians may, however, prescribe medication for any reason they believe to be medically indicated for the welfare of the person. This clarification is important in view of the increasing regulation of clinicians by federal, state, and local governmental agencies.

Off-label drug use for treatment of mental disorders most frequently occurs when a patient has repeatedly failed to experience an adequate response to, or could not tolerate, standard therapies. A good example of recent off-label drug use involves utilization of drugs that are believed to act on the glutamate system. A growing body of evidence suggests that glutamate (glutamic acid), the most abundant excitatory neurotransmitter in the brain, is involved in the pathophysiology of several disorders. The most notable example, glutamate-modulating drug therapy, is the use of ketamine infusions to treat treatment-refractory depression. Another is the use of riluzole (Rilutek) in cases of severe obsessive-compulsive disorder (OCD). Other glutamatergic drugs being used outside of their FDA-approved indication include topiramate (Topamax) for weight loss, pregabalin (Lyrica) for anxiety, and memantine (Namenda) for depression. At the moment, the degree to which any of these drugs benefit a large number of patients in need of an unconventional pharmacologic intervention remains to be determined. With all of these drugs, symptom severity and a history of failure of conventional pharmacotherapy typically determine whether it is decided to use these agents.

When using a drug for an unapproved indication or in a dose outside the usual range, the clinician should document the reason for these treatment decisions in the person's chart. If a clinician is in doubt about a treatment plan, he or she should consult a colleague or suggest that the person under treatment obtain a second opinion.

PRECAUTIONS AND ADVERSE EFFECTS
Overall, psychotropic drugs are remarkably safe, especially during short-term use. Only a few drugs—such as lithium, clozapine (Clozaril), valproic acid (Depakene), and carbamazepine (Tegretol)—require close laboratory monitoring. It has also become evident that the newer antipsychotic agents require regular blood tests to monitor changes in blood glucose and lipid levels.

Precautions
Before use of a drug, it is important to be prepared to safely manage any expected adverse effects. Clinicians should be fully aware of any warnings and precautions in the product literature and should anticipate how to respond at least to the more common adverse effects listed.

Adverse Effects

Adverse effects are an unavoidable risk of medication treatment. Although it is impossible to have an encyclopedic knowledge of all possible adverse drug effects, prescribing clinicians should be familiar with the more common adverse effects as well as those with serious medical consequences. Even though the FDA requires that product information contain the results of clinical trials, many of the listed adverse effects are not actually causally associated with use of the drug, and it is common for adverse effects to be missed during clinical trials. It is thus important for clinicians to follow reports of treatment-associated adverse events during the postmarketing period. No single text or document, including the product information, contains a complete list of possible treatment-emergent events.

It is always best to anticipate expected adverse effects, as well as rare but potentially problematic adverse effects, and to consider whether those effects will be unacceptable to the patient. For example, sexual dysfunction, weight gain, daytime sedation, sweating, nausea, and constipation may predictably cause some patients to discontinue treatment. It is thus important to discuss potential adverse effects with the patient and to determine if a problem with compliance is likely to arise. Persons generally have decreased trouble with adverse effects if they have been warned to expect them.

Drug adverse effects can largely be explained by their interactions with several neurotransmitter systems, both in the brain and in the peripheral nervous system. Older psychotherapeutic drugs, for example, commonly cause anticholinergic effects (Table 1–5) or bind to dopaminergic, histaminergic, and adrenergic receptors, resulting in the adverse effects listed in Table 1–6.

Newer agents tend to have either more specific neurotransmitter activity or combinations of effects that make them better tolerated than older agents. Nevertheless, some of the adverse effects of the newer agents remain problematic (Table 1–7), and in some cases—such as nausea, weight gain, and sexual dysfunction, all the result of serotonergic activity—these effects are more common than with the older drugs. It is usually not possible to predict which persons will not tolerate a serotonergic agent.

Table 1–5
Potential Adverse Effects Caused by Blockade of Muscarinic Acetylcholine Receptors

Blurred vision
Constipation
Decreased salivation
Decreased sweating
Delayed or retrograde ejaculation
Delirium
Exacerbation of asthma (through decreased bronchial secretions)
Hyperthermia (through decreased sweating)
Memory problems
Narrow-angle glaucoma
Photophobia
Sinus tachycardia
Urinary retention

Table 1–6
Potential Adverse Effects of Psychotherapeutic Drugs and Associated Neurotransmitter Systems

Antidopaminergic	Antihistaminergic
Endocrine dysfunction	Hypotension
Hyperprolactinemia	Sedation
Menstrual dysfunction	Weight gain
Sexual dysfunction	Multiple neurotransmitter systems
Movement disorders	Agranulocytosis (and other blood dyscrasias)
Akathisia	Allergic reactions
Dystonia	Anorexia
Parkinsonism	Cardiac conduction abnormalities
Tardive dyskinesia	Nausea and vomiting
Antiadrenergic (primarily α)	Seizures
Dizziness	
Postural hypotension	
Reflex tachycardia	

Treatment of Common Adverse Effects

Psychotherapeutic drugs may cause a wide range of adverse effects. The management of a particular adverse effect is similar, regardless of which psychotherapeutic drug the person is taking. If possible, another drug with similar benefits but fewer adverse effects should be used instead. In each drug section in this text, common adverse effects and their treatments are described in detail.

Sexual Dysfunction. Some degree of sexual dysfunction may occur with the use of many psychotropic drugs. This is by far the most common adverse effect associated with the use of SSRIs. About 50% to 80% of persons taking an SSRI report some sexual dysfunction, such as decreased libido, impaired ejaculation and erection, or inhibition of female orgasm.

As a rule, the best approach to pharmacologic management of sexual dysfunction involves either switching from the SSRI to mirtazapine (Remeron) or bupropion (Wellbutrin), drugs that are unlikely to cause sexual dysfunction. If it is thought that use of an SSRI is indicated, adding a prosexual agent such as bupropion may be enough to reverse the sexual inhibition caused by SSRIs. The best tolerated and most potent prosexual drugs currently available are the phosphodiesterases (PDEs), such as sildenafil (Viagra).

Anxiety, Akathisia, Agitation, and Insomnia. Many persons initiating treatment with serotonergic antidepressants (e.g., fluoxetine) experience an increase in psychomotor activation in the first 2 to 3 weeks of use. The agitating effects of SSRIs modestly increase the risk of acting out suicidal impulses in persons at risk for suicide. During the initial period of SSRI treatment, persons at risk for self-injury should maintain close contact with the clinician or should be hospitalized, depending on the clinician's assessment of the risk for suicide.

The insomnia and anxiety associated with use of serotonergic drugs can be counteracted by administration of a benzodiazepine or trazodone (Desyrel) for the first several weeks. If the agitation is extreme or persists beyond the initial 3-week period, another type of antidepressant drug, such as mirtazapine or a tricyclic agent, should be considered. Both typical and atypical antipsychotic medications are associated with movement disorders.

Table 1-7
Common Adverse Effects Associated with Newer Psychotropic Drugs

Movement disorders
First-generation antipsychotics (the DRAs) are the most common cause of medication-induced movement disorders. The introduction of SDAs has greatly reduced the incidence of these adverse effects, but varying degrees of dose-related parkinsonism, akathisia, and dystonia still occur. Risperidone (Risperdal) most closely resembles the older agents in terms of these adverse effects. Olanzapine (Zyprexa) also causes more EPS than clinical trials suggested. There have been rare reports of SSRI-induced movement disorders, ranging from akathisia to tardive dyskinesia.

Sexual dysfunction
The use of psychiatric drugs may be associated with sexual dysfunction—decreased libido, impaired ejaculation and erection, and inhibition of female orgasm. In clinical trials with the SSRIs, the extent of sexual adverse effects was grossly underestimated because data were based on spontaneous reports by patients. The rate of sexual dysfunction in the original fluoxetine (Prozac) product information, e.g., was <5%. In subsequent studies in which information about sexual adverse effects was elicited by specific questions, the rate of SSRI-associated sexual dysfunction was found to be between 35% and 75%. In clinical practice, patients are not likely to report sexual dysfunction spontaneously to the physician, so it is important to ask about this adverse effect. In addition, some forms of sexual dysfunction may be related to the primary psychiatric disorder. Nevertheless, if sexual dysfunction emerges after pharmacotherapy has begun and the primary response to treatment has been positive, it may be worthwhile to attempt to treat the symptoms. Long lists of possible antidotes to these adverse effects have evolved, but few interventions are consistently effective, and few have more than anecdotal evidence to support their use. The clinician and patient should consider the possibility of sexual adverse effects with a patient when selecting a drug and switching treatment to another drug that is less or not at all associated with sexual dysfunction if this adverse effect is not acceptable to the patient.

Weight gain
Weight gain accompanies the use of many psychotropic drugs as a result of retained fluid, increased caloric intake, decreased exercise, or altered metabolism. Weight gain may also occur as a symptom of disorder, as in bulimia or atypical depression, or as a sign of recovery from an episode of illness. Treatment-emergent increase in body weight is a common reason for noncompliance with a drug regimen. No specific mechanisms have been identified as causing weight gain, and it appears that the histamine and serotonin systems mediate changes in weight associated with many drugs used to treat depression and psychosis. Metformin (Glucophage) has been reported to facilitate weight loss among patients whose weight gain is attributed to use of serotonin–dopamine reuptake inhibitors and valproic acid (Depakene). Valproate and olanzapine have been linked to the development of insulin resistance, which could induce appetite increase, with subsequent weight increase.

Weight gain is a noteworthy adverse effect of clozapine (Clozaril) and olanzapine. Genetic factors that regulate body weight, as well as the related problem of diabetes mellitus, seem to involve the $5-HT_{2C}$ receptor. There is a genetic polymorphism of the promoter region of this receptor, with significantly less weight gain in patients with the variant allele than in those without this allele. Drugs with a strong $5-HT_{2C}$ affinity would be expected to have a greater effect on body weight of patients with a polymorphism of the $5-HT_{2C}$ receptor promoter region.

Weight loss
Initial weight loss is associated with SSRI treatment but is usually transient, with most weight being regained within the first few months. Bupropion (Wellbutrin) has been shown to cause modest weight loss that is sustained. When combined with diet and lifestyle changes, bupropion can facilitate more significant weight loss. Topiramate (Topamax) and zonisamide (Zonegran), marketed as treatments for epilepsy, produce sometimes substantial, sustained loss of weight.

Glucose changes
Increased risk of glucose abnormalities, including diabetes mellitus, is associated with weight increase during psychotropic drug therapy. Data are not conclusive, but olanzapine is associated with more frequent reports than other SDAs of abnormalities in fasting glucose levels, as well as in reported cases of hyperosmolar diabetes and ketoacidosis.

Hyponatremia
Hyponatremia is associated with oxcarbazepine (Trileptal) and SSRI treatment, especially in elderly patients. Confusion, agitation, and lethargy are common symptoms.

(continued)

Table 1-7—*continued*
Common Adverse Effects Associated with Newer Psychotropic Drugs

Cognitive
  Cognitive impairment means a disturbance in the capacity to think. Some agents, such as
    the benzodiazepine agonists, are recognized as causes of cognitive impairment. However,
    other widely used psychotropics, such as the SSRIs, lamotrigine (Lamictal), gabapentin
    (Neurontin), lithium (Eskalith), TCAs, and bupropion, are also associated with varying degrees of
    memory impairment and word-finding difficulties. In contrast to the benzodiazepine-induced
    anterograde amnesia, these agents cause a more subtle type of absent-mindedness. Drugs
    with anticholinergic properties are likely to worsen memory performance.
Sweating
  Severe perspiration unrelated to ambient temperature is associated with TCAs, SSRIs, and
    venlafaxine (Effexor). This adverse effect is often socially disabling. Attempts can be made to
    treat this adverse effect with α agents, such as terazosin (Hytrin) and oxybutynin (Ditropan).
Cardiovascular
  Newer agents are less prone to having direct cardiac effects. Many older agents, such as TCAs
    and phenothiazines, affected blood pressure and cardiac conduction. The drug thioridazine
    (Mellaril), which has been in use for decades, has been shown to prolong the QTc interval in
    a dose-related manner and may increase the risk of sudden death by delaying ventricular
    repolarization and causing torsades de pointes. Newer drugs are now routinely scrutinized for
    evidence of cardiac effects. A promising treatment for psychosis, sertindole (Serlect), was not
    marketed because the FDA would have required a black box warning. Slight QTc effects noted
    with ziprasidone (Geodon) delayed the marketing of that drug. High-normal and high-dose
    olanzapine may cause prolongation of the PR interval and atrioventricular conduction delay.
    The management of specific adverse effects for individual drugs is covered in their respective
    chapters.
Rash
  Any medication is a potential source of a drug rash. Some psychotropics, such as
    carbamazepine (Tegretol) and lamotrigine, have been linked to an increased risk of serious
    exfoliative dermatitis, so patients should be informed about the seriousness of widespread
    lesions that occur above the neck and involve the mucous membranes. If such symptoms
    manifest, a patient should be instructed at the time the medication is prescribed to go
    immediately to an emergency department and not to first attempt to contact the prescribing
    psychiatrist.

BP, blood pressure; DRA, dopamine receptor antagonist; EPS, extrapyramidal side effects; FDA, Food and Drug Administration; 5-HT$_{2C}$, serotonin type 2C; QTc, quick test corrected for heart rate; SDA, serotonin-dopamine antagonist; SSRI, selective serotonin reuptake inhibitor; TCA, tricyclic antidepressant.

Gastrointestinal Upset and Diarrhea.   Most of the body's serotonin is in the GI tract, and serotonergic drugs, particularly sertraline (Zoloft), venlafaxine (Effexor), and fluvoxamine (Luvox), may therefore produce mildly to moderately severe stomach pain, nausea, and diarrhea, usually only for the first few weeks of therapy. Sertraline is most likely to cause loose stools, and fluvoxamine is most likely to cause nausea.

These symptoms may be minimized by initiating treatment with a very small dosage and administering the drug after eating. Dietary alteration, such as the BRAT diet (*b*ananas, *r*ice, *a*pples, and *t*oast), may reduce loose stools. These symptoms usually abate over time, but some persons never accommodate and must switch to another drug.

Gastrointestinal Bleeding.   Drugs that inhibit the serotonin reuptake transporter, most notably the SSRIs and SNRIs, are associated with increased tendency toward bleeding. Most commonly, this involves GI bleeding. Patients who are taking anticoagulant drugs or who use aspirin or nonsteroidal anti-inflammatory drugs are most at risk and should be monitored for this adverse effect, and those agents should be used only if needed.

Headache.   A small fraction of persons initiating therapy with any psychotherapeutic drug may experience mildly to moderately severe headache. These headaches often respond to over-the-counter analgesics, but it may be necessary for some persons to switch to another medication.

Anorexia.   SSRIs may produce a short-term suppression of appetite. The same is true of bupropion. In patients who are already dangerously underweight, these agents should be used with caution and treatment closely monitored. Fluoxetine (60 mg per day) in the context of a comprehensive program of behavioral management is an approved treatment for bulimia and is also useful for treatment of anorexia nervosa. Unless a comprehensive therapeutic program is available, SSRIs should be used cautiously by persons with eating disorders.

Weight Gain.   Most commonly used drugs cause weight gain. The mechanisms can be as diverse as fluid retention, stimulation of appetite, or alteration in metabolism. Olanzapine (Zyprexa), clozapine, and mirtazapine are associated with early, frequent, and sometimes extreme or persistent increases in body weight. SSRIs may be associated with more gradual or late-emergent weight gain that may be resistant to weight loss through diet and exercise. In these instances, some form of diet and exercise regimen should be attempted to salvage an otherwise effective treatment regimen. No drug has yet been shown to suppress the appetite safely in all persons. The most effective appetite suppressants, the amphetamines, are not used generally because of concerns about abuse. The addition of topiramate, 25 to 200 mg daily, or zonisamide (Zonegran), 50 to 150 mg daily, may help to reverse drug-induced weight gain that results from increased caloric intake.

Edema can be treated by elevating the affected body parts or by administering a diuretic. If the person adds a diuretic to a regimen of lithium or cardiac medications, the clinician must monitor blood concentrations, blood chemistries, and vital signs.

Orlistat (Xenical) does not suppress appetite; instead, it blocks absorption of fat from the intestine. Therefore, it reduces caloric intake from fatty foods but not from carbohydrates or proteins. Because orlistat causes retention of dietary fats in the intestines, it frequently causes excessive flatulence.

Somnolence.   Many psychotropic drugs cause sedation. Some persons may self-medicate this adverse effect with caffeine, but this practice may worsen orthostatic hypotension.

It is important for the clinician to alert the patient to the possibility of sedation and to document that the person was advised not to drive or operate dangerous equipment if sedated by medications. Fortunately, some of newer generations of antidepressant and antipsychotic drugs are much less likely to cause sedation than were their predecessors, and the newer drugs should be substituted for the sedating medications when possible. Modafinil (Provigil) can be added to counteract residual sedative effects of psychotropic drugs.

Dry Mouth. Dry mouth is caused by the blockade of muscarinic acetylcholine receptors. When persons attempt to relieve the dry mouth by constantly sucking on sugar-containing hard candies, they increase their risk for dental cavities. They can avoid the problem by chewing sugarless gum or sucking on sugarless hard candies.

Some clinicians recommend the use of a 1% solution of pilocarpine (Salagen), a cholinergic agonist, as a mouthwash three times daily. Other clinicians suggest bethanechol tablets, another cholinergic agonist, 10 to 30 mg once or twice daily. It is best to start with 10 mg once a day and to increase the dose slowly. Adverse effects of cholinomimetic drugs, such as bethanechol, include tremor, diarrhea, abdominal cramps, and excessive eye watering.

Blurred Vision. The blockage of muscarinic acetylcholine receptors causes mydriasis (pupillary dilation) and cycloplegia (ciliary muscle paresis), resulting in blurred vision. The symptom can be relieved by cholinomimetic eye drops. A 1% solution of pilocarpine can be prescribed as one drop, four times daily. Alternatively, bethanechol can be used as it is used for dry mouth. Topiramate, an anticonvulsant often used to treat drug-induced weight gain, can cause glaucoma and subsequent blindness. Patients should be informed to immediately report any change in vision when using topiramate.

Urinary Retention. The anticholinergic activity of many psychotherapeutic drugs can lead to urinary hesitation, dribbling, urinary retention, and increased urinary tract infections. Elderly persons with prostatic enlargement are at increased risk for these adverse effects. Ten to 30 mg of bethanechol three to four times daily is usually effective in the treatment of the urologic adverse effects.

Constipation. The anticholinergic activity of psychotherapeutic drugs can cause constipation. The first line of treatment involves the prescribing of bulk laxatives, such as Citrucel, FiberCon, Konsyl, or Metamucil. If this treatment fails, cathartic laxatives, such as Milk of Magnesia, or other laxative preparations can be tried. Prolonged use of cathartic laxatives can result in a loss of their effectiveness. Bethanechol, 10 to 30 mg three to four times daily, can also be used.

Orthostatic Hypotension. Orthostatic hypotension is caused by the blockade of α_1-adrenergic receptors. Elderly people are at particular risk for development of orthostatic hypotension. The risk of hip fractures from falls is significantly elevated in persons who are taking psychotherapeutic drugs.

Most simply, the person can be instructed to get up slowly and to sit down immediately if dizziness is experienced. Treatments for orthostatic hypotension include avoidance of caffeine, intake of at least 2 L of fluid per day, addition of salt to food (unless prescribed by a physician), reassessment of the dosages of any antihypertensive medications, and wearing support hose. Fludrocortisone (Florinef) is rarely needed.

Overdose

An extreme adverse effect of drug treatment is an attempt by a person to commit suicide by overdosing on a psychotherapeutic drug. Clinicians should be aware of the risk and attempt to prescribe the safest possible drugs.

It is good clinical practice to write nonrefillable prescriptions for small quantities of drugs when suicide is a consideration. In extreme cases, an attempt should be made to verify that persons are taking the medication and not hoarding the pills for a later overdosage attempt. Persons may attempt suicide just as they are beginning to get better. Clinicians, therefore, should continue to be careful about prescribing large quantities of medication until the person has almost completely recovered, and such patients should be seen at least weekly.

Another consideration for clinicians is the possibility of an accidental overdose, particularly by children in the household. Persons should be advised to keep psycho-therapeutic medications in a safe place.

Discontinuation (Withdrawal) Syndromes

The transient emergence of mild symptoms upon discontinuation or reduction of dosage is associated with a number of drugs, including paroxetine, venlafax-ine, duloxetine (Cymbalta), sertraline, fluvoxamine, and the tricyclic and tetra-cyclic drugs. More severe discontinuation symptoms are associated with lithium (rebound mania), DRAs (tardive dyskinesias), and benzodiazepines (anxiety and insomnia).

Signs and symptoms of the discontinuation syndrome after SSRI use consist of agitation, nausea, dysequilibrium, and dysphoria. The syndrome is more likely to occur if the plasma half-life of the agent is brief, if the drug is taken for at least 2 months, or if higher dosages are used and if the drug is stopped abruptly. The symptoms are time limited and can be minimized by a gradual reduction of the dosage.

DOSAGE AND CLINICAL GUIDELINES

Diagnosis and the Identification of Target Symptoms

Treatment with psychotherapeutic drugs begins with formation of a therapeutic bond between the doctor and the person seeking treatment. The initial interview is devoted to defining the clinical problem as comprehensively as possible, with spe-cial attention paid to the identification of specific target symptoms whose improve-ment will indicate that the drug therapy is effective.

Medication History. Past and present medication history discusses the use of all prescription, nonprescription, herbal, and illicit drugs ever taken, including caf-feine, ethanol, and nicotine; the sequence in which the drugs were used; the dosages used; the therapeutic effects; the adverse effects; details of any overdosages; and the reasons for discontinuing any drug.

Persons and their families are often ignorant about what drugs have been used before, in what dosages, and for how long. This ignorance may reflect the ten-dency of clinicians not to explain drug trials before writing prescriptions. Clini-cians should provide written records of drug trials for each person to present to future caregivers.

A caveat to obtaining a history of drug response from persons is that because of their mental disorders, they may inaccurately report the effects of a previous drug trial. If possible, therefore, the persons' medical records should be obtained to con-firm their reports.

Explaining Rationale, Risks, Benefits, and Treatment Alternatives

The use of psychotropic drugs should not be oversimplified into a one diagnosis–one pill approach. Many variables impinge on a person's psychological response to drug treatment. Some persons may view a drug as a panacea, and other persons may view a drug as an assault. Compliance with the dosing regimen is improved by providing a person with ample opportunities to ask questions at the time of prescribing, distributing written material that reinforces proper use of the medication, streamlining the medication regimen to the extent possible, and ensuring that office visits begin at the scheduled appointment time.

Choice of Drug

Previous Drug History. A specific drug should be selected according to the patient's history of drug response (compliance, therapeutic response, and adverse effects), the person's family history of drug response, and the profile of adverse effects expected for that particular person. If a drug has previously been effective in treating a person or a family member, the same drug should be used again unless there is some specific reason not to use the drug.

Adverse Effect Profile. Psychotropic drugs of a single class are equally efficacious but do differ in their adverse effect profile. A drug should be selected that is least likely to exacerbate any pre-existing disorders, whether medical or psychiatric, and that has probable adverse effects that are acceptable to the patient. Nevertheless, idiosyncratic reactions may occur.

Assessment of Outcome

Clinical improvements that occur during the course of drug treatment may not necessarily be related to the pharmacologic effects of the drug. For example, psychological distress often improves with the simple reassurances of a medical caregiver. Many disorders remit spontaneously, so "feeling better" may be the result of coincidence rather than medication. Therefore, it is important to identify unambiguously the nature and expected time course of clinical improvements caused by the pharmacologic effects of the medications.

In clinical practice, a person's subjective impression of a beneficial drug effect is the single most consistent indicator of future response to that drug. Assessments of clinical outcome in randomized, double-blind, placebo-controlled clinical trials rely on quantitative psychiatric rating scales, such as the Brief Psychiatric Rating Scale, Positive and Negative Syndrome Scale, Montgomery–Asberg Depression Rating Scale, Hamilton Rating Scale for Depression, Hamilton Anxiety Rating Scale, or Global Assessment of Functioning Scale.

Therapeutic Trials. A common question a patient typically asks is, "How long do I need to take the medication?" Patients can be given a reasonable explanation of the probabilities but told that it is best to first see if the medication works for him or her and whether the adverse effects are acceptable. Any more definitive discussion of duration of treatment can be held for when the degree of success is clear. Even patients with a philosophical aversion to the use of psychotropic drugs may elect to stay on medication indefinitely if the magnitude of improvement is great.

Treatment is conceptually broken down into three phases: the initial therapeutic trial, the continuation, and the maintenance phase. The initial period of treatment should last at least 4 to 6 weeks because of the delay in therapeutic effects that characterizes most classes of psychotropic drugs. The required duration of a "therapeutic trial" of a drug should be discussed at the outset of treatment so the patient does not have unrealistic expectations of an immediate improvement in symptoms. Unfortunately, patients are more likely to experience adverse effects in the course of pharmacotherapy earlier than any relief from their disorder. In some cases, medication may even exacerbate some symptoms. Patients should be counseled that a poor initial reaction to medication is not an indicator of the ultimate outcome of treatment. For instance, many patients with panic disorder develop jitteriness or an increase in panic attacks after starting on tricyclic or SSRI treatment. Benzodiazepine agonists are an exception to the rule that there is a delay in clinical onset. In most cases, their hypnotic and antianxiety effects are evident immediately.

Ongoing use of medication does not provide absolute protection against relapse. However, continuation therapy may provide significant protective effects against relapse.

Possible Reasons for Therapeutic Failures

The failure of a specific drug trial should prompt the clinician to consider a number of possibilities.

First, was the original diagnosis correct? This consideration should include the possibility of an undiagnosed coexisting disorder or illicit drug or alcohol abuse.

Second, did the person take the drug as directed?

Third, was the drug administered in sufficient dosage for an appropriate period of time? Persons can have varying drug absorption and metabolic rates for the same drug, and, if available, plasma drug concentrations should be obtained to assess this variable.

Fourth, did the drug's adverse effects produce signs and symptoms unrelated to the original disease? If so, did these effects counteract any therapeutic response? Antipsychotic drugs, for example, can produce akinesia, which resembles psychotic withdrawal; akathisia and neuroleptic malignant syndrome resemble increased psychotic agitation. SSRIs can produce fatigue, insomnia, and emotional blunting, symptoms that resemble manifestations of depression.

Fifth, did a pharmacokinetic or pharmacodynamic interaction with another drug the person was taking reduce the efficacy of the psychotherapeutic drug?

Regardless of optimal drug selection and use, some patients fail to respond to repeated trials of medication.

Poorly understood is the phenomenon of drug "poop out," in which patients who have been taking a drug for long periods of time, with good effect, suddenly have a return of symptoms. A number of possibilities have been suggested as causing loss of therapeutic effect. These include:

• Pharmacodynamic or pharmacokinetic tolerance (tachyphylaxis)
• Side effects (apathy, anhedonia, and emotional blunting)
• Onset of a comorbid medical disorder
• Increase in disease severity or change in disease pathogenesis (progression)

- Depletion of effector substance (neurotransmitter?)
- Serum drug levels that have drifted below or above that drug's therapeutic window
- Accumulation of detrimental metabolites
- Initial misdiagnosis
- Loss of placebo response
- Lack of bioequivalence when compared to a generic version.

Strategies for Increasing Efficacy

The most fruitful initial strategy for increasing the efficacy of a psychotherapeutic drug is to review whether the drug is being taken correctly. A fresh clinical evaluation of the psychiatric symptoms and the rationale of the drug therapy is one of the psychopharmacologist's most valuable tools for revealing previously unappreciated impediments to drug efficacy.

Adding a drug with another indication is termed *augmentation.* Augmentation often entails use of a drug that is not primarily considered a psychotropic. For example, in treating depression, it is common to add thyroid hormone to an approved antidepressant. In a typical scenario, a patient has little or no response to a medication, so the physician adds a second agent to induce a better response. In some cases, the use of multiple medications is the rule. Almost all patients with bipolar disorder take more than one psychotropic agent. Combination treatment with drugs that treat depression has long been held as preferable in patients with psychotic depression. Similarly, SSRIs typically produce partial improvement in patients with OCD, so the addition of a serotonin–dopamine antagonist (SDA) may be helpful.

In addition, drugs may be combined to counteract side effects, to treat specific symptoms, and as a temporary measure to transition from one drug to another. It is common practice to add a new agent without the discontinuation of a prior drug, particularly when the first drug has provided partial benefit. This can be done as part of a plan to transition from an agent that is not producing a satisfactory response or as an attempt to maintain the patient on combined therapy.

One limitation of augmentation is increased noncompliance and adverse effects, and the clinician may not be able to determine whether it was the second drug alone or the combination of drugs that resulted in a therapeutic success or a particular adverse effect. Combining drugs can create a broad-spectrum effect and change the ratio of metabolites.

The merits of going to a single drug with a different pharmacologic profile include a lower risk of drug–drug interactions, simplicity, and lower cost. It is less burdensome to take one medication than two or three and is less likely to meet resistance from the patient. Many patients are ambivalent about taking even one medication, let alone two.

COMBINED PSYCHOTHERAPY AND PHARMACOTHERAPY

Many patients are best treated with a combination of medication and psychotherapy. In many cases, the results of combined therapy are superior to those of either type of therapy alone. For example, pharmacotherapy alleviates the depression that often interferes with the introspection and focus that are needed for psychotherapy. Conversely, patients who are engaged in ongoing therapy are more likely to continue taking medication.

Duration of Treatment

Use of the Correct Dosage. Subtherapeutic dosages and incomplete trials should not be prescribed solely to assuage the clinician's anxiety about the development of adverse effects. The prescription of drugs for mental disorders must be made by a knowledgeable practitioner and requires continuous clinical observation. Treatment response and the emergence of adverse effects must be monitored closely. The dosage of the drug must be adjusted accordingly, and appropriate treatments for emergent adverse effects must be instituted as quickly as possible.

Long-Term Maintenance Therapy. Persons with mood, anxiety, and schizophrenic disorders live with an increased risk for relapse into illness at virtually any phase of their lives. Although some patients discontinue treatment because drugs are ineffective or poorly tolerated, many patients stop their medication because they are feeling well. This might be the result of effective treatment or simply naturally occurring remission. Clinicians should anticipate and alert persons to the natural variations of psychiatric illnesses. For example, a person who has taken medication to treat an acute psychotic episode may soon thereafter experience a relatively symptom-free period and may then impulsively discontinue taking the medication without informing his or her physician.

Long-term data show that persons who stop their medications after resolution of an acute episode of mental illness markedly increase their risk of relapse during the subsequent year compared with persons who remain on maintenance drug therapy. The fact is, most psychiatric disorders are chronic or recurrent. With disorders such as bipolar disorder, schizophrenia, or depression associated with suicide attempts, the consequences of relapse can be severe.

Treating clinicians are obliged to provide continuous educational review and reinforcement of the importance of taking medication. By comparing psychiatric illnesses with common chronic medical conditions, such as hypertension and diabetes mellitus, clinicians can help patients to understand that psychotropic drugs do not cure the disorders but rather keep their manifestations from causing distress or disability.

Special Populations

Children. Other than attention-deficit/hyperactivity disorder (ADHD) and OCD, commonly used psychotropic drugs have no labeling for pediatric use. When drugs are used to treat children and adolescents, results are extrapolated from adult studies. This should be done with caution. For example, the smaller volume of distribution suggests the use of lower dosages than in adults, but children's higher rate of metabolism indicates that higher ratios of milligrams of drug to kilograms of body weight might be required.

In practice, it is best to begin with a small dose and to increase it until clinical effects are observed. However, the clinician may use adult doses in children if they are effective and the adverse effects are acceptable.

Geriatric Patients. Cardiac rhythm disturbances, hypotension, cognitive disturbances, and falls are major concerns when treating geriatric persons. Elderly people may also metabolize drugs slowly (Table 1–8) and thus require low doses of

Table 1–8
Pharmacokinetics and Aging

Phase	Change	Effect
Absorption	Gastric pH increases Decreased surface villi Decreased gastric motility and delayed gastric emptying Intestinal perfusion decreases	Absorption is slowed but just as complete
Distribution	Total body water and lean body mass decrease Increased total body fat, more marked in women than in men	Vd increases for lipid-soluble drugs, decreases for water-soluble drugs
	Albumin decreased, γ globulin increased, α, acid glycoprotein unchanged	The free or unbound percentage of albumin-bound drugs increases
Metabolism	Renal: renal blood flow and glomerular filtration rates decreaseHepatic: decreased enzyme activity and perfusion	Decreased metabolism leads to prolonged half-lives, if Vd remains the same
Total body weight	Decreases	Think on a mg/kg basis
Receptor sensitivity	May increase	Increased effect

Vd, volume of distribution.
From Guttmacher LB. *Concise Guide to Somatic Therapies in Psychiatry.* Washington, DC: American Psychiatric Press, 1988:126, with permission.

medication. Another concern is that geriatric persons often take other medications, thereby requiring clinicians to consider the possible drug interactions.

In practice, clinicians should begin treating geriatric persons with low doses, usually about one-half the usual dose. The dose should be raised in small amounts, more slowly than for middle-aged adults, until either a clinical benefit is achieved or unacceptable adverse effects appear. Although many geriatric persons require low doses of medication, many others require the usual adult dose.

Pregnant and Nursing Women. Physicians who are considering the use of psychotropic drugs during pregnancy should weigh known risks or the lack of available information against the risks of nontreatment. The basic rule is to avoid administering any drug to a woman who is pregnant (particularly during the first trimester) or who is breastfeeding a child, unless the mother's mental disorder is severe. In 2014, the FDA announced that it was replacing its previous classification system for safety of specific drug use during pregnancy. The new system removes the pregnancy letter categories A, B, C, D and X, and combines sections pertaining to pregnancy and lactation. It is now required that drug labels be updated when information becomes outdated.

If a drug associated with the risk of birth defects needs to be used during pregnancy, the risks and benefits of the treatment, as well as therapeutic abortion, should be discussed. The most teratogenic psychotropic drugs are valproate (Depakote, Depakene); carbamazepine; and, to a lesser degree, lithium. Valproate exposure is associated with significant risk of spina bifida and midline craniofacial abnormalities, and carbamazepine exposure causes similar midline defects. Prophylactic folic acid supplementation may reduce the risk of spina bifida. Lithium exposure during pregnancy is associated with a small risk of Ebstein's anomaly, a serious abnormality in cardiac development.

The administration of psychotherapeutic drugs at or near delivery may cause neonatal sedation and respiratory depression, possibly requiring mechanical ventilatory support, or physical dependence on the drug, requiring detoxification and the treatment of a withdrawal syndrome.

Virtually all psychotropic drugs are secreted in the milk of nursing mothers.

Persons with Hepatic or Renal Insufficiency. Persons with hepatocellular insufficiency of any cause, including cirrhosis, hepatitis, metabolic disorders, and bile duct obstruction, are at risk of accumulating elevated concentrations of hepatically metabolized drugs. Drugs that are excreted by the kidneys may accumulate to toxic concentrations in persons with renal insufficiency of any cause, including atherosclerosis, nephrosis, nephritis, infiltrative disorders, and outflow obstruction. The presence of hepatocellular or renal insufficiency requires administration of a reduced dosage, usually half of the recommended dosage for healthy persons. Clinicians should be particularly alert to signs and symptoms of adverse drug effects in persons with hepatic or renal disorders. If available, monitoring of plasma drug concentrations may help guide dosage adjustments.

Persons with Other Medical Illnesses. Medical disorders should be ruled out as the cause of psychiatric symptoms. Considerations in the use of psychotropic drugs in medically ill persons include a potentially increased sensitivity to the drug's adverse effects, either increased or decreased metabolism and excretion of the drug, and interactions with other medications. As with children and geriatric persons, the most reasonable clinical practice is to begin with a low dose, increase it slowly, and watch for both clinical and adverse effects. Special caution is needed with potential drug–disease interactions. Patients with diabetes, for example, should not be treated with drugs such as mirtazapine or olanzapine, which risk causing weight gain, or drugs such as olanzapine or valproate, which cause insulin resistance. Patients with seizure disorders should not receive bupropion, maprotiline (Ludiomil), or clomipramine (Anafranil), which lower the seizure threshold.

Laboratory Monitoring

For most commonly used psychotropic drugs, routine testing is not required. However, serious complications of treatment with certain drugs can be prevented through laboratory monitoring of either plasma drug concentrations or laboratory indicators of organ dysfunction. Apart from drugs that require monitoring, laboratory testing and therapeutic blood monitoring should be based on clinical circumstances. Lithium and clozapine treatment require ongoing monitoring. Given the increased use of antidepressant and atypical antipsychotic drugs in combination it is prudent to obtain baseline and follow-up electrocardiography EKG studies. Further information on monitoring is found in the chapter in which each drug is discussed.

2

α_2-Adrenergic Receptor Agonists, α_1-Adrenergic Receptor Antagonists: Clonidine, Guanfacine, Prazosin, and Yohimbine

INTRODUCTION

Clonidine (Catapres) is an α_2-adrenergic receptor agonist that affects plasma nor-epinephrine and other neurotransmitters. More recently guanfacine (Tenex), another α_2-adrenergic receptor agonist, has been preferentially used because its differential affinity for certain α_2-adrenergic receptor subtypes results in less sedation and hypotension. Clonidine extended release (Kapvay) and guanfacine extended release (Intuniv) are FDA approved in the treatment of attention-deficit/hyperactivity disorder (ADHD) as monotherapy and as adjunctive therapy to stimulant medication in children and adults. Immediate-release clonidine and guanfacine are FDA approved only for the treatment of hypertension as monotherapy or in combination with other antihypertensive medications. These drugs have also been studied in and used to treat neurologic and psychiatric conditions, other than ADHD. These include Tourette's syndrome (TS) and other tic disorders, opiate and alcohol withdrawal, and posttraumatic stress disorder (PTSD).

Prazosin (Minipress) is an α_1 postsynaptic antagonist. It reduces blood pressure (BP) through vasodilation. Prazosin has shown benefits in treating sleep disorders associated with PTSD.

CLONIDINE AND GUANFACINE

Pharmacologic Actions

Guanfacine is an agonist on presynaptic α_2-receptors. It inhibits sympathetic outflow and causes vasodilation of blood vessels, lowering BP. It is more selective and less potent than clonidine. Immediate-release clonidine and guanfacine are well absorbed from the gastrointestinal tract and reach peak plasma levels 1 to 3 hours after oral administration. The half-life of clonidine is 6 to 20 hours and that of guanfacine is 10 to 30 hours.

The agonist effects of clonidine and guanfacine on presynaptic α_2-adrenergic receptors in the sympathetic nuclei of the brain result in a decrease in the amount of norepinephrine released from the presynaptic nerve terminals. This serves generally to reset the body's sympathetic tone at a lower level and decrease arousal.

Therapeutic Indications

There is recent interest in the use of guanfacine for the same indications that respond to clonidine, due to guanfacine's longer half-life and relative lack of sedative effects.

Table 2–1
Oral Clonidine Protocols for Opioid Detoxification

Clonidine 0.1–0.2 mg PO four times a day; hold for systolic BP <90 mm Hg or bradycardia; stabilize for 2–3 days, then taper over 5–10 days

OR

Clonidine 0.1–0.2 mg PO q4–6h as needed for withdrawal signs or symptoms; stabilize for 2–3 days, then taper over 5–10 days

OR

Test dose with clonidine 0.1–0.2 mg PO or SL (for patients weighing over 200 lb); check BP after 1 hour. If diastolic BP >70 mm Hg and no symptoms of hypotension, begin treatment as follows:

Weight (lb)	Number of Clonidine Patches
<110	1 patch
110–160	2 patches
160–200	2 patches
>200	2 patches

OR

Test dose of oral clonidine 0.1 mg; check BP after 1 hour (if systolic BP <90 mm Hg, do not give patch)

Place two TTS-2 clonidine patches (or three patches if patient weighs >150 lb) on hairless area of upper body; then

For first 23 hours after patch application, give oral clonidine 0.2 mg q6h; then

For next 24 hours, give oral clonidine 0.1 mg q6h

Change patches weekly

After 2 weeks of two patches, switch to one patch (or two patches if patient weighs >150 lb)

After 1 week of one patch, discontinue patches

BP, blood pressure; PO, oral; q, every; SL, sublingual; TTS, through the skin.
From American Society of Addiction Medicine. Detoxification: principle and protocols. In: *The Principles Update Series: Topics in Addiction Medicine, section 11.* American Society of Addiction, 1997, with permission.

Withdrawal from Opioids, Alcohol, or Nicotine. Clonidine and guanfacine are effective in reducing the autonomic symptoms of rapid opioid withdrawal (e.g., hypertension, tachycardia, dilated pupils, sweating, lacrimation, and rhinorrhea) but not the associated subjective sensations. Clonidine administration (0.1 to 0.2 mg two to four times a day) is initiated before detoxification and is then tapered off over 1 to 2 weeks (Table 2–1).

Clonidine and guanfacine can reduce symptoms of alcohol withdrawal, including anxiety, diarrhea, and tachycardia. Clonidine and guanfacine can reduce craving, anxiety, and the irritability symptoms of nicotine withdrawal. The transdermal patch formulation of clonidine is associated with better long-term compliance for purposes of detoxification than is the tablet formulation.

Tourette's Disorder. Clonidine and guanfacine are effective drugs for the treatment of Tourette's disorder. Most clinicians begin treatment for Tourette's disorder with the standard dopamine receptor antagonists, such as haloperidol (Haldol) and serotonin–dopamine antagonists, such as risperidone (Risperdal) and olanzapine (Zyprexa). However, if concerned about the adverse effects of these drugs, the clinician may begin treatment with clonidine or guanfacine. The starting dose of clonidine for children is 0.05 mg a day; it can be increased to 0.3 mg a day in divided doses. Up to 3 months are needed before the beneficial effects of clonidine can be seen in patients with Tourette's disorder. The response rate has been reported to be up to 70%.

Other Tic Disorders. Clonidine and guanfacine reduce the frequency and severity of tics in persons with tic disorder with or without comorbid ADHD.

Hyperactivity and Aggression in Children. Clonidine and guanfacine can be useful alternatives for the treatment of ADHD. They are used in place of sympathomimetics and antidepressants, which may produce paradoxical worsening of hyperactivity in some children with intellectual disability, aggression, or features on the spectrum of autism. Clonidine and guanfacine can improve mood, reduce activity level, and improve social adaptation. Some impaired children may respond favorably to clonidine, but others may simply become sedated. The starting dose is 0.05 mg a day; it can be raised to 0.3 mg a day in divided doses. The efficacy of clonidine and guanfacine for control of hyperactivity and aggression often diminishes over several months of use.

Clonidine and guanfacine can be combined with methylphenidate (Ritalin) or dextroamphetamine (Dexedrine) to treat hyperactivity and inattentiveness, respectively. A small number of cases have been reported of sudden death of children taking clonidine together with methylphenidate; however, it has not been conclusively demonstrated that these medications contributed to these deaths. The clinician should explain to the family that the efficacy and safety of this combination have not been investigated in controlled trials. Periodic cardiovascular assessments, including vital signs and electrocardiograms, are warranted if this combination is used.

Posttraumatic Stress Disorder. Acute exacerbations of PTSD may be associated with hyperadrenergic symptoms such as hyperarousal, exaggerated startle response, insomnia, vivid nightmares, tachycardia, agitation, hypertension, and perspiration. Preliminary reports suggested that these symptoms may respond to the use of clonidine or, especially for overnight benefit, to the use of guanfacine. More recent studies have failed to demonstrate that guanfacine and clonidine produce an improvement in PTSD symptoms.

Precautions and Adverse Reactions

The most common adverse effects associated with clonidine are dry mouth and eyes, fatigue, sedation, dizziness, nausea, hypotension, and constipation, which result in discontinuation of therapy by about 10% of all persons taking the drug. Some persons also experience sexual dysfunction. Tolerance may develop to these adverse effects. A similar but milder adverse profile is seen with guanfacine, especially in doses of 3 mg or more per day. Clonidine and guanfacine should not be taken by adults with BP below 90/60 mm Hg or with cardiac arrhythmias, especially bradycardia. Development of bradycardia warrants gradual, tapered discontinuation of the drug. Clonidine in particular is associated with sedation, and tolerance does not usually develop to this adverse effect. Uncommon central nervous system (CNS) adverse effects of clonidine include insomnia, anxiety, and depression; rare CNS adverse effects include vivid dreams, nightmares, and hallucinations. Fluid retention associated with clonidine treatment can be treated with diuretics.

The transdermal patch formulation of clonidine may cause local skin irritation, which can be minimized by rotating the sites of application.

Use in Pregnancy and Lactation.   There are limited controlled data on clonidine in human pregnancy, so risk cannot be ruled out. The drug passes the placental barrier, possibly lowering the fetal heart rate. It should not be used while breastfeeding. Guanfacine, while not linked to any specific birth defects, is not well studied and should also be avoided during pregnancy and by nursing mothers.

Overdose.   Persons who take an overdose of clonidine may present with coma and constricted pupils, symptoms similar to those of an opioid overdose. Other symptoms of overdose are decreased BP, pulse, and respiratory rate. Guanfacine overdose produces a milder version of these symptoms. Elderly persons are more sensitive to the drug than are younger adults. Children are susceptible to the same adverse effects as are adults.

Withdrawal.   Abrupt discontinuation of clonidine can cause anxiety, restlessness, perspiration, tremor, abdominal pain, palpitations, headache, and a dramatic increase in BP. These symptoms may appear about 20 hours after the last dose of clonidine and these may be seen if one or two doses are skipped. A similar set of symptoms occasionally occurs 2 to 4 days after discontinuation of guanfacine, but the usual course is gradual return to baseline BP over 2 to 4 days. Because of the possibility of discontinuation symptoms, dosages of clonidine and guanfacine should be tapered slowly.

Drug Interactions

Clonidine and guanfacine cause sedation, especially early in therapy, and when administered with other centrally active depressants, such as barbiturates, alcohol, and benzodiazepines, the potential for additive sedative effects should be considered. Dose reduction may be required in patients receiving agents that interfere with atrioventricular (AV) node and sinus node conduction such as β-blockers, calcium channel blockers, and digitalis. This combination increases the risk of AV block and bradycardia. Clonidine should not be given with tricyclic antidepressants, which can inhibit the hypotensive effects of clonidine.

Laboratory Interferences

No known laboratory interferences are associated with the use of clonidine or guanfacine.

Dosage and Clinical Guidelines

Clonidine is available in 0.1-, 0.2-, and 0.3-mg tablets, 0.1- and 0.2-mg extended-release tablets. The usual starting dosage for the immediate release is 0.1 mg orally twice a day; the dosage can be raised by 0.1 mg a day to an appropriate level (up to 1.2 mg/day). Clonidine must always be tapered when it is discontinued to avoid rebound hypertension, which may occur about 20 hours after the last clonidine dose. A weekly transdermal formulation of clonidine is available at doses of 0.1, 0.2, and 0.3 mg/day. The usual starting dosage is the 0.1-mg-a-day patch, which is changed each week for adults and every 5 days for children; the dose can be increased, as needed, every 1 to 2 weeks. Transition from the oral to the transdermal formulations should be accomplished gradually by overlapping them for 3 to 4 days.

Guanfacine is available in 1- and 2-mg tablets. The usual starting dose is 1 mg before sleep, and this can be increased to 2 mg before sleep after 3 to 4 weeks, if necessary. Regardless of the indication for which clonidine or guanfacine is being used, the drug should be withheld if a person becomes hypotensive (BP below 90/60 mm Hg).

Extended-release guanfacine should be dosed once daily. Tablets should not be crushed, chewed, or broken before swallowing because this will increase the rate of guanfacine release. It should not be administered with high-fat meals, due to increases in peak plasma levels. The extended-release formulation should not be substituted for immediate-release guanfacine tablets on an mg-per-mg basis, because of differing pharmacokinetic profiles. If switching from immediate-release guanfacine, discontinue that treatment, and titrate with extended-release guanfacine according to the following recommended schedule:

1. Begin at a dose of 1 mg/day, and adjust in increments of no more than 1 mg/wk, for both monotherapy and adjunctive therapy to a psychostimulant.
2. Maintain the dose within the range of 1 mg to 4 mg once daily, depending on clinical response and tolerability, for both monotherapy and adjunctive therapy to a psychostimulant. In clinical trials, patients were randomized or dose optimized to doses of 1, 2, 3, or 4 mg and received extended-release guanfacine once daily in the morning in monotherapy trials and once daily in the morning or evening in the adjunctive therapy trial.
3. In monotherapy trials, clinically relevant improvements were observed beginning at doses in the range 0.05 to 0.08 mg/kg once daily. Efficacy increased with increasing weight-adjusted dose (mg/kg). If well tolerated, doses up to 0.12 mg/kg once daily may provide additional benefit. Doses above 4 mg/day have not been systematically studied in controlled clinical trials.
4. In the adjunctive trial, the majority of subjects reached optimal doses in the 0.05 to 0.12 mg/kg/day range.

In clinical trials, there were dose-related and exposure-related risks for several clinically significant adverse reactions (e.g., hypotension, bradycardia, sedative events). Thus, consideration should be given to dosing an extended-release preparation of guanfacine on an mg/kg basis in order to balance the exposure-related potential benefits and risks of treatment. The safety of clonidine in pregnancy is uncertain, and well-controlled studies of risks to the fetus do not exist. Studies of guanfacine in humans have shown no evidence of risk to the fetus.

Yohimbine

Yohimbine is an α_2-adrenergic receptor antagonist that is available without a prescription as a nutritional supplement. It is derived from an alkaloid found in *Rubiaceae* and related trees and in the *Rauwolfia serpentina* plant. It has been studied and is promoted as a treatment for both idiopathic and medication-induced erectile disorder and as a "fat burner." There is not sufficient evidence supporting its effectiveness for either of these roles.

Precautions

The side effects of yohimbine include anxiety, elevated BP and heart rate, increased psychomotor activity, irritability, tremor, headache, skin flushing, dizziness, urinary frequency, nausea, vomiting, and sweating. Yohimbine should be used judiciously in psychiatric patients because it may have an adverse effect on their mental status. Patients with panic disorder show heightened sensitivity to yohimbine and experience increased anxiety, increased BP, and increased plasma 3-methoxy-4-hydroxyphenylglycol (MHPG).

Yohimbine should be used with caution in female patients and should not be used in patients with renal disease, cardiac disease, glaucoma, or a history of gastric or duodenal ulcer.

Pregnancy and Lactation.   Yohimbine was never assigned to a pregnancy category under the old FDA classification system and animal studies have not been done. Due to the lack of controlled data, yohimbine should not be used during pregnancy and lactation.

Drug Interactions

Yohimbine blocks the effects of clonidine, guanfacine, and other α_2-receptor agonists.

Laboratory Interferences

No known laboratory interferences are associated with yohimbine use.

Dosage and Clinical Guidelines

Yohimbine is available in 5.4-mg tablets. The dosage of yohimbine when used in the treatment of erectile disorder is approximately 18 mg a day, given in dosages that range from 2.7 to 5.4 mg three times a day. In the event of significant adverse effects, dosage should first be reduced and then gradually increased again. Yohimbine should be used judiciously in psychiatric patients because it may have an adverse effect on their mental status.

PRAZOSIN

Prazosin (Minipress) is a quinazoline derivative used as an antihypertensive. It is an α_1-adrenergic receptor antagonist as opposed to the drugs mentioned above, which are α_2-blockers.

Pharmacologic Actions

The exact mechanism of the hypotensive action of prazosin is unknown, particularly as it effects nightmare suppression. Prazosin causes a decrease in total peripheral resistance that is related to its action as an α_1-adrenergic receptor antagonist. BP is lowered in both the supine and standing positions. This effect is most pronounced on the diastolic BP. After oral administration, human plasma concentrations reach a peak at about 3 hours with a plasma half-life of 2 to 3 hours. The drug is highly bound to plasma protein. Tolerance has not been observed to develop with long-term therapy.

Therapeutic Action

Prazosin is used in psychiatry to suppress nightmares, particularly those associated with PTSD. Nightmares return when the drug is discontinued.

Precautions and Adverse Reactions

During clinical trials and subsequent marketing experience, the most frequent reactions were dizziness, 10.3%; headache, 7.8%; drowsiness, 7.6%; lack of energy, 6.9%; weakness, 6.5%; palpitations, 5.3%; and nausea, 4.9%. In most instances, side effects disappeared with continued therapy or have been tolerated with no decrease in dose of drug.

Use in Pregnancy and Lactation

Prazosin should not be used in nursing mothers or during pregnancy.

Drug Interactions

No adverse drug interactions have been reported.

Laboratory Interferences

None reported.

Dosage and Clinical Guidelines

The drug is supplied in 1-, 2-, and 5-mg capsules and a nasal spray. The therapeutic dosages most commonly used have ranged from 6 to 15 mg daily, given in

Table 2–2
α_2-Adrenergic Receptor Agonists Used in Psychiatry[a]

Drug	Preparations	Usual Child Starting Dosage	Usual Child Dosage Range	Usual Adult Starting Dosage	Usual Adult Dosage
Clonidine tablets (Catapres)	0.1, 0.2, 0.3 mg	0.05 mg a day	Up to 0.3-mg-a-day tablets in divided doses	0.1–0.2 mg two to four times a day (0.2–0.8 mg a day)	0.3–1.2 mg a day two to three times a day (1.2 mg a day maximal dosage)
Clonidine transdermal system (Catapres-TTS)	0.1, 0.2, 0.3 mg/day	0.05 mg a day	Up to 0.3 mg a day patch every 5 days (0.5 mg a day every 5 days maximal dosage)	0.1 mg a day every 7 days	0.1 mg a day patch per week 0.6 mg a day every 7 days
Clonidine extended release (Kapvay)	0.1- and 0.2-mg tablets	0.1 mg a day	Up to 0.2 mg twice a day	0.1 mg twice a day	0.2 mg twice a day
Guanfacine (Tenex)	1- and 2-mg tablets	1 mg a day at bedtime	1–2 mg a day at bedtime (3 mg a day maximal dosage)	1 mg a day at bedtime	1–2 mg at bedtime (3 mg a day maximal dosage)
Guanfacine extended release (Intuniv)	1-, 2-, 3-, 4-mg tablets	1 mg a day	1–4 mg a day	1 mg a day	0.005–0.12 mg/kg/day (1–7 mg a day maximal dose)

[a]Dosages for medical indications, such as hypertension, vary.

divided doses. Doses higher than 20 mg do not increase efficacy. When adding a diuretic or other antihypertensive agent, the dose should be reduced to 1 or 2 mg three times a day and retitration then carried out. Concomitant use with a PDE-5 inhibitor can result in additive BP-lowering effects and symptomatic hypotension; therefore, PDE-5 inhibitor therapy should be initiated at the lowest dose in patients taking prazosin.

Table 2–2 provides a summary of α_2-adrenergic receptor agonists used in psychiatry.

3
β-Adrenergic Receptor Antagonists

INTRODUCTION

β-Adrenergic receptors are ubiquitously distributed throughout the body including the heart, lung, autonomic, and CNS. Although β-adrenergic receptor antagonists are not currently FDA approved for use in any psychiatric disorder, these agents have been used to treat disparate psychiatric conditions such as performance anxiety, posttraumatic stress disorder (PTSD), panic attacks, major depressive disorder, aggressive and violent behavior, behavioral symptoms associated with dementia, alcohol and cocaine withdrawal, lithium-induced postural tremor, antipsychotic-induced akathisia, and migraine. The five β-adrenergic receptor antagonists most frequently studied for psychiatric application are propranolol (Inderal), metoprolol (Lopressor, Toprol XL), atenolol (Tenormin), nadolol (Corgard), and pindolol (Visken).

PHARMACOLOGIC ACTIONS

The β-receptor antagonists differ with regard to lipophilicities, metabolic routes, β-receptor selectivity, and half-lives (Table 3–1). The absorption of the β-receptor antagonists from the gastrointestinal tract is variable. The agents that are most soluble in lipids (i.e., are lipophilic) are likely to cross the blood–brain barrier and enter the brain; those agents that are least lipophilic are less likely to enter the brain. When CNS effects are desired, a lipophilic drug may be preferred; when only peripheral effects are desired, a less lipophilic drug may be indicated.

Whereas propranolol, nadolol, pindolol, and labetalol (Normodyne, Trandate) have essentially equal potency at both the β_1- and β_2-receptors, metoprolol and atenolol have greater affinity for the β_1-receptor than for the β_2-receptor. Relative β_1-selectivity confers few pulmonary and vascular effects of these drugs, although they must be used with caution in persons with asthma because the drugs retain some activity at the β_2-receptors.

Pindolol has sympathomimetic effects in addition to its β-antagonist effects, which has permitted its use for augmentation of antidepressant drugs. Pindolol, propranolol, and nadolol possess some antagonist activity at the serotonin 5-HT$_{1A}$ receptors.

THERAPEUTIC INDICATIONS
Anxiety Disorders

Propranolol is useful for the treatment of social phobia, primarily of the performance type (e.g., disabling anxiety before a musical performance). Data are also available for its use in treatment of panic disorder, PTSD, and generalized anxiety disorder. In social phobia, the common treatment approach is to take 10 to 40 mg of propranolol 20 to 30 minutes before the anxiety-provoking situation. The β-receptor antagonists are less effective for the treatment of panic disorder than are benzodiazepines or selective serotonin reuptake inhibitors (SSRIs).

Table 3-1

β-Adrenergic Drugs Used in Psychiatry

Drug	Trade Name	Protein Binding (%)	Lipophilic	ISA	Metabolism	Receptor Selectivity	Half-Life (hours)	Usual Starting Dosage (mg)	Usual Maximal Dosage (mg)
Atenolol (Tenormin)	Tenormin	6-16	No		Renal	$\beta_1 > \beta_2$	6-9	50 OD	50-100 OD
Metoprolol (Lopressor)	Lopressor	5-10	Yes		Hepatic	$\beta_1 > \beta_2$	3-4	50 BID	75-150 BID
Nadolol (Corgard)	Corgard	30	No		Renal	$\beta_1 = \beta_2$	14-24	40 OD	80-240 OD
Propranolol (Inderal)	Inderal	>90	Yes		Hepatic	$\beta_1 = \beta_2$	3-6	10-20 BID/TID	80-140 TID
Pindolol (Visken)	Visken	40	Yes	Minimal	Hepatic	$\beta_1 > \beta_2$	3-4	5 TID/QID	60 BID/TID

ISA, intrinsic sympathomimetic activity.

Lithium-Induced Postural Tremor

The β-receptor antagonists are beneficial for lithium-induced postural tremor and other medication-induced postural tremors—for example, those induced by tricycle antidepressants (TCAs) and valproate (Depakene). The initial approach to this movement disorder includes lowering the dose of lithium, eliminating aggravating factors, such as caffeine, and administering lithium at bedtime. If these interventions are inadequate, however, propranolol in the range of 20 to 160 mg a day given two or three times daily is generally effective for the treatment of lithium-induced postural tremor.

Neuroleptic-Induced Acute Akathisia

Many studies have shown that β-receptor antagonists can be effective in the treatment of neuroleptic-induced acute akathisia. They are generally more effective for this indication than are anticholinergics and benzodiazepines. The β-receptor antagonists are not effective in the treatment of such neuroleptic-induced movement disorders as acute dystonia and parkinsonism.

Aggression and Violent Behavior

The β-receptor antagonists may be effective in reducing the number of aggressive and violent outbursts in persons with impulse disorders, schizophrenia, and aggression associated with brain injuries such as trauma, tumors, anoxic injury, encephalitis, alcohol dependence, and degenerative disorders (e.g., Huntington's disease).

Alcohol Withdrawal

Propranolol is reported to be useful as an adjuvant to benzodiazepines but not as a sole agent in the treatment of alcohol withdrawal. The following dose schedule is suggested: no propranolol for a pulse rate below 50 beats/min; 50 mg propranolol for a pulse rate between 50 and 79 beats/min; and 100 mg propranolol for a pulse rate of 80 beats/min or above.

Antidepressant Augmentation

Pindolol has been studied as augmentation to hasten the antidepressant effects of SSRIs, tricyclic drugs, and electroconvulsive therapy. Evidence of its effectiveness in this role is not well established. Because the β-receptor antagonists may possibly induce depression in some persons, augmentation strategies with these drugs need to be further clarified in controlled trials.

Other Disorders

β-receptor antagonists have also been used in some cases of stuttering (Table 3–2).

PRECAUTIONS AND ADVERSE REACTIONS

The β-receptor antagonists are contraindicated for use in people with asthma, insulin-dependent diabetes, congestive heart failure, significant vascular disease, persistent angina, and hyperthyroidism. The contraindication in diabetic persons is because of the drugs' antagonizing the normal physiologic response to hypoglycemia. The β-receptor antagonists can worsen atrioventricular (AV) conduction defects and

Table 3–2
Psychiatric Uses for β-Adrenergic Receptor Antagonists

Definitely effective
Performance anxiety
Lithium-induced tremor
Neuroleptic-induced akathisia
Probably effective
Adjunctive therapy for alcohol withdrawal and other substance-related disorders
Adjunctive therapy for aggressive or violent behavior
Possibly effective
Antipsychotic augmentation
Antidepressant augmentation

lead to complete AV heart block and death. If the clinician decides that the risk-to-benefit ratio warrants a trial of a β-receptor antagonist in a person with one of these coexisting medical conditions, a β_1-selective agent should be the first choice, and the patient should be monitored. All currently available β-receptor antagonists are excreted in breast milk and should be administered with caution to nursing women.

The most common adverse effects of β-receptor antagonists are hypotension and bradycardia. In persons at risk for these adverse effects, a test dosage of 20 mg a day of propranolol can be given to assess reaction to the drug. Depression has been associated with lipophilic β-receptor antagonists, such as propranolol, but it is probably rare. Nausea, vomiting, diarrhea, and constipation can also be caused by treatment with these agents. The β-receptor antagonists may blunt cognition in some people. Serious CNS adverse effects (e.g., agitation, confusion, and hallucinations) are rare.

Use in Pregnancy and Lactation
There are no proven risks associated with use of β-receptor antagonists during pregnancy and lactation. There have been reports of possible fetal growth retardation when these drugs are used early in pregnancy.

Table 3–3 lists the possible adverse effects of β-receptor antagonists.

DRUG INTERACTIONS
Concomitant administration of propranolol results in increases in plasma concentrations of antipsychotics, anticonvulsants, theophylline (Theo-Dur, Slo-Bid), and levothyroxine sodium (Synthroid). Other β-receptor antagonists may have similar effects. The β-receptor antagonists that are eliminated by the kidneys may have similar effects on drugs that are also eliminated by the renal route. Barbiturates, phenytoin (Dilantin), and cigarette smoking increase the elimination of β-receptor antagonists that are metabolized by the liver. Several reports have associated hypertensive crises and bradycardia with the coadministration of β-receptor antagonists and monoamine oxidase inhibitors. Depressed myocardial contractility and AV nodal conduction can occur from concomitant administration of a β-receptor antagonist and calcium channel inhibitors.

LABORATORY INTERFERENCES
The β-receptor antagonists do not interfere with standard laboratory tests.

Table 3–3
Adverse Effects and Toxicity of β-Adrenergic Receptor Antagonists

Cardiovascular
  Hypotension
  Bradycardia
  Congestive heart failure (in patients with compromised myocardial function)
Respiratory
  Asthma (less risk with β₁-selective drugs)
Metabolic
  Worsened hypoglycemia in diabetic patients on insulin or oral agents
Gastrointestinal
  Nausea
  Diarrhea
  Abdominal pain
Sexual function
  Impotence
Neuropsychiatric
  Lassitude
  Fatigue
  Dysphoria
  Insomnia
  Vivid nightmares
  Depression (rare)
  Psychosis (rare)
Other (rare)
  Raynaud's phenomenon
  Peyronie's disease
Withdrawal syndrome
  Rebound worsening of pre-existing angina pectoris when β-adrenergic receptor antagonists are
  discontinued

DOSAGE AND CLINICAL GUIDELINES

Propranolol is available in 10-, 20-, 40-, 60-, 80-, and 90-mg tablets; 4-, 8-, and 80-mg/mL solutions; and 60-, 80-, 120-, and 160-mg sustained-release capsules. Nadolol is available in 20-, 40-, 80-, 120-, and 160-mg tablets. Pindolol is available in 5- and 10-mg tablets. Metoprolol is available in 50- and 100-mg tablets and 50-, 100-, and 200-mg sustained-release tablets. Atenolol is available in 25-, 50-, and 100-mg tablets. Acebutolol is available in 200- and 400-mg capsules.

For the treatment of chronic disorders, propranolol administration is usually initiated at 10 mg by mouth three times a day or 20 mg by mouth twice daily. The dosage can be raised from 20 to 30 mg a day until a therapeutic effect emerges. The dosage should be leveled off at the appropriate range for the disorder under treatment. The treatment of aggressive behavior sometimes requires dosages up to 80 mg a day, and therapeutic effects may not be seen until the person has been receiving the maximal dosage for 4 to 8 weeks. For the treatment of social phobia, primarily the performance type, the patient should take 10 to 40 mg of propranolol 20 to 30 minutes before the performance.

Pulse and blood pressure (BP) readings should be taken regularly, and the drug should be withheld if the pulse rate is below 50 beats/min or the systolic BP is below 90 mm Hg. The drug should be temporarily discontinued if it produces severe dizziness, ataxia, or wheezing. Treatment with β-receptor antagonists should never be discontinued abruptly. Propranolol should be tapered by 60 mg a day until a dosage of 60 mg a day is reached, after which the drug should be tapered by 10 to 20 mg a day every 3 or 4 days.

The clinical guidelines for the other drugs listed in this chapter are similar to propranolol taking into consideration the different doses used. For example, if propranolol is prescribed initially at the lowest available dose (e.g., 10 mg) then metoprolol should be prescribed at its lowest available dose (e.g., 50 mg).

4
Anticholinergic Agents

INTRODUCTION

Anticholinergic drugs block the binding of acetylcholine to its receptor. They block the effects of atropine. In psychiatry, the anticholinergic drugs are primarily used to treat medication-induced movement disorders, particularly neuroleptic-induced parkinsonism, neuroleptic-induced acute dystonia, and medication-induced postural tremor. It is commonly used to treat asthma and motion sickness.

ANTICHOLINERGICS
Pharmacologic Actions

All anticholinergic drugs are well absorbed from the gastrointestinal (GI) tract after oral administration, and all are sufficiently lipophilic to enter the central nervous system (CNS). Trihexyphenidyl (Artane) and benztropine (Cogentin) reach peak plasma concentrations in 2 to 3 hours after oral administration, and their duration of action is 1 to 12 hours. Benztropine is absorbed equally rapidly by intramuscular (IM) and intravenous (IV) administration; IM administration is preferred because of its low risk for adverse effects.

All six anticholinergic drugs listed (Table 4–1) in this section block muscarinic acetylcholine receptors, and benztropine also has some antihistaminergic effects. None of the available anticholinergic drugs have any effects on the nicotinic acetylcholine receptors. Of these drugs, trihexyphenidyl is the most stimulating agent, perhaps acting through dopaminergic neurons, and benztropine is the least stimulating and thus is least associated with abuse potential.

Therapeutic Indications

The primary indication for the use of anticholinergics in psychiatric practice is for the treatment of *neuroleptic-induced parkinsonism*, characterized by tremor, rigidity, cogwheeling, bradykinesia, sialorrhea, stooped posture, and festination. All of the available anticholinergics are equally effective in the treatment of parkinsonian symptoms. Neuroleptic-induced parkinsonism is most common in elderly persons and is most frequently seen with high-potency dopamine receptor antagonists (DRAs), for example, haloperidol (Haldol). The onset of symptoms usually occurs after 2 or 3 weeks of treatment. The incidence of neuroleptic-induced parkinsonism is lower with the newer generation of antipsychotic drugs of the serotonin–dopamine antagonist (SDA) class.

Another indication is for the treatment of *neuroleptic-induced acute dystonia*, which is most common in young men. The syndrome often occurs early in the course of treatment; is commonly associated with high-potency DRAs (e.g., haloperidol); and most commonly affects the muscles of the neck, tongue, face, and back.

Table 4–1
Anticholinergic Drugs

Generic Name	Brand Name	Tablet Size	Injectable	Usual Daily Oral Dosage	Short-Term Intramuscular or Intravenous Dosage
Benztropine	Cogentin	0.5, 1, 2 mg	1 mg/mL	1–4 mg one to three times	1–2 mg
Biperiden	Akineton	2 mg	5 mg/mL	2 mg one to three times	2 mg
Ethopropazine	Parsidol	10, 50 mg	—	50–100 mg one to three times	—
Orphenadrine	Norflex, Disipal	100 mg	30 mg/mL	50–100 mg three times	60 mg IV given over 5 minutes
Procyclidine hydrochloride	Kemadrin	5 mg	—	2, 5–5 mg three times	—
Trihexyphenidyl	Artane, Trihexane, Trihexy-5	2, 5 mg elixir 2 mg/5 mL	—	2–5 mg two to four times	—

IV, intravenous.

Anticholinergic drugs are effective both in the short-term treatment of dystonias and in prophylaxis against neuroleptic-induced acute dystonias.

Akathisia is characterized by a subjective and objective sense of restlessness, anxiety, and agitation. Although a trial of anticholinergics for the treatment of neuroleptic-induced acute akathisia is reasonable, these drugs are not generally considered as effective as the β-adrenergic receptor antagonists, the benzodiazepines, and clonidine (Catapres).

Precautions and Adverse Reactions

The adverse effects of the anticholinergic drugs result from blockade of muscarinic acetylcholine receptors. Anticholinergic drugs should be used cautiously, if at all, by persons with prostatic hypertrophy, urinary retention, and narrow-angle glaucoma. The anticholinergics are occasionally used as drugs of abuse because of their mild mood-elevating properties, most notably, trihexyphenidyl.

The most serious adverse effect associated with anticholinergic toxicity is anticholinergic intoxication, which can be characterized by delirium, coma, seizures, agitation, hallucinations, severe hypotension, supraventricular tachycardia, and peripheral manifestations (flushing, mydriasis, dry skin, hyperthermia, and decreased bowel sounds). Treatment should begin with the immediate discontinuation of all anticholinergic drugs. The syndrome of anticholinergic intoxication can be diagnosed and treated with physostigmine (Antilirium, Eserine), an inhibitor of anticholinesterase, 1 to 2 mg IV (1 mg every 2 minutes) or IM every 30 or 60 minutes. Treatment with physostigmine should be used only in severe cases and only when emergency cardiac monitoring and life-support services are available because physostigmine can lead to severe hypotension and bronchial constriction.

Use in Pregnancy and Lactation

There are no proven risks associated with use of anticholinergics during pregnancy and lactation, but caution is advised because of possible cases of neonatal paralytic ileus and of decreases in milk production.

Drug Interactions

The most common drug–drug interactions with the anticholinergics occur when they are coadministered with psychotropics that also have high anticholinergic activity, such as DRAs, tricyclic and tetracyclic drugs, and monoamine oxidase inhibitors (MAOIs). Many other prescription drugs and over-the-counter cold preparations also induce significant anticholinergic activity. The coadministration of those drugs can result in a life-threatening anticholinergic intoxication syndrome. Anticholinergic drugs can also delay gastric emptying, thereby decreasing the absorption of drugs that are broken down in the stomach and usually absorbed in the duodenum (e.g., levodopa [Larodopa] and DRAs).

Laboratory Interferences

No known laboratory interferences have been associated with anticholinergics.

Dosage and Clinical Guidelines

The three most commonly used anticholinergic drugs discussed in this chapter are available in a range of preparations (Table 4–1).

Neuroleptic-Induced Parkinsonism.   For the treatment of neuroleptic-induced parkinsonism, the equivalent of 1 to 3 mg of benztropine should be given one to two times daily. The anticholinergic drug should be administered for 4 to 8 weeks, and then it should be discontinued to assess whether the person still requires the drug. Anticholinergic drugs should be tapered over a period of 1 to 2 weeks.

Treatment with anticholinergics as prophylaxis against the development of neuroleptic-induced parkinsonism is usually not indicated because the onset of its symptoms are usually sufficiently mild and gradual to allow the clinician to initiate treatment only after it is clearly indicated. In young men, prophylaxis may be indicated, however, especially if a high-potency DRA is being used. The clinician should attempt to discontinue the antiparkinsonian agent in 4 to 6 weeks to assess whether its continued use is necessary.

Neuroleptic-Induced Acute Dystonia.   For the short-term treatment and prophylaxis of neuroleptic-induced acute dystonia, 1 to 2 mg of benztropine or its equivalent in another drug should be given IM. The dose can be repeated in 20 to 30 minutes, as needed. If the person still does not improve in another 20 to 30 minutes, a benzodiazepine (e.g., 1 mg IM or IV lorazepam [Ativan]) should be given. Laryngeal dystonia is a medical emergency and should be treated with benztropine, up to 4 mg in a 10-minute period, followed by 1 to 2 mg of lorazepam, administered slowly by the IV route.

Prophylaxis against dystonias is indicated in persons who have had one episode or in persons at high risk (young men taking high-potency DRAs). Prophylactic treatment is given for 4 to 8 weeks and then gradually tapered over 1 to 2 weeks to allow assessment of its continued need. The prophylactic use of anticholinergics in persons requiring antipsychotic drugs has largely become a moot issue because of the availability of SDAs, which are relatively free of parkinsonian effects.

Akathisia.   As mentioned, anticholinergics are not the drugs of choice for this syndrome. The β-adrenergic receptor antagonists (Chapter 3) and perhaps the benzodiazepines (Chapter 8) and clonidine (Chapter 2) are preferable drugs to try initially.

5

Anticonvulsants

INTRODUCTION

The newer anticonvulsants described in this section were developed for the treatment of epilepsy but were also found to have beneficial effects in psychiatric disorders. They are also used as skeletal muscle relaxants and in neurogenic pain. These drugs have a variety of mechanisms including increasing γ-aminobutyric acid (GABAergic) function or decreasing glutamatergic function. This chapter includes five anticonvulsants that are sometimes used in treating psychiatric disorders: gabapentin (Neurontin), levetiracetam (Keppra), pregabalin (Lyrica), tiagabine (Gabitril), topiramate (Topamax), and zonisamide (Zonegran), as well as one of the first used anticonvulsants, phenytoin (Dilantin). The drugs carbamazepine (Tegretol), valproate (Depakene, Depakote), lamotrigine (Lamictal), and oxcarbazepine (Trileptal) are discussed in separate sections, because with the exception of oxcarbazepine, those drugs are approved by the FDA for treatment of bipolar disorder.

The Food and Drug Administration (FDA) has issued a warning that anticonvulsant drugs may increase the risk of suicidal ideation or act in some persons compared with placebo; however, in clinical trials, the relative risk for suicidality was higher in patients with epilepsy compared with those with psychiatric disorders. However, some published data contradict the warning by the FDA regarding the use of anticonvulsants and the risk of suicidal thoughts. These studies suggest that anticonvulsants may have a protective effect on suicidal thoughts in bipolar disorder. Considering the inherent increased risk of suicide in persons with bipolar disorder, clinicians should be aware of these warnings.

GABAPENTIN

Gabapentin was first introduced as an antiepileptic medication and was found to have sedative effects that were useful in some psychiatric disorders, especially insomnia. It was also found to be beneficial in reducing neuropathic pain, including postherpetic neuralgia. It is used in anxiety disorders (social phobia and panic disorder), but not as a main intervention in mania or treatment-resistant mood disorders.

Pharmacologic Actions

Gabapentin circulates in the blood largely unbound and is not appreciably metabolized in humans. It is eliminated unchanged by renal excretion and can be removed by hemodialysis. Food only moderately affects the rate and extent of absorption. Clearance is decreased in elderly persons, requiring dosage adjustments. Gabapentin appears to increase cerebral GABA and may inhibit glutamate synthesis as well. It increases human whole blood serotonin concentrations and modulates calcium channels to reduce monoamine release. It has antiseizure as well as antispastic activity and antinociceptive effects in pain.

Therapeutic Indications

In neurology, gabapentin is used for the treatment of both general and partial seizures. It is effective in reducing the pain of postherpetic neuralgia and other pain syndromes associated with diabetic neuropathy, neuropathic cancer pain, fibromyalgia, meralgia paresthetica, amputation, and headache. It has been found to be effective in some cases of chronic pruritus.

In psychiatry, gabapentin is used as a hypnotic agent because of its sedating effects. It has anxiolytic properties and benefits patients with social anxiety and panic disorder. It may decrease the craving for alcohol in some patients and improve mood as well; hence, it may have some use in depressed patients. Some bipolar patients have benefited when gabapentin is used adjunctively with mood stabilizers.

Precautions and Adverse Reactions

Adverse effects are mild with the most common being daytime somnolence, ataxia, and fatigue, which are usually dose related. Overdose (over 45 g) has been associated with diplopia, slurred speech, lethargy, and diarrhea, but all patients recovered.

Use in Pregnancy and Lactation

Gabapentin use and risk to the fetus has not been ruled out since it is excreted in breast milk, so it is best to avoid gabapentin in pregnant women and nursing mothers.

Drug Interactions

Gabapentin bioavailability may decrease as much as 20% when administered with antacids. In general, there are no drug interactions. Chronic use does not interfere with lithium administration.

Laboratory Interferences

Gabapentin does not interfere with any laboratory tests, although spontaneous reports of false-positive or positive drug toxicology screenings for amphetamines, barbiturates, benzodiazepines, and marijuana have been reported.

Dosages and Clinical Guidelines

Gabapentin is well tolerated, and the dosage can be increased to the maintenance range within a few days. A general approach is to start with 300 mg on day 1, increase to 600 mg on day 2, 900 mg on day 3, and subsequently increase up to 1,800 mg per day in divided doses as needed to relieve symptoms. Final total daily doses tend to be between 1,200 and 2,400 mg per day but occasionally results may be achieved with dosages as low as 200 to 300 mg per day, especially in elderly persons. Sedation is usually the limiting factor in determining the dosage. Some patients have taken dosages as high as 4,800 mg per day.

Gabapentin is available as 100-, 300-, and 400-mg capsules and as 600- and 800-mg tablets. A 250-mg/5-mL oral solution is also available. Although abrupt discontinuation of gabapentin does not cause withdrawal effects, use of all anticonvulsant drugs should be gradually tapered.

TOPIRAMATE

Topiramate (Topamax) was developed as an anticonvulsant and was found useful in migraine prevention, treatment of obesity, bulimia, binge eating, and alcohol dependence.

Pharmacologic Actions

Topiramate has GABAergic effects and increases cerebral GABA in humans. It has 80% oral bioavailability and is not significantly altered by food. It is 15% protein bound, and about 70% of the drug is eliminated by renal excretion. With renal insufficiency topiramate clearance decreases about 50%, so the dosage needs to be decreased. It has a half-life of around 24 hours.

Therapeutic Indications

Topiramate is used mainly as an antiepileptic medication and has been found superior to placebo as monotherapy in patients with seizure disorders. It is also used in the prevention of migraine, smoking cessation, pain syndromes (e.g., low back pain), posttraumatic stress disorder (PTSD), and essential tremor. The drug has been associated with weight loss, and that fact has been used to counteract the weight gain caused by many psychotropic drugs. It has also been used in general obesity and in the treatment of bulimia and binge-eating disorder. Self-mutilating behavior may be decreased in borderline personality disorder. It is of little or no benefit in the treatment of psychotic disorders. The combination of topiramate bupropion (Wellbutrin) has been used for weight loss.

Precautions and Adverse Reactions

The most common adverse effects of topiramate include paresthesias, weight loss, somnolence, anorexia, dizziness, and memory problems. Sometimes disturbances in the sense of taste occur. In many cases, the adverse effects are mild to moderate and can be attenuated by decreasing the dose. No deaths have been reported during overdose. The drug affects acid–base balance (low serum bicarbonate), which can be associated with cardiac arrhythmias, and the formation of renal calculi in about 1.5% of cases. Patients taking the drug should be encouraged to drink plenty of fluids.

Use in Pregnancy and Lactation

Use of topiramate during the first trimester is associated with an increased risk of oral clefts. Since there is positive risk of birth defects, it should be avoided during pregnancy. Topiramate is carried in breast milk.

Drug Interactions

Topiramate has few drug interactions with other anticonvulsant drugs. Topiramate may increase phenytoin concentrations up to 25% and valproic acid up to 11%; it does not affect the concentration of carbamazepine, phenobarbital (Luminal), or primidone. Topiramate concentrations are decreased by 40% to 48% with concomitant administration of carbamazepine or phenytoin. Topiramate should not be combined with other carbonic anhydrase inhibitors, such as acetazolamide (Diamox) or dichlorphenamide (Daranide), because this could increase the risk of nephrolithiasis or heat-related problems (oligohidrosis and hyperthermia).

Laboratory Interferences
Topiramate does not interfere with any laboratory tests.

Dosages and Clinical Guidelines
Topiramate is available as unscored 25-, 100-, and 200-mg tablets. To reduce the risk of adverse cognitive and sedative effects, topiramate dosage is titrated gradually over 8 weeks to a maximum of 200 mg twice a day. Off-label topiramate is typically used adjunctively, starting with 25 mg at bedtime and increasing weekly by 25 mg as necessary and tolerated. Final doses in efforts to promote weight loss are often between 75 and 150 mg per day at bedtime. Doses higher than 400 mg are not associated with increased efficacy. All of the dose can be given at bedtime to take advantage of the sedative effects. Persons with renal insufficiency should reduce doses by half.

TIAGABINE
Tiagabine was introduced as a treatment for epilepsy in 1997 and was found to have efficacy in some psychiatric conditions, including acute mania. However, safety concerns (see later) along with a lack of controlled data have limited the use of tiagabine in disorders other than epilepsy.

Pharmacologic Actions
Tiagabine is well absorbed with a bioavailability of about 90% and is extensively (96%) bound to plasma proteins. Tiagabine is a CYP3A substrate and is extensively transformed into inactive 5-oxo-tiagabine and glucuronide metabolites, with only 2% being excreted unchanged in the urine. The remainder is excreted as metabolites in the feces (65%) and the urine (25%). Tiagabine blocks uptake of the inhibitory amino acid neurotransmitter GABA into neurons and glia, enhancing the inhibitory action of GABA at both $GABA_A$ and $GABA_B$ receptors, putatively yielding anticonvulsant and antinociceptive effects, respectively. It has mild blocking effects on histamine 1 (H_1), serotonin type 1B ($5-HT_{1B}$), benzodiazepine, and chloride channel receptors.

Therapeutic Indications
Tiagabine is rarely used for psychiatric disorders and then it is only used for generalized anxiety disorder and insomnia. Its main indication is in generalized epilepsy.

Precautions and Adverse Reactions
Tiagabine may cause withdrawal seizures, cognitive or neuropsychiatric problems (impaired concentration, speech or language problems, somnolence, and fatigue), status epilepticus, and sudden unexpected death in epilepsy. Acute oral overdoses of tiagabine have been associated with seizures, status epilepticus, coma, ataxia, confusion, somnolence, drowsiness, impaired speech, agitation, lethargy, myoclonus, stupor, tremors, disorientation, vomiting, hostility, temporary paralysis, and respiratory depression. Deaths have been reported in polydrug overdoses involving tiagabine. Cases of serious rash may occur, including Stevens–Johnson syndrome.

Use in Pregnancy and Lactation
Tiagabine has been linked to fetal loss and teratogenicity has been demonstrated in animals. The drug is excreted in breast milk. Pregnant women and nursing mothers should not be given the drug.

Laboratory Tests

Tiagabine does not interfere with any laboratory tests.

Dosage and Administration

Tiagabine should not be rapidly loaded or rapidly initiated because of the risk of serious adverse effects. In adults and adolescents 12 years of age or older with epilepsy who are also taking enzyme inducers, tiagabine should be initiated at 4 mg per day and increased weekly by 4 mg per day during the first month and then increased weekly by 4 to 8 mg per day for weeks 5 and 6, yielding 24 to 32 mg per day administered in two to four divided doses by week 6. In adults (but not adolescents), tiagabine doses may be further increased weekly by 4 to 8 mg per day to as high as 56 mg per day. Plasma concentrations in epilepsy patients commonly range between 20 and 100 ng/mL but do not appear to be systematically related to antiseizure effects and thus are not routinely monitored.

LEVETIRACETAM

Initially developed as a nootropic (memory enhancing) drug, levetiracetam proved to be a potent anticonvulsant and marketed as a treatment for partial seizures. It has been used to treat acute mania and anxiety and to augment antidepressant drug therapy.

Pharmacologic Actions

The central nervous system (CNS) effects are not well understood, but it appears to indirectly enhance GABA inhibition. It is rapidly and completely absorbed, and peak concentrations are reached in 1 hour. Food delays the rate of absorption and decreases the amount of absorption. Levetiracetam is not significantly plasma protein bound and is not metabolized through the hepatic CYP system. Its metabolism involves hydrolysis of the acetamide group. Serum concentrations are not correlated with therapeutic effects.

Therapeutic Indications

The major indication is for the treatment in convulsive disorders, including partial onset seizures, myoclonic seizures, and idiopathic generalized epilepsy. In psychiatry, it has been used off label to treat acute mania, as an add-on treatment for major depression, and as an anxiolytic agent.

Precautions and Adverse Reactions

The most common side effects of levetiracetam include drowsiness, dizziness, ataxia, diplopia, memory impairment, apathy, and paresthesias. Some patients develop behavioral disturbances during treatment, and hallucinations may occur. Suicidal patients may become agitated.

Use in Pregnancy and Lactation

There are no proven risks associated with use of levetiracetam during pregnancy, but risk cannot be ruled out. Even though very little of the medication gets into breast milk, the product labeling says it should not be used in lactating women.

Drug Interactions

There are few if any interactions with other drugs, including other anticonvulsants. There is no interaction with lithium.

Laboratory Interferences

No laboratory interferences have been reported.

Dosages and Clinical Guidelines

The drug is available as 250-, 500-, 750-, and 1,000-mg tablets, 500-mg extended-release tablets; a 100-mg/mL oral solution, and a 100-mg/mL intravenous solution. In epilepsy, the typical adult daily dose is 1,000 mg.

In view of its renal clearance, dosages should be reduced in patients with impaired renal function.

ZONISAMIDE

Used originally as an anticonvulsant for the treatment of seizure disorders, zonisamide was also found to be useful in bipolar disorder, obesity, and binge-eating disorder.

Pharmacologic Actions

Zonisamide blocks sodium channels and may weakly potentiate dopamine and serotonin activity. It also inhibits carbonic anhydrase. Some evidence suggests that it may block calcium channels. Zonisamide is metabolized by the hepatic CYP4503A system, so enzyme-inducing agents, such as carbamazepine, alcohol, and phenobarbital, increase the clearance and reduce the availability of the drug. Zonisamide does not affect the metabolism of other drugs. It has a long half-life of 60 hours, so it is easily dosed once daily, preferably at nighttime.

Therapeutic Indications

Its main use is in the treatment of generalized seizure disorders and in refractory partial seizures. In psychiatry, controlled studies found it to be of use in obesity and binge-eating disorder. Uncontrolled trials have found it useful in bipolar disorder, particularly mania; however, further studies are warranted for this indication.

Precautions and Adverse Reactions

Zonisamide is a sulfonamide and thus may cause fatal rash and blood dyscrasias, although these events are rare. About 4% of patients develop kidney stones. The most common side effects are drowsiness, cognitive impairment, insomnia, ataxia, nystagmus, paresthesia, speech abnormalities, constipation, diarrhea, nausea, and dry mouth. Weight loss is also a common side effect, which has been exploited as a therapy for patients who have gained weight during treatment with psychotropics or, as mentioned above, have ongoing difficulty controlling their eating.

Use in Pregnancy and Lactation

Zonisamide should not be used in pregnant women or breastfeeding mothers. Fetal abnormalities or embryofetal deaths have been reported in animal tests at doses and maternal plasma levels similar to, or less than human therapeutic concentrations.

Drug Interactions

Zonisamide does not inhibit CYP450 isoenzymes and does not instigate drug inter-actions. It is important not to combine carbonic anhydrase inhibitors with zon-isamide because of an increased risk of nephrolithiasis related to increased blood levels of urea.

Laboratory Interferences

Zonisamide can elevate hepatic alkaline phosphatase and increase blood urea nitro-gen and creatinine.

Dosages and Clinical Guidelines

Zonisamide is available in 100- and 200-mg capsules. In epilepsy, the dosage range is 100 to 400 mg per day, with side effects becoming more pronounced at doses above 300 mg. Because of its long half-life, zonisamide can be given once a day.

PREGABALIN

Pregabalin is pharmacologically similar to gabapentin. It is believed to work by inhibiting the release of excess excitatory neurotransmitters. It increases neuronal GABA levels, its binding affinity is six times greater than that of gabapentin, and it has a longer half-life.

Pharmacologic Actions

Pregabalin exhibits linear pharmacokinetics. It is extremely and rapidly absorbed in proportion to its dose. The time to maximal plasma concentration is about 1 hour and that to steady state is within 24 to 48 hours. Pregabalin demonstrates high bio-availability, and it has a mean elimination half-life of about 6.5 hours. Food does not affect absorption. Pregabalin does not bind to plasma proteins and is excreted virtually unchanged (<2% metabolism) by the kidneys. It is not subject to hepatic metabolism and does not induce or inhibit liver enzymes such as the CYP450 sys-tem. Dose reduction may be necessary in patients with creatinine clearance (CLcr) less than 60 mL per minute. Daily doses should be further reduced by approxi-mately 50% for each additional 50% decrease in CLcr. Pregabalin is highly cleared by hemodialysis, so additional doses may be needed for patients on chronic hemodi-alysis treatment after each hemodialysis treatment.

Therapeutic Indications

Pregabalin is approved for the management of diabetic peripheral neuropathy and postherpetic neuralgia and for adjunctive treatment of partial onset seizures. It has been found to be of benefit to some patients with generalized anxiety disorder. In studies, no consistent dose–response relationship was found, although 300 mg of pregabalin per day was more effective than 150 or 450 mg. Some patients with panic disorder or social anxiety disorder may benefit from pregabalin, but little evidence supports its routine use in treating persons with these disorders. It was most recently approved for the treatment of fibromyalgia.

Precautions and Adverse Reactions

The most common adverse events associated with pregabalin use are dizziness, somnolence, blurred vision, peripheral edema, amnesia or loss of memory, and tremors. Pregabalin potentiates sedating effects of alcohol, antihistamines, benzodiazepines, and other CNS depressants. It remains to be seen if pregabalin is associated with benzodiazepine-type withdrawal symptoms.

Use in Pregnancy and Lactation

Prenatal pregabalin use is associated with an increased risk of major birth defects. These include heart defects and CNS abnormalities.

Drug Interactions

In view of the absence of hepatic metabolism, pregabalin lacks metabolic drug interactions.

Laboratory Interferences

There are no effects on laboratory tests.

Dosage and Clinical Guidelines

The recommended dose for postherpetic neuralgia is 50 or 100 mg orally three times a day. The recommended dose for diabetic peripheral neuropathy is 100 to 200 mg orally three times a day. Patients with fibromyalgia may require up to 450 to 600 mg per day given in divided doses. Pregabalin is available as 25-, 50-, 75-, 100-, 150-, 200-, 225-, and 300-mg capsules.

PHENYTOIN

Phenytoin sodium (Dilantin) is an antiepileptic drug and is related to the barbiturates in chemical structure. It is indicated for the control of generalized tonic–clonic (grand mal) and complex partial (psychomotor, temporal lobe) seizures and prevention and treatment of seizures occurring during or after neurosurgery. Studies have shown comparable efficacy of phenytoin to other anticonvulsants in bipolar disorder, but clinicians should take into account the danger of gingival hyperplasia, leukopenia, or anemia and the danger of toxicity caused by nonlinear pharmacokinetics.

Pharmacologic Action

Similar to other anticonvulsants, phenytoin causes blockade of voltage-activated sodium channels and hence is efficacious as an antimanic agent. The plasma half-life after oral administration averages 22 hours, with a range of 7 to 42 hours. Steady-state therapeutic levels are achieved at least 7 to 10 days (5 to 7 half-lives) after initiation of therapy with recommended doses of 300 mg per day. Serum level should be obtained at least 5 to 7 half-lives after treatment initiation. Phenytoin is excreted in the bile, which is then reabsorbed from the intestinal tract and excreted in the urine. Urinary excretion of phenytoin occurs partly with glomerular filtration and by tubular secretion. Small incremental doses of phenytoin may increase the half-life and produce very substantial increases in serum levels. Patients should adhere strictly to the prescribed dosage, and serial monitoring of phenytoin levels is recommended.

Therapeutic Indications

Apart from its indication in generalized tonic–clonic (grand mal) and complex partial (psychomotor, temporal lobe) seizures, phenytoin is also used for the treatment of acute mania in bipolar disorder.

Precautions and Adverse Reactions

The most common adverse reactions reported with phenytoin therapy are usually dose related and include nystagmus, ataxia, slurred speech, decreased coordination, and mental confusion. Other side effects include dizziness, insomnia, transient nervousness, motor twitching, and headaches. There have been rare reports of phenytoin-induced dyskinesias, similar to those induced by phenothiazine and other neuroleptic drugs. More serious side effects include thrombocytopenia, leukopenia, agranulocytosis, and pancytopenia with or without bone marrow suppression.

A number of reports have suggested the development of lymphadenopathy (local or generalized), including benign lymph node hyperplasia, pseudolymphoma, lymphoma, and Hodgkin's disease. Hyperglycemia has been reported, and it may also increase the serum glucose level in diabetic patients.

Use in Pregnancy and Lactation

There is positive evidence that prenatal exposure to phenytoin may increase the risks for birth defects. The most severe is fetal hydantoin syndrome, which is characterized by mental and physical birth defects. In addition to congenital malformations, newborns exposed to phenytoin in utero may develop a potentially life-threatening bleeding disorder related to decreased levels of vitamin K–dependent clotting factors. Deficiencies in vitamins K and D, as well as folate, may cause megaloblastic anemia.

Drug Interactions

Acute alcohol intake, amiodarone, chlordiazepoxide, cimetidine, diazepam, disulfiram, estrogens, fluoxetine, H_2-antagonists, isoniazid, methylphenidate, phenothiazines, salicylates, and trazodone may increase phenytoin serum levels. Drugs that may lower phenytoin levels include carbamazepine, chronic alcohol abuse, and reserpine.

Laboratory Interferences

Phenytoin may decrease serum concentrations of thyroxine. It may cause increased serum levels of glucose, alkaline phosphatase, and γ-glutamyl transpeptidase.

Dosage and Clinical Guidelines

Patients may be started on one 100-mg extended oral capsule three times daily and the dosage then adjusted to suit individual requirements. Patients may then be switched to once-a-day daily dosing, which is more convenient. In this case, extended-release capsules may be used. Serial monitoring of phenytoin levels is recommended, and the normal range is usually 10 to 20 mcg/mL.

INTRODUCTION

Antihistamines are frequently used in the treatment of a variety of psychiatric disorders. First- and second-generation antihistamines, which target the H_1 receptor, can be sedating or nonsedating. Some antihistamines with less arrhythmogenic potential (e.g., fexofenadine [Allegra], loratadine [Claritin], desloratadine [Clarinex], and cetirizine [Zyrtec]) have been referred to as third-generation antihistamines and are not commonly used in psychiatric practice.

Antihistamines are used to treat neuroleptic-induced parkinsonism and neuroleptic-induced acute dystonia and as hypnotics and anxiolytics. Diphenhydramine (Benadryl) is used to treat neuroleptic-induced parkinsonism and neuroleptic-induced acute dystonia and sometimes as a hypnotic. Hydroxyzine hydrochloride (Atarax) and hydroxyzine pamoate (Vistaril) are used as anxiolytics. Promethazine (Phenergan) is used for its sedative and anxiolytic effects. Cyproheptadine (Periactin) has been used for the treatment of anorexia nervosa and inhibited male and female orgasms caused by serotonergic agents. The antihistamines most commonly used in psychiatry are listed in Table 6–1. The newer H_2-receptor antagonists, such as cimetidine, work primarily on gastric mucosa, inhibiting gastric secretion.

Table 6–2 lists antihistaminic drugs not used in psychiatry but that may have psychiatric adverse effects or drug–drug interactions.

PHARMACOLOGIC ACTIONS

The H_1 antagonists used in psychiatry are well absorbed from the gastrointestinal (GI) tract. The antiparkinsonian effects of intramuscular (IM) diphenhydramine have their onset in 15 to 30 minutes, and the sedative effects of diphenhydramine peak in 1 to 3 hours. The sedative effects of hydroxyzine and promethazine begin after 20 to 60 minutes and last for 4 to 6 hours. Because all three drugs are metabolized in the liver, persons with hepatic disease, such as cirrhosis, may attain high plasma concentrations with long-term administration. Cyproheptadine is well absorbed after oral administration, and its metabolites are excreted in the urine.

Activation of H_1 receptors stimulates wakefulness; therefore, receptor antagonism causes sedation. All four agents also possess some antimuscarinic cholinergic activity. Cyproheptadine is unique among the drugs because it has both potent antihistamine and serotonin $5\text{-}HT_2$–receptor antagonist properties.

THERAPEUTIC INDICATIONS

Antihistamines are useful as a treatment for neuroleptic-induced parkinsonism, neuroleptic-induced acute dystonia, and neuroleptic-induced akathisia. They are

Table 6–1
Antihistamines Commonly Used in Psychiatry

Generic Name	Trade Name	Duration of Action (hours)
Diphenhydramine	Benadryl	4–6
Hydroxyzine	Atarax, Vistaril	6–24
Promethazine	Phenergan	4–6
Cyproheptadine	Periactin	4–6

an alternative to anticholinergics and amantadine for these purposes. The antihistamines are relatively safe hypnotics, but they are not superior to the benzodiazepines, which have been much better studied in terms of efficacy and safety. The antihistamines have not been proven effective for long-term anxiolytic therapy; therefore, the benzodiazepines, buspirone (BuSpar), or selective serotonin reuptake inhibitors (SSRIs) are preferable for such treatment. Cyproheptadine is sometimes used to treat impaired orgasms, especially delayed orgasm resulting from treatment with serotonergic drugs.

Because it promotes weight gain, cyproheptadine may be of some use in the treatment of eating disorders, such as anorexia nervosa. Cyproheptadine can reduce recurrent nightmares with posttraumatic themes. The antiserotonergic activity of cyproheptadine may counteract the serotonin syndrome caused by concomitant use of multiple serotonin-activating drugs, such as SSRIs and monoamine oxidase inhibitors.

PRECAUTIONS AND ADVERSE REACTIONS

Antihistamines are commonly associated with sedation, dizziness, and hypotension, all of which can be severe in elderly persons, who are also likely to experience the anticholinergic effects of those drugs. Paradoxical excitement and agitation is an adverse effect seen in a small number of persons. Poor motor coordination can result in accidents; therefore, persons should be warned about driving and operating dangerous machinery. Other common adverse effects include epigastric distress, nausea, vomiting, diarrhea, and constipation. Because of mild anticholinergic activity, some people experience dry mouth, urinary retention, blurred vision, and constipation. For this reason also, antihistamines should be used only at very low doses, if at all, by persons with narrow-angle glaucoma or obstructive GI, prostate, or bladder

Table 6–2
Other Antihistamines

Class	Generic Name	Trade Name
Third-generation antihistamines	Cetirizine	Zyrtec
	Loratadine	Claritin
	Fexofenadine	Allegra
H$_2$ receptor antagonists	Nizatidine	Axid
	Famotidine	Pepcid
	Ranitidine	Zantac
	Cimetidine	Tagamet

conditions. A central anticholinergic syndrome with psychosis may be induced by either cyproheptadine or diphenhydramine. The use of cyproheptadine in some persons has been associated with weight gain, which may contribute to its reported efficacy in some persons with anorexia nervosa.

In addition to the above adverse effects, antihistamines have some potential for abuse. The coadministration of antihistamines and opioids can increase the euphoria experienced by persons with substance dependence. Overdoses of antihistamines can be fatal.

Use in Pregnancy and Lactation

Because of some potential for teratogenicity, pregnant women should avoid the use of antihistamines. Antihistamines are excreted in breast milk, so these should be used only if necessary by nursing mothers.

DRUG INTERACTIONS

The sedative property of antihistamines can be additive with other central nervous system depressants, such as alcohol, other sedative-hypnotic drugs, and many psychotropic drugs, including tricyclic drugs and dopamine receptor antagonists (DRAs). Anticholinergic activity can also be additive with that of other anticholinergic drugs and may sometimes result in severe anticholinergic symptoms or intoxication.

LABORATORY INTERFERENCES

H_1 antagonists may eliminate the wheal and induration that form the basis of allergy skin tests. Promethazine may interfere with pregnancy tests and may increase blood glucose concentrations. Diphenhydramine may yield a false-positive urine test result for phencyclidine (PCP). Hydroxyzine use can falsely elevate the results of certain tests for urinary 17-hydroxycorticosteroids.

DOSAGE AND CLINICAL GUIDELINES

The antihistamines are available in a variety of preparations (Table 6–3). IM injections should be deep because superficial administration can cause local irritation.

Intravenous (IV) administration of 25 to 50 mg of diphenhydramine is an effective treatment for neuroleptic-induced acute dystonia, which may immediately disappear. Treatment with 25 mg three times a day—up to 50 mg four times a day, if necessary—can be used to treat neuroleptic-induced parkinsonism, akinesia, and buccal movements. Diphenhydramine can be used as a hypnotic at a 50-mg dose for mild transient insomnia. Doses of 100 mg have not been shown to be superior to doses of 50 mg, but they produce more anticholinergic effects than doses of 50 mg.

Hydroxyzine is most commonly used as a short-term anxiolytic. Hydroxyzine should not be given IV because it is irritating to the blood vessels. Dosages of 50 to 100 mg given orally four times a day for long-term treatment or 50 to 100 mg IM every 4 to 6 hours for short-term treatment are usually effective.

SSRI-induced anorgasmia may be reversed sometimes with 4 to 16 mg a day of cyproheptadine taken by mouth 1 or 2 hours before anticipated sexual activity. A number of case reports and small studies have also reported that cyproheptadine

Table 6-3
Dosage and Administration of Common Histamine Antagonists

Medication	Route	Preparation	Common Dosage
Diphenhydramine (Benadryl)	PO	Capsules and tablets: 25 mg, 50 mg	Adults: 25–50 mg three to four times per day
		Liquid: 12.5 mg/ 5.0 mL	Children: 5 mg/kg three to four times per day, not to exceed 300 mg/day
	Deep IM or IV	Solution: 10 or 50 mg/mL	Same as oral
Hydroxyzine Hydrochloride (Atarax)	PO	Tablets: 10, 25, 50, and 100 mg	Adults: 50–100 mg three to four times daily
		Syrup: 10 mg/5 mL	Children younger than 6 years of age: 2 mg/kg/day in divided doses
			Children older than 6 years of age: 12.5–25.0 mg three to four times daily
	IM	Solution: 25 or 50 mg/mL	Same as oral
Pamoate (Vistaril)	PO	Suspension: 25 mg/mL	Same as dosages for hydrochloride
		Capsules: 25, 50, and 100 mg	
Promethazine (Phenergan)	PO	Tablets: 15.2, 25.0, and 50.0 mg	Adults: 50–100 mg three to four times daily for sedation
		Syrup: 3.25 mg/5 mL	Children: 12.5–25.0 mg at night for sedation
	Rectal	Suppositories: 12.5, 25.0, and 50.0 mg	
	IM	Solution: 25 and 50 mg/mL	
Cyproheptadine (Periactin)	PO	Tablets: 4 mg	Adults: 4–20 mg/day
		Syrup: 2 mg/5 mL	Children 2–7 years of age: 2 mg two to three times daily (maximum, 12 mg/day)
			Children 7–14 years of age: 4 mg two to three times daily (maximum of 16 mg/day)

IM, intramuscular; IV, intravenous; PO, oral.

may be of some use in the treatment of eating disorders, such as anorexia nervosa. Cyproheptadine is available in 4-mg tablets and a 2-mg/5-mL solution. Children and elderly patients are more sensitive to the effects of antihistamines than are young adults.

Barbiturates and Similarly Acting Drugs

INTRODUCTION

The first barbiturate to be used in medicine was barbital (Veronal), which was introduced in 1903. It was followed by phenobarbital (Luminal), amobarbital (Amytal), pentobarbital (Nembutal), secobarbital (Seconal), and thiopental (Pentothal). Many others have been synthesized, but only a handful has been used clinically (Table 7–1). Many problems are associated with these drugs, including high abuse and addiction potential, a narrow therapeutic range with low therapeutic index, and unfavorable side effects. The use of barbiturates and similar compounds such as meprobamate (Miltown) has practically been eliminated by the benzodiazepines and hypnotics, such as zolpidem (Ambien), eszopiclone (Lunesta), and zaleplon (Sonata), which have a lower abuse potential and a higher therapeutic index than the barbiturates. Nevertheless, the barbiturates still have an important role in the treatment of certain mental and convulsive disorders.

PHARMACOLOGIC ACTIONS

The barbiturates are well absorbed after oral administration. The binding of barbiturates to plasma proteins is high, but lipid solubility varies. The individual barbiturates are metabolized by the liver and excreted by the kidneys. The half-lives of specific barbiturates range from 1 to 120 hours. The barbiturates may also induce hepatic enzymes (CYP450), thereby reducing the levels of both the barbiturate and any other concurrently administered drugs metabolized by the liver. The mechanism of action of barbiturates involves the γ-aminobutyric acid (GABA) receptor–benzodiazepine receptor–chloride ion channel complex.

THERAPEUTIC INDICATIONS

Electroconvulsive Therapy

Methohexital (Brevital) is commonly used as an anesthetic agent for electroconvulsive therapy (ECT). It has lower cardiac risks than other barbiturate anesthetics. Used intravenously (IV), methohexital produces rapid unconsciousness, and because of its rapid redistribution, it has a brief duration of action (5 to 7 minutes). Typical dosing for ECT is 0.7 to 1.2 mg/kg. Methohexital can also be used to abort prolonged seizures in ECT or to limit postictal agitation.

Seizures

Phenobarbital (Solfoton, Luminal), the most commonly used barbiturate for treatment of seizures, has indications for the treatment of generalized tonic–clonic and simple partial seizures. Parenteral barbiturates are used in the emergency management of seizures independent of cause. IV phenobarbital should be administered slowly at 10 to 20 mg/kg for status epilepticus.

Table 7–1
Barbiturate Dosages (Adult)

Drug	Trade Name	Available Preparations	Hypnotic Dose Range	Anticonvulsant Dose Range
Amobarbital	Amytal	200 mg	50–300 mg	65–500 mg IV
Aprobarbital	Alurate	40-mg/5-mL elixir	40–120 mg	Not established
Butabarbital	Butisol	15-, 30-, and 50-mg tablets 30-mg/5-mL elixir	45–120 mg	Not established
Mephobarbital	Mebaral	32-, 50-, and 100-mg tablets	100–200 mg	200–600 mg
Methohexital	Brevital	500 mg/50 cc	1 mg/kg for electroconvulsive therapy	Not established
Pentobarbital	Nembutal	50- and 100-mg capsules 50-mg/mL injection or elixir 30-, 60-, 120-, and 200-mg suppository	100–200 mg	100 mg IV, each minute up to 500 mg
Phenobarbital	Luminal	Tablets range from 15–100 mg 20-mg/5-mL elixir 30- to 130-mg/mL injection	30–150 mg	100–300 mg IV, up to 600 mg/day
Secobarbital	Seconal	100-mg capsule, 50-mg/mL injection	100 mg	5.5 mg/kg IV

IV, intravenous.

Narcoanalysis

Amobarbital (Amytal) has been used historically as a diagnostic aid in a number of clinical conditions, including conversion reactions, catatonia, hysterical stupor, and unexplained muteness, and to differentiate stupor of depression, schizophrenia, and structural brain lesions.

The *Amytal interview* is performed by placing the patient in a reclining position and administering amobarbital IV at 50 mg a minute. Infusion is continued until lateral nystagmus is sustained or drowsiness is noted, usually at 75 to 150 mg. After this, 25 to 50 mg can be administered every 5 minutes to maintain narcosis. The patient should be allowed to rest for 15 to 30 minutes after the interview before attempting to walk.

Because of the risk of laryngospasm with IV amobarbital diazepam has become the drug of choice for narcoanalysis.

Sleep

The barbiturates reduce sleep latency and the number of awakenings during sleep, although tolerance to these effects generally develops within 2 weeks. Discontinuation of barbiturates often leads to rebound increases on electroencephalographic measures of sleep and a worsening of the insomnia.

WITHDRAWAL FROM SEDATIVE-HYPNOTICS

Barbiturates are sometimes used to determine the extent of tolerance to barbiturates or other hypnotics to guide detoxification. After intoxication has resolved, a test dose of pentobarbital (200 mg) is given orally. One hour later, the patient is examined. Tolerance and dose requirements are determined by the degree to which the patient is affected. If the patient is not sedated, another 100 mg of pentobarbital can be administered every 2 hours, up to three times (maximum, 500 mg over 6 hours). The amount needed for mild intoxication corresponds to the approximate daily dose of barbiturate used. Phenobarbital (30 mg) may then be substituted for each 100 mg of pentobarbital. This daily dose requirement can be administered in divided doses and gradually tapered by 10% a day, with adjustments made according to withdrawal signs.

PRECAUTIONS AND ADVERSE REACTIONS

Some adverse effects of barbiturates are similar to those of benzodiazepines, including paradoxical dysphoria, hyperactivity, and cognitive disorganization. Rare adverse effects associated with barbiturate use include the development of Stevens–Johnson syndrome, megaloblastic anemia, and neutropenia.

Prior to the advent of benzodiazepines, the widespread use of barbiturates as hypnotics and anxiolytics made them the most common cause of acute porphyria reactions. Severe attacks of porphyria have decreased largely because barbiturates are now seldom used and are contraindicated in patients with the disease.

A major difference between the barbiturates and the benzodiazepines is the low therapeutic index of the barbiturates. An overdose of barbiturates can easily prove fatal. In addition to narrow therapeutic indexes, the barbiturates are associated with a significant risk of abuse potential and the development of tolerance and dependence. Barbiturate intoxication is manifested by confusion, drowsiness, irritability, hyporeflexia or areflexia, ataxia, and nystagmus. The symptoms of barbiturate withdrawal are similar to, but more marked than, those of benzodiazepine withdrawal.

Ten times the daily dose or 1 g of most barbiturates causes severe toxicity; 2 to 10 g generally proves fatal. Manifestations of barbiturate intoxication may include delirium, confusion, excitement, headache, central nervous system (CNS), and respiratory depression ranging from somnolence to coma. Other adverse reactions include Cheyne–Stokes respiration, shock, miosis, oliguria, tachycardia, hypotension, hypothermia, irritability, hyporeflexia or areflexia, ataxia, and nystagmus. Treatment of overdose includes induction of emesis or lavage, activated charcoal, and saline cathartics; supportive treatment, including maintaining airway and respiration and treating shock as needed; maintaining vital signs and fluid balance; alkalinizing the urine which increases excretion; forced diuresis if renal function is normal, or hemodialysis in severe cases.

Barbiturates should be used with caution by patients with a history of substance abuse, depression, diabetes, hepatic impairment, renal disease, severe anemia, pain, hyperthyroidism, or hypoadrenalism. Barbiturates are also contraindicated in patients with acute intermittent porphyria, impaired respiratory drive, or limited respiratory reserve.

Use in Pregnancy and Lactation

Because of some evidence of teratogenicity, barbiturates should not be used by pregnant women or women who are breastfeeding.

DRUG INTERACTIONS

The primary area for concern about drug interactions is the potentially dangerous effects of respiratory depression. Barbiturates should be used with great caution with other prescribed CNS drugs (including antipsychotic and antidepressant drugs) and nonprescribed CNS agents (e.g., alcohol). Caution must also be exercised when prescribing barbiturates to patients who are taking other drugs that are metabolized in the liver, especially cardiac drugs and anticonvulsants. Because individual patients have a wide range of sensitivities to barbiturate-induced enzyme induction, it is not possible to predict the degree to which the metabolism of concurrently administered medications may be affected. Drugs that have their metabolism enhanced by barbiturate administration include opioids, antiarrhythmic agents, antibiotics, anticoagulants, anticonvulsants, antidepressants, β-adrenergic receptor antagonists, dopamine receptor antagonists, contraceptives, and immunosuppressants.

LABORATORY INTERFERENCES

No known laboratory interferences are associated with the administration of barbiturates.

DOSE AND CLINICAL GUIDELINES

Barbiturates and other drugs described later begin to act within 1 to 2 hours of administration. The doses of barbiturates vary, and treatment should begin with low doses that are increased to achieve a clinical effect. Children and older people are more sensitive to the effects of the barbiturates than are young adults. The most commonly used barbiturates are available in a variety of dose forms. Barbiturates with half-lives in the 15 to 40-hour range are preferable because long-acting drugs tend to accumulate in the body. Clinicians should instruct patients clearly about the adverse effects and the potential for dependence associated with barbiturates.

Although determining plasma concentrations of barbiturates is rarely necessary in psychiatry, monitoring of phenobarbital concentrations is standard practice when the drug is used as an anticonvulsant. The therapeutic blood concentrations for phenobarbital in this indication range from 15 to 40 mg/L, although some patients may experience significant adverse effects in that range.

Barbiturates are contained in combination products with which the clinician should be familiar.

OTHER SIMILARLY ACTING DRUGS

A number of agents that act similarly to the barbiturates have been used in the treatment of anxiety and insomnia. Three such available drugs are paraldehyde (Paral), meprobamate, and chloral hydrate (Noctec). These drugs are rarely used because of their abuse potential and potential toxic effects.

Paraldehyde

Paraldehyde is a cyclic ether and was first used in 1882 as a hypnotic. It has also been used to treat epilepsy, alcohol withdrawal symptoms, and delirium tremens. Because of its low therapeutic index, it has been supplanted by the benzodiazepines and other anticonvulsants.

Pharmacologic Actions. Paraldehyde is rapidly absorbed from the gastrointestinal (GI) tract and from intramuscular (IM) injections. It is primarily metabolized to acetaldehyde by the liver, and unmetabolized drug is expired by the lungs. Reported half-lives range from 3.4 to 9.8 hours. The onset of action is 15 to 30 minutes.

Therapeutic Indications. Paraldehyde is not indicated as an anxiolytic or a hypnotic and has little place in current psychopharmacology.

Precautions and Adverse Reactions. Paraldehyde frequently causes foul breath because of expired unmetabolized drug. It can inflame pulmonary capillaries and cause coughing. It can also cause local thrombophlebitis with IV use. Patients may experience nausea and vomiting with oral use. Overdose leads to metabolic acidosis and decreased renal output. There is risk of abuse among drug addicts.

Use in Pregnancy and Lactation. Paraldehyde should not be used during pregnancy or lactation.

Drug Interactions. Disulfiram (Antabuse) inhibits acetaldehyde dehydrogenase and reduces metabolism of paraldehyde, leading to possible toxic concentration of paraldehyde. Paraldehyde has addictive sedating effects in combination with other CNS depressants such as alcohol or benzodiazepines.

Laboratory Interferences. Paraldehyde can interfere with the metyrapone, phentolamine, and urinary 17-hydroxycorticosteroid tests.

Dosing and Clinical Guidelines. Paraldehyde is available in 30-mL vials for oral, IV, or rectal use. For seizures in adults, up to 12 mL (diluted to a 10% solution) can be administered by gastric tube every 4 hours. For children, the oral dose is 0.3 mg/kg.

Meprobamate

Meprobamate, a carbamate, was introduced shortly before the benzodiazepines, specifically to treat anxiety. It is also used for muscle relaxant effects.

Pharmacologic Actions. Meprobamate is rapidly absorbed from the GI tract and from IM injections. It is primarily metabolized by the liver, and a small portion is excreted unchanged in urine. The plasma half-life is approximately 10 hours.

Therapeutic Indications. Meprobamate is indicated for short-term treatment of anxiety disorders. It has also been used as a hypnotic and is prescribed as a muscle relaxant.

Precautions and Adverse Reactions. Meprobamate can cause CNS depression and death in overdose and carries the risk of abuse by patients with drug or alcohol dependence. Abrupt cessation after long-term use can lead to withdrawal syndrome, including seizures and hallucinations. Meprobamate can exacerbate acute intermittent porphyria. Other rare side effects include hypersensitivity reactions, wheezing, hives, paradoxical excitement, and leukopenia. It should not be used in patients with hepatic compromise.

Use in Pregnancy and Lactation.   An increased risk of congenital malformations, especially when used in the first trimester, has been suggested. Use during breastfeeding is not recommended.

Drug Interactions.   Meprobamate has additive sedating effects in combination with other CNS depressants, such as alcohol, barbiturates, or benzodiazepines.

Laboratory Interferences.   Meprobamate can interfere with the metyrapone, phentolamine, and urinary 17-hydroxycorticosteroid tests.

Dosing and Clinical Guidelines.   Meprobamate is available in 200-, 400-, and 600-mg tablets; 200- and 400-mg extended-release capsules; and various combinations, for example, aspirin, 325 mg and 200 mg of meprobamate (Equagesic) for oral use. For adults, the usual dose is 400 to 800 mg twice daily. Elderly patients and children aged 6 to 12 years require half the adult dose.

Chloral Hydrate
Chloral hydrate is a hypnotic agent rarely used in psychiatry because numerous safer options, such as benzodiazepines, are available.

Pharmacologic Actions.   Chloral hydrate is well absorbed from the GI tract. The parent compound is metabolized within minutes by the liver to the active metabolite trichloroethanol, which has a half-life of 8 to 11 hours. A dose of chloral hydrate induces sleep in about 30 to 60 minutes and maintains sleep for 4 to 8 hours. It probably potentiates GABAergic neurotransmission, which suppresses neuronal excitability.

Therapeutic Indications.   The major indication for chloral hydrate is to induce sleep. It should be used for no more than 2 or 3 days because longer-term treatment is associated with an increased incidence and severity of adverse effects. Tolerance develops to the hypnotic effects of chloral hydrate after 2 weeks of treatment. The benzodiazepines are superior to chloral hydrate for all psychiatric uses.

Precautions and Adverse Reactions.   Chloral hydrate has adverse effects on the CNS, GI system, and skin. High doses (>4 g) may be associated with stupor, confusion, ataxia, falls, or coma. The GI effects include nonspecific irritation, nausea, vomiting, flatulence, and an unpleasant taste. With long-term use and overdose, gastritis and gastric ulceration can develop. In addition to the development of tolerance, dependence on chloral hydrate can occur, with symptoms similar to those of alcohol dependence. With a lethal dose between 5,000 and 10,000 mg, chloral hydrate is a particularly poor choice for potentially suicidal persons.

Use in Pregnancy and Lactation.   Chloral hydrate should not be prescribed to pregnant women and can pass through the breast milk and harm the infant.

Drug Interactions.   Because of metabolic interference, chloral hydrate should be strictly avoided with alcohol, a notorious concoction known as a *Mickey Finn.* Chloral hydrate may displace warfarin (Coumadin) from plasma proteins and enhance anticoagulant activity; this combination should be avoided.

Laboratory Interferences.   Chloral hydrate administration can lead to false-positive results for urine glucose determinations that use cupric sulfate (e.g., Clinitest) but not in tests that use glucose oxidase (e.g., Clinistix and Tes-Tape). Chloral hydrate can also interfere with the determination of urinary catecholamines in 17-hydroxycorticosteroids.

Dosing and Clinical Guidelines.   Chloral hydrate is available in 500-mg capsules; 500-mg/5-mL solution; and 324-, 500-, and 648-mg rectal suppositories. The standard dose of chloral hydrate is 500 to 2,000 mg at bedtime. Because the drug is a GI irritant, it should be administered with excess water, milk, other liquids, or antacids to decrease gastric irritation.

Propofol

Propofol (Diprivan) is a GABA$_A$ agonist that is used as an anesthetic. In psychiatry it is sometimes used in place of barbiturates in narcoanalysis. It induces presynaptic release of GABA and dopamine (the latter possibility through an action on GABA$_B$ receptors) and is a partial agonist at dopamine D$_2$ and NMDA receptors. Because it is very lipid soluble, it crosses the blood–brain barrier readily and induces anesthesia in less than 1 minute. Rapid redistribution out of the CNS results in offset of action within 3 to 8 minutes after the infusion is discontinued. It is well tolerated when used for conscious sedation, but it has a potential for acute adverse effects, including respiratory depression, apnea, and bradyarrhythmias, and prolonged infusion can cause acidosis and mitochondrial myopathies. The carrier used for the infusion is a soybean emulsion that can be a culture medium for various organisms. The carrier also can impair macrophage function and cause hematologic and lipid abnormalities and anaphylactic reactions.

Etomidate

Etomidate is a carboxylated imidazole that acts at the β_2 and β_3 subunits of the GABA$_A$ receptor. It has a rapid onset (1 minute) and short duration (less than 5 minutes) of action. The propylene glycol vehicle has been linked to hyperosmolar metabolic acidosis. It has both proconvulsant and anticonvulsant properties, and it inhibits cortisol release, with possible adverse consequences after long-term use.

8

Benzodiazepines and Drugs Acting on GABA Receptors

INTRODUCTION

The first benzodiazepine to be introduced was chlordiazepoxide (Librium), in 1959. In 1963, diazepam (Valium) became available. Over the next three decades, superior safety and tolerability helped the benzodiazepines replace the older antianxiety and hypnotic medications, such as the barbiturates and meprobamate (Miltown). Dozens of benzodiazepines and drugs acting on benzodiazepine receptors have been synthesized and marketed worldwide. Many of these agents are not in the United States, and some benzodiazepines have been discontinued because of lack of use. Table 8–1 lists agents currently available in the United States.

The benzodiazepines derive their name from their molecular structure. They share a common effect on receptors that have been termed benzodiazepine receptors, which in turn modulate γ-aminobutyric acid (GABA) activity. Nonbenzodiazepine agonists, such as zolpidem (Ambien), zaleplon (Sonata), and eszopiclone (Lunesta)—the so-called "Z drugs"—are discussed in this chapter because their clinical effects result from binding domains located close to benzodiazepine receptors. Flumazenil (Romazicon), a benzodiazepine receptor antagonist used to reverse benzodiazepine-induced sedation and in emergency care of benzodiazepine overdosage, is also covered here.

Because benzodiazepines have a rapid anxiolytic sedative effect, they are most commonly used for acute treatment of insomnia, anxiety, agitation, or anxiety associated with any psychiatric disorder. In addition, the benzodiazepines are used as anesthetics, anticonvulsants, and muscle relaxants and as the preferred treatment for catatonia. Because of the risk of psychological and physical dependence associated with long-term use of benzodiazepines, ongoing assessment should be made as to the continued clinical need for these drugs in treating patients. In most patients, given the nature of their disorders, it is often best if benzodiazepine agents are used in conjunction with psychotherapy and in cases where alternative agents have been tried and proven ineffective or poorly tolerated. In many forms of chronic anxiety disorders, antidepressant drugs such as the selective serotonin reuptake inhibitors (SSRIs) and serotonin–norepinephrine reuptake inhibitors (SNRIs) are now used as primary treatments, with benzodiazepines used as adjuncts. Benzodiazepine abuse is rare, usually found in patients who abuse multiple prescription and recreational drugs.

PHARMACOLOGIC ACTIONS

All benzodiazepines except clorazepate (Tranxene) are completely absorbed after oral administration and reach peak serum levels within 30 minutes to 2 hours. Metabolism of clorazepate in the stomach converts it to desmethyldiazepam, which is then completely absorbed.

Table 8–1
Preparations and Doses of Medications Acting on the Benzodiazepine Receptor Available in the United States

Medication	Brand Name	Dose Equivalent	Usual Adult Dose (mg)	How Supplied
Diazepam	Valium	5	2.5–40.0	2-, 5-, and 10-mg tablets 15-mg slow-release tablets
Clonazepam	Klonopin	0.25	0.5–4.0	0.5-, 1.0-, and 2.0-mg tablets
Alprazolam	Xanax	0.5	0.5–6.0	0.25-, 0.5-, 1.0-, and 2.0-mg tablets 1.5-mg sustained-release tablet
Lorazepam	Ativan	1	0.5–6.0	0.5-, 1.0-, and 2.0-mg tablets 4 mg/mL parenteral
Oxazepam	Serax	15	15–120	7.5-, 10.0-, 15.0-, and 30.0-mg capsules 15-mg tablets
Chlordiazepoxide	Librium	25	10–100	5-, 10-, and 25-mg capsules and tablets
Clorazepate	Tranxene	7.5	15–60	3.75-, 7.50-, and 15.0-mg tablets 11.25- and 22.50-mg slow-release tablets
Midazolam	Versed	0.25	1–50	5 mg/mL parenteral 1-, 2-, 5-, and 10-mL vials
Flurazepam	Dalmane	15	15–30	15- and 30-mg capsules
Temazepam	Restoril	15	7.5–30.0	7.5-, 15.0-, and 30.0-mg capsules
Triazolam	Halcion	0.125	0.125–0.250	0.125- and 0.250-mg tablets
Estazolam	ProSom	1	1–2	1- and 2-mg tablets
Quazepam	Doral	5	7.5–15.0	7.5- and 15.0-mg tablets
Zolpidem	Ambien	10	5–10	5- and 10-mg tablets
	Ambien CR	5	6.25–12.5	6.25- and 12.5-mg tablets
Zaleplon	Sonata	10	5–20	5- and 10-mg capsules
Eszopiclone	Lunesta	1	1–3	1-, 2- and 3-mg tablets
Flumazenil	Romazicon	0.05	0.2–0.5 per min	0.1 mg/mL 5- and 10-mL vials

The absorption, the attainment of peak concentrations, and the onset of action are quickest for diazepam (Valium), lorazepam (Ativan), alprazolam (Xanax), triazolam (Halcion), and estazolam (ProSom). The rapid onset of effects is important to persons who take a single dose of a benzodiazepine to calm an episodic burst of anxiety or to fall asleep rapidly. Several benzodiazepines are effective after intravenous (IV) injection, but only lorazepam and midazolam (Versed) have rapid and reliable absorption after intramuscular (IM) administration.

Diazepam, chlordiazepoxide, clonazepam (Klonopin), clorazepate, flurazepam (Dalmane), and quazepam (Doral) have plasma half-lives of 30 hours to more than 100 hours and are technically described as long-acting benzodiazepines. The plasma half-lives of these compounds can be as high as 200 hours in persons whose metabolism is genetically slow. Because the attainment of steady-state plasma concentrations of the drugs can take up to 2 weeks, persons may experience symptoms and signs of toxicity after only 7 to 10 days of treatment with a dosage that seemed initially to be in the therapeutic range.

Clinically, half-life alone does not necessarily determine the duration of therapeutic action for most benzodiazepines. The fact that all benzodiazepines are lipid soluble to varying degrees means that benzodiazepines and their active metabolites bind to plasma proteins. The extent of this binding is proportional to their lipid solubility. The amount of protein binding varies from 70% to 99%. Distribution, onset, and termination of action after a single dose are thus largely determined by benzodiazepine lipid solubility, not elimination half-life. Preparations with high lipid solubility, such as diazepam and alprazolam, are absorbed rapidly from the gastrointestinal (GI) tract and distribute rapidly to the brain by passive diffusion along a concentration gradient, resulting in a rapid onset of action. However, as the concentration of the medication increases in the brain and decreases in the bloodstream, the concentration gradient reverses itself, and these medications leave the brain rapidly, resulting in fast cessation of drug effect. Drugs with longer elimination half-lives, such as diazepam, may remain in the bloodstream for a substantially longer period of time than their actual pharmacologic action at benzodiazepine receptors because the concentration in the brain decreases rapidly below the level necessary for a noticeable effect. In contrast, lorazepam, which has a shorter elimination half-life than diazepam but is less lipid soluble, has a slower onset of action after a single dose because the drug is absorbed and enters the brain more slowly. However, the duration of action after a single dose is longer because it takes longer for lorazepam to leave the brain and for brain levels to decrease below the concentration that produces an effect. In chronic dosing, some of these differences are not as apparent because brain levels are in equilibrium with higher and more consistent steady-state blood levels, but additional doses still produce a more rapid but briefer action with diazepam than with lorazepam. Benzodiazepines are distributed widely in adipose tissue. As a result, medications may persist in the body after discontinuation longer than would be predicted from their elimination half-lives. In addition, the dynamic half-life (i.e., duration of action on the receptor) may be longer than the elimination half-life.

The advantages of long–half-life drugs over short–half-life drugs include less frequent dosing, less variation in plasma concentration, and less severe withdrawal phenomena. The disadvantages include drug accumulation, increased risk of daytime psychomotor impairment, and increased daytime sedation.

The half-lives of lorazepam, oxazepam (Serax), temazepam (Restoril), and estazolam are between 8 and 30 hours. Alprazolam has a half-life of 10 to 15 hours, and triazolam has the shortest half-life (2 to 3 hours) of all the orally administered benzodiazepines. Rebound insomnia and anterograde amnesia are thought to be more of a problem with the short–half-life drugs than with the long–half-life drugs.

Because administration of medications more frequently than the elimination half-life leads to drug accumulation, medications such as diazepam and flurazepam accumulate with daily dosing, eventually resulting in increased daytime sedation.

Some benzodiazepines (e.g., oxazepam) are conjugated directly by glucuronidation and are excreted. Most benzodiazepines are oxidized first by CYP3A4 and CYP2C19, often to active metabolites. These metabolites may then be hydroxylated to another active metabolite. For example, diazepam is oxidized to desmethyldiazepam, which, in turn, is hydroxylated to produce oxazepam. These products undergo glucuronidation to inactive metabolites. A number of benzodiazepines (e.g., diazepam, chlordiazepoxide) have the same active metabolite (desmethyldiazepam), which has an elimination half-life of more than 120 hours. Flurazepam (Dalmane), a lipid-soluble benzodiazepine used as a hypnotic that has a short elimination half-life, has an active metabolite (desalkylflurazepam) with a half-life greater than 100 hours. This is another reason that the duration of action of a benzodiazepine may not correspond to the half-life of the parent drug.

Zaleplon, zolpidem, and eszopiclone are structurally distinct and vary in their binding to the GABA receptor subunits. Benzodiazepines activate all three specific GABA–benzodiazepine (GABA–BZ) binding sites of the $GABA_A$-receptor, which opens chloride channels and reduces the rate of neuronal and muscle firing. Zolpidem, zaleplon, and eszopiclone have selectivity for certain subunits of the GABA receptor. This may account for their selective sedative effects and relative lack of muscle relaxant and anticonvulsant effects.

Zolpidem, zaleplon, and eszopiclone are rapidly and well absorbed after oral administration, although absorption can be delayed by as much as 1 hour if they are taken with food. Zolpidem reaches peak plasma concentrations in 1.6 hours and has a half-life of 2.6 hours. Zaleplon reaches peak plasma concentrations in 1 hour and has a half-life of 1 hour. If taken immediately after a high-fat or heavy meal, the peak is delayed by approximately 1 hour, reducing the effects of eszopiclone on sleep onset. The terminal-phase elimination half-life is approximately 6 hours in healthy adults. Eszopiclone is weakly bound to plasma protein (52% to 59%).

The rapid metabolism and lack of active metabolites of zolpidem, zaleplon, and eszopiclone avoid the accumulation of plasma concentrations compared to the long-term use of benzodiazepines.

THERAPEUTIC INDICATIONS
Insomnia
Because insomnia may be a symptom of a physical or psychiatric disorder, hypnotics should not be used for more than 7 to 10 consecutive days without a thorough investigation of the cause of the insomnia. However, in fact, many patients have long-standing sleep difficulties and benefit greatly from long-term use of hypnotic agents. Temazepam, flurazepam, and triazolam are benzodiazepines with a sole indication for insomnia. Zolpidem, zaleplon, and eszopiclone are also indicated only for insomnia. Although these "Z drugs" are not usually associated with rebound insomnia after the discontinuation of their use for short periods, some patients experience increased sleep difficulties the first few nights after discontinuing their use. Use of zolpidem, zaleplon, and eszopiclone for periods longer than 1 month is not associated with the delayed emergence of adverse effects. No development of tolerance to any parameter of sleep measurement was observed over 6 months in clinical trials of eszopiclone.

Flurazepam, temazepam, quazepam, estazolam, and triazolam are the benzodiazepines approved for use as hypnotics. The benzodiazepine hypnotics differ principally in their half-lives; flurazepam has the longest half-life, and triazolam has the shortest. Flurazepam may be associated with minor cognitive impairment on the day after its administration, and triazolam may be associated with mild rebound anxiety and antero-grade amnesia. Quazepam may be associated with daytime impairment when used for a long time. Temazepam or estazolam may be a reasonable compromise for most adults. Estazolam produces rapid onset of sleep and a hypnotic effect for 6 to 8 hours.

γ-Hydroxybutyrate (GHB, Xyrem), which is approved for the treatment of narcolepsy and improves slow-wave sleep, is also an agonist at the $GABA_A$ receptor, where it binds to specific GHB receptors. GHB has the capacity both to reduce drug craving and to induce dependence, abuse, and absence seizures as a result of complex actions on tegmental dopaminergic systems.

Anxiety Disorders

Generalized Anxiety Disorder. Benzodiazepines are highly effective for the relief of anxiety associated with generalized anxiety disorder. Most persons should be treated for a predetermined, specific, and relatively brief period. However, because generalized anxiety disorder is a chronic disorder with a high rate of recurrence, some persons with generalized anxiety disorder may warrant long-term maintenance treatment with benzodiazepines.

Panic Disorder. Alprazolam and clonazepam, both high-potency benzodiazepines, are commonly used medications for panic disorder with or without agoraphobia. Although the SSRIs are also indicated for treatment of panic disorder, the benzodiazepines have the advantage of working quickly and not causing significant sexual dysfunction and weight gain. However, the SSRIs are still often preferred because they target common comorbid conditions, such as depression or obsessive–compulsive disorder. Benzodiazepines and SSRIs can be initiated together to treat acute panic symptoms; use of the benzodiazepine can be tapered after 3 to 4 weeks after the therapeutic benefits of the SSRI have emerged.

Social Phobia. Clonazepam has been shown to be an effective treatment for social phobia. In addition, several other benzodiazepines (e.g., diazepam) have been used as adjunctive medications for treatment of social phobia.

Other Anxiety Disorders. Benzodiazepines are used adjunctively for treatment of adjustment disorder with anxiety, pathologic anxiety associated with life events (e.g., after an accident), obsessive–compulsive disorder, and posttraumatic stress disorder.

Anxiety Associated with Depression. Depressed patients often experience significant anxiety, and antidepressant drugs may cause initial exacerbation of these symptoms. Accordingly, benzodiazepines are indicated for the treatment of anxiety associated with depression.

Bipolar I and II Disorders

Clonazepam, lorazepam, and alprazolam are effective in the management of acute manic episodes and as an adjuvant to maintenance therapy in lieu of antipsychotics. As an adjuvant to lithium (Eskalith) or lamotrigine (Lamictal), clonazepam may result in an increased time between cycles and fewer depressive episodes. Benzodiazepines may help patients with bipolar disorder sleep better.

Catatonia

Lorazepam, sometimes in low doses (less than 5 mg per day), and sometimes in very high doses (12 mg per day or more), is regularly used to treat acute catatonia, which is more frequently associated with bipolar disorder than with schizophrenia. Other benzodiazepines have also been said to be helpful. However, there are no valid controlled trials of benzodiazepines in catatonia. Chronic catatonia does not respond as well to benzodiazepines. The definitive treatment for catatonia is electroconvulsive therapy.

Akathisia

The first-line drug for akathisia is most commonly a β-adrenergic receptor antagonist. However, benzodiazepines are also effective in treating some patients with akathisia.

Parkinson's Disease

A small number of persons with idiopathic Parkinson's disease respond to long-term use of zolpidem with reduced bradykinesia and rigidity. Zolpidem dosages of 10 mg four times daily may be tolerated without sedation for several years.

Other Psychiatric Indications

Chlordiazepoxide (Librium) and clorazepate (Tranxene) are used to manage the symptoms of alcohol withdrawal. The benzodiazepines (especially IM lorazepam) are used to manage substance induced and psychotic agitation in the emergency department. Benzodiazepines have been used instead of amobarbital (Amytal) for drug-assisted interviewing.

Flumazenil for Benzodiazepine Overdosage

Flumazenil is used to reverse the adverse psychomotor, amnestic, and sedative effects of benzodiazepine receptor agonists, including benzodiazepines, zolpidem, and zaleplon. Flumazenil is administered IV and has a half-life of 7 to 15 minutes. The most common adverse effects of flumazenil are nausea, vomiting, dizziness, agitation, emotional lability, cutaneous vasodilation, injection-site pain, fatigue, impaired vision, and headache. The most common serious adverse effect associated with the use of flumazenil is the precipitation of seizures, which is especially likely to occur in persons with seizure disorders, those who are physically dependent on benzodiazepines, and those who have ingested large quantities of benzodiazepines. Flumazenil alone may impair memory retrieval.

In mixed-drug overdosage, the toxic effects (e.g., seizures and cardiac arrhythmias) of other drugs (e.g., tricyclic antidepressants) may emerge with the reversal of the benzodiazepine effects of flumazenil. For example, seizures caused by an overdosage of tricyclic antidepressants may have been partially treated in a person who had also taken an overdosage of benzodiazepines. With flumazenil treatment, the tricyclic-induced seizures or cardiac arrhythmias may appear and result in a fatal outcome. Flumazenil does not reverse the effects of ethanol, barbiturates, or opioids.

For the initial management of a known or suspected benzodiazepine overdosage, the recommended initial dosage of flumazenil is 0.2 mg (2 mL) administered IV over 30 seconds. If the desired consciousness is not obtained after 30 seconds, a further dose of 0.3 mg (3 mL) can be administered over 30 seconds. Further doses of 0.5 mg (5 mL) can be administered over 30 seconds at 1-minute intervals up to a cumulative dose of 3.0 mg. The clinician should not rush the administration of flumazenil. A secure airway and IV access should be established before the administration of the drug. Persons should be awakened gradually.

Most persons with a benzodiazepine overdosage respond to a cumulative dose of 1 to 3 mg of flumazenil; doses above 3 mg of flumazenil do not reliably produce additional effects. If a person has not responded 5 minutes after receiving a cumulative dose of 5 mg of flumazenil, the major cause of sedation is probably not benzodiazepine receptor agonists, and additional flumazenil is unlikely to have an effect.

Sedation can return in 1% to 3% of persons treated with flumazenil. It can be prevented or treated by giving repeated dosages of flumazenil at 20-minute intervals. For repeat treatment, no more than 1 mg (given as 0.5 mg a minute) should be given at any one time, and no more than 3 mg should be given in any 1 hour.

PRECAUTIONS AND ADVERSE REACTIONS

The most common adverse effect of the benzodiazepines is drowsiness, which occurs in about 10% of all persons. Because of this adverse effect, persons should be advised to be careful while driving or using dangerous machinery when taking the drugs. Drowsiness can be present during the day after the use of a benzodiazepine for insomnia the previous night, the so-called residual daytime sedation. Some persons also experience ataxia (fewer than 2%) and dizziness (less than 1%). These symptoms can result in falls and hip fractures, especially in elderly persons. The most serious adverse effects of the benzodiazepines occur when other sedative substances, such as alcohol, are taken concurrently. These combinations can result in marked drowsiness, disinhibition, or even respiratory depression. Infrequently, benzodiazepine receptor agonists cause mild cognitive deficits that may impair job performance. Persons taking benzodiazepine receptor agonists should be advised to exercise additional caution when driving or operating dangerous machinery.

High-potency benzodiazepines, especially triazolam can cause anterograde amnesia. A paradoxical increase in aggression has been reported in persons with pre-existing brain damage. Allergic reactions to the drugs are rare, but a few studies report maculopapular rashes and generalized itching. The symptoms of benzodiazepine intoxication include confusion, slurred speech, ataxia, drowsiness, dyspnea, and hyporeflexia.

Triazolam has received significant attention in the media because of an alleged association with serious aggressive behavioral manifestations. Therefore, the manufacturer recommends that the drug be used for no more than 10 days for treatment of insomnia and that physicians carefully evaluate the emergence of any abnormal thinking or behavioral changes in persons treated with triazolam, giving appropriate consideration to all potential causes. Triazolam was banned in Great Britain in 1991.

Zolpidem (Ambien) has also been associated with automatic behavior and amnesia.

Persons with hepatic disease and elderly persons are particularly likely to have adverse effects and toxicity from the benzodiazepines, including hepatic coma, especially when the drugs are administered repeatedly or in high dosages. Benzodiazepines can produce clinically significant impairment of respiration in persons with chronic obstructive pulmonary disease and sleep apnea. Alprazolam may exert a direct appetite stimulant effect and may cause weight gain. The benzodiazepines should be used with caution by persons with a history of substance abuse, cognitive disorders, renal disease, hepatic disease, porphyria, central nervous system (CNS) depression, or myasthenia gravis.

Zolpidem and zaleplon are generally well tolerated. At zolpidem dosages of 10 mg per day and zaleplon dosages above 10 mg per day, a small number of persons will experience dizziness, drowsiness, dyspepsia, or diarrhea. Zolpidem and zaleplon are secreted in breast milk and are therefore contraindicated for use by nursing mothers. The dosage of zolpidem and zaleplon should be reduced in elderly persons and persons with hepatic impairment.

In rare cases, zolpidem may cause hallucinations and behavioral changes. The coadministration of zolpidem and SSRIs may extend the duration of hallucinations in susceptible patients.

Eszopiclone exhibits a dose–response relationship in elderly adults for the side effects of pain, dry mouth, and unpleasant taste.

USE IN PREGNANCY AND LACTATION

The benzodiazepines are commonly used during pregnancy with no ill effects. The drugs are secreted in the breast milk.

Tolerance, Dependence, and Withdrawal

When benzodiazepines are used for short periods (1 to 2 weeks) in moderate dosages, they usually cause no significant tolerance, dependence, or withdrawal effects. The short-acting benzodiazepines (e.g., triazolam) may be an exception to this rule because some persons have reported increased anxiety the day after taking a single dose of the drug and then stopping its use. Some persons also report a tolerance for the anxiolytic effects of benzodiazepines and require increased doses to maintain the clinical remission of symptoms.

The appearance of a withdrawal syndrome, also called a discontinuation syndrome, depends on the length of time the person has been taking a benzodiazepine, the dosage the person has been taking, the rate at which the drug is tapered, and the half-life of the compound. Benzodiazepine withdrawal syndrome consists of anxiety, nervousness, diaphoresis, restlessness, irritability, fatigue, light-headedness, tremor, insomnia, and weakness (Table 8–2). Abrupt discontinuation of benzodiazepines, particularly those with short half-lives, is associated with severe withdrawal symptoms, which may include depression, paranoia, delirium, and seizures. These severe symptoms are more likely to occur if flumazenil is used for rapid reversal of the benzodiazepine receptor agonist effects. Some features of the syndrome may

Table 8–2
Signs and Symptoms of Benzodiazepine Withdrawal

Anxiety	Tremor
Irritability	Depersonalization
Insomnia	Hyperesthesia
Hyperacusis	Myoclonus
Nausea	Delirium
Difficulty concentrating	Seizures

occur in as many as 90% of persons treated with the drugs. The development of a severe withdrawal syndrome is seen only in persons who have taken high dosages for long periods. The appearance of the syndrome may be delayed for 1 or 2 weeks in persons who had been taking benzodiazepines with long half-lives. Alprazolam seems to be particularly associated with an immediate and severe withdrawal syndrome and should be tapered gradually.

When the medication is to be discontinued, the drug must be tapered slowly (25% a week); otherwise, recurrence or rebound of symptoms is likely. Monitoring of any withdrawal symptoms (possibly with a standardized rating scale) and psychological support of the person are helpful in the successful accomplishment of benzodiazepine discontinuation. Concurrent use of carbamazepine (Tegretol) during benzodiazepine discontinuation has been reported to permit a more rapid and better-tolerated withdrawal than does a gradual taper alone. The dosage range of carbamazepine used to facilitate withdrawal is 400 to 500 mg a day. Some clinicians report particular difficulty in tapering and discontinuing alprazolam, especially in persons who have been receiving high dosages for long periods. There have been reports of successful discontinuation of alprazolam by switching to clonazepam, which is then gradually withdrawn.

Zolpidem and zaleplon can produce a mild withdrawal syndrome lasting 1 day after prolonged use at higher therapeutic dosages. Rarely, a person taking zolpidem has self-titrated up the daily dosage to 30 to 40 mg a day. Abrupt discontinuation of such a high dosage of zolpidem may cause withdrawal symptoms for 4 or more days. Tolerance does not develop to the sedative effects of zolpidem and zaleplon.

DRUG INTERACTIONS

The most common and potentially serious benzodiazepine receptor agonist interaction is excessive sedation and respiratory depression occurring when benzodiazepines, zolpidem, or zaleplon are administered concomitantly with other CNS depressants, such as alcohol, barbiturates, tricyclic and tetracyclic drugs, dopamine receptor antagonists, opioids, and antihistamines. Ataxia and dysarthria may be likely to occur when lithium, antipsychotics, and clonazepam are combined. The combination of benzodiazepines and clozapine (Clozaril) has been reported to cause delirium and should be avoided. Cimetidine (Tagamet), disulfiram (Antabuse), isoniazid, estrogen, and oral contraceptives increase the plasma concentrations of diazepam, chlordiazepoxide, clorazepate, and flurazepam. Cimetidine increases the plasma concentrations of zaleplon. However, antacids may reduce GI absorption of benzodiazepines. The plasma concentrations of triazolam and alprazolam are increased to potentially toxic concentrations by nefazodone (Serzone) and fluvoxamine (Luvox). The manufacturer of nefazodone recommends that the dosage of triazolam be lowered by 75% and the dosage of alprazolam lowered by 50% when given concomitantly with nefazodone. Over-the-counter preparations of kava plant, advertised as a "natural tranquilizer," can potentiate the action of benzodiazepine receptor agonists through synergistic overactivation of GABA receptors. Carbamazepine can lower the plasma concentration of alprazolam. Antacids and food may decrease the plasma concentrations of benzodiazepines, and smoking may increase the metabolism of benzodiazepines. Rifampin (Rifadin), phenytoin (Dilantin), carbamazepine, and phenobarbital (Solfoton, Luminal) significantly increase the metabolism of zaleplon. The benzodiazepines may increase the plasma concentrations of phenytoin and digoxin (Lanoxin). The SSRIs may prolong and exacerbate the severity of zolpidem-induced hallucinations. Deaths have been reported when parental lorazepam is given with parental olanzapine.

The CYP3A4 and CYP2E1 enzymes are involved in the metabolism of eszopiclone. Eszopiclone did not show any inhibitory potential on CYP450 1A2, 2A6, 2C9, 2C19, 2D6, 2E1, and 3A4 in cryopreserved human hepatocytes. Coadministration of 3 mg of eszopiclone to subjects receiving 400 mg of ketoconazole, a potent inhibitor of CYP3A4, resulted in a 2.2-fold increase in exposure to eszopiclone.

LABORATORY INTERFERENCES

No known laboratory interferences are associated with the use of the benzodiazepines, zolpidem, and zaleplon.

DOSAGE AND CLINICAL GUIDELINES

The clinical decision to treat an anxious person with a benzodiazepine should be carefully considered. Medical causes of anxiety (e.g., thyroid dysfunction, caffeinism, and prescription medications) should be ruled out. Benzodiazepine use should be started at a low dosage, and the person should be instructed regarding the drug's sedative properties and abuse potential. An estimated length of therapy should be decided at the beginning of therapy, and the need for continued therapy should be reevaluated at least monthly because of the problems associated with long-term use. However, certain persons with anxiety disorders are unresponsive to treatments other than benzodiazepines in long-term use.

Benzodiazepines are available in a wide range of formulations. Clonazepam is available in a wafer formulation that facilitates its use in patients who have trouble swallowing pills. Alprazolam is available in an extended-release form, which reduces the frequency of dosing. Some benzodiazepines are more potent than others in that one compound requires a relatively smaller dosage than another compound to achieve the same effect. For example, clonazepam requires 0.25 mg to achieve the same effect as 5 mg of diazepam; thus, clonazepam is considered a high-potency benzodiazepine. Conversely, oxazepam has an approximate dosage equivalence of 15 mg and is a low-potency drug.

Zaleplon is available in 5- and 10-mg capsules. A single 10-mg dose is the usual adult dose. The dose can be increased to a maximum of 20 mg as tolerated. A single dose of zaleplon can be expected to provide 4 hours of sleep with minimal residual impairment. For persons older than age 65 or persons with hepatic impairment, an initial dose of 5 mg is advised.

Eszopiclone is available in 1-, 2-, and 3-mg tablets. The starting dose should not exceed 1 mg in patients with severe hepatic impairment or those taking potent CYP3A4 inhibitors. The recommended dosing to improve sleep onset or maintenance is 2 or 3 mg for adult patients (ages 18 to 64 years) and 2 mg for older adult patients (ages 65 years and older). The 1-mg dose is for sleep onset in older adult patients whose primary complaint is difficulty falling asleep.

Table 8–1 lists preparations and doses of medications discussed in this chapter.

SUVOREXANT (BELSOMRA)

The FDA has approved a new hypnotic agent, suvorexant (Belsomra); but as of early 2015, the drug was still not available for clinical use due to ongoing efforts to establish prescribing guidelines for the drug. This is mainly due to the fact that in clinical trials, residual daytime sedation was the most commonly reported side effect. This effect appears to be related to dose. The FDA has approved suvorexant in four different strengths: 5, 10, 15, and 20 milligrams. Suvorexant is an orexin receptor antagonist. The chemical orexin functions in the brain to keep people awake and alert; a medication that blocks its action has the potential to promote sleep. In this respect, suvorexant differs from other commonly prescribed sleep aids that cause sleepiness by enhancing GABA or melatonin activity.

9

Bupropion

INTRODUCTION

Bupropion (Wellbutrin, Wellbutrin SR, Wellbutrin XL, Zyban) is an antidepressant drug that inhibits the reuptake of norepinephrine and, possibly, dopamine. Most significantly, it does not act on the serotonin system like SSRI antidepressants. Consequently, its side-effect profile is characterized by minimal risks of sexual dysfunction and sedation and with modest weight loss during acute and long-term treatment. No withdrawal syndrome has been linked to discontinuation of bupropion. Although increasingly used as first-line monotherapy, a significant percentage of bupropion use occurs as add-on therapy to other antidepressants, usually SSRIs. Bupropion has been marketed under the name Zyban for use in smoking cessation regimens, so clinicians should not combine these two formulations as this may increase the risk of adverse effects, particularly seizures. A bupropion/naltrexone combination (Contrave) is FDA approved for weight loss. Bupropion also has the unique clinical distinction of being the only antidepressant approved by the FDA as a proven treatment for seasonal affective disorder (SAD).

PHARMACOLOGIC ACTIONS

Three formulations of bupropion are available: immediate release (taken three times daily), sustained release (taken twice daily), and extended release (taken once daily). The different versions of the drug contain the same active ingredient but differ in their pharmacokinetics and dosing. There have been reports of inconsistencies in bioequivalence between various branded and generic versions of bupropion. Any changes with this drug in tolerability or clinical efficacy in a patient who had been doing well should prompt an inquiry about whether these changes correspond to a switch to a new formulation.

Immediate-release bupropion is well absorbed from the gastrointestinal (GI) tract. Peak plasma concentrations of bupropion are usually reached within 2 hours of oral administration, and peak levels of the sustained-release version are seen after 3 hours. The mean half-life of the compound is 12 hours, ranging from 8 to 40 hours. Peak levels of extended-release bupropion occur 5 hours after ingestion. This provides a longer time to maximum plasma concentration (t_{max}) but comparable peak and trough plasma concentrations. The 24-hour exposure occurring after administration of the extended-release version of 300 mg once daily is equivalent to that provided by sustained release of 150 mg twice daily. Clinically, this permits the drug to be taken once a day in the morning. Plasma levels are also reduced in the evening, making it less likely for some patients to experience treatment-related insomnia.

The mechanism of action for the antidepressant effects of bupropion is presumed to involve the inhibition of dopamine and norepinephrine reuptake. Bupropion binds to the dopamine transporter in the brain. The effects of bupropion on smoking cessation may be related to its effects on dopamine reward pathways or to inhibition of nicotinic acetylcholine receptors.

THERAPEUTIC INDICATIONS

Depression

Although overshadowed by the SSRIs as first-line treatment for major depression, the therapeutic efficacy of bupropion in depression is well established in both outpatient and inpatient settings. Observed rates of response and remission are comparable to those seen with the SSRIs. Bupropion has been found to prevent seasonal major depressive episodes in patients with a history of seasonal pattern or affective disorder.

Smoking Cessation

As the brand name Zyban, bupropion is indicated for use in combination with behavioral modification programs for smoking cessation. It is intended to be used in patients who are highly motivated and who receive some form of structured behavioral support. Bupropion is most effective when combined with nicotine substitutes (Nicoderm, Nicotrol).

Bipolar Disorders

Bupropion is less likely than tricyclic antidepressants to precipitate mania in persons with bipolar I disorder and less likely than other antidepressants to exacerbate or induce rapid cycling bipolar II disorder; however, the evidence about use of bupropion in the treatment of patients with bipolar disorder is limited.

Attention-Deficit/Hyperactivity Disorder

Bupropion is used as a second-line agent, after the sympathomimetics, for treatment of attention-deficit/hyperactivity disorder (ADHD). It has not been compared with proven ADHD medications such as methylphenidate (Ritalin) or atomoxetine (Strattera) for childhood and adult ADHD. Bupropion is an appropriate choice for persons with comorbid ADHD and depression or persons with comorbid ADHD, conduct disorder, or substance abuse. It may also be considered for use in patients who develop tics when treated with psychostimulants.

Cocaine Detoxification

Bupropion may be associated with a euphoric feeling; thus, it may be contraindicated in persons with histories of substance abuse. However, because of its dopaminergic effects, bupropion has been explored as a treatment to reduce the cravings for cocaine in persons who have withdrawn from the substance. Results have been inconclusive, with some patients showing a reduction in drug craving and others finding their cravings increased.

Hypoactive Sexual Desire Disorder

Bupropion is often added to drugs such as SSRIs to counteract sexual side effects and may be helpful as a treatment for nondepressed individuals with hypoactive sexual desire disorder. Bupropion may improve sexual arousal, orgasm completion, and sexual satisfaction.

Weight Loss

Although bupropion can cause modest weight loss, when combined with naltrexone, it can produce clinically significant weight loss. Naltrexone is an opioid receptor antagonist. They are available as Contrave, an extended-release 8/90-mg tablet. It is labeled as an adjunct to increased physical activity and reduced calorie diet.

PRECAUTIONS AND ADVERSE REACTIONS

Headache, insomnia, dry mouth, tremor, and nausea are the most common side effects. Restlessness, agitation, and irritability may also occur. Patients with severe anxiety or panic disorder should not be prescribed bupropion. Most likely because of its potentiating effects on dopaminergic neurotransmission, bupropion can cause psychotic symptoms, including hallucinations, delusions, and catatonia, as well as delirium. Most notable about bupropion is the absence of significant drug-induced orthostatic hypotension, weight gain, daytime drowsiness, and anticholinergic effects. Some persons, however, may experience dry mouth or constipation and weight loss. Hypertension may occur in some patients, but bupropion causes no other significant cardiovascular or clinical laboratory changes. Bupropion exerts indirect sympathomimetic activity, producing positive inotropic effects in human myocardium, an effect that may reflect catecholamine release. Some patients experience cognitive impairment, most notably word-finding difficulties.

Concern about seizure has deterred some physicians from prescribing bupropion. The risk of seizure is dose dependent. Studies show that at dosages of 300 mg a day or less of sustained-release bupropion, the incidence of seizures is 0.05%, which is no worse than the incidence of seizures with other antidepressants. The risk of seizures increases to about 0.1% with dosages of 400 mg a day.

Changes in electroencephalographic (EEG) waveforms have been reported to be associated with bupropion use. About 20% of individuals treated with bupropion exhibit spike waves, sharp waves, and focal slowing. The likelihood of females having sharp waves is higher than males. The presence of these waveforms in individuals taking a medication known to lower the seizure threshold may be a risk factor for developing seizures. Other risk factors for seizures include a history of seizures, use of alcohol, recent benzodiazepine withdrawal, organic brain disease, head trauma, or pretreatment epileptiform discharges on EEG.

The use of bupropion by pregnant women is not associated with specific risk of increased rate of birth defects. Bupropion is secreted in breast milk, so the use of bupropion in nursing women should be based on the clinical circumstances of the patient and the judgment of the clinician.

Few deaths have been reported after overdoses of bupropion. Poor outcomes are associated with cases of huge doses and mixed-drug overdoses. Seizures occur in about one-third of all overdoses and are dose dependent, with those having seizures ingesting a significantly higher median dose. Fatalities can involve uncontrollable seizures, sinus bradycardia, and cardiac arrest. Symptoms of poisoning most often involve seizures, sinus tachycardia, hypertension, GI symptoms, hallucinations, and agitation. All seizures are typically brief and self-limited. In general, however, bupropion is safer in overdose cases than are other antidepressants, except perhaps SSRIs.

USE IN PREGNANCY AND LACTATION

There is insufficient information about the safety of bupropion use in pregnancy. It is excreted in breast milk.

DRUG INTERACTIONS

Given the fact that bupropion is frequently combined with SSRIs or venlafaxine, potential interactions are significant. Bupropion has been found to have an effect on the pharmacokinetics of venlafaxine. One study noted a significant increase in venlafaxine levels and a consequent decrease in its main metabolite O-desmethylvenlafaxine during combined treatment with sustained-release bupropion. Bupropion hydroxylation is weakly inhibited by venlafaxine. No significant changes in plasma levels of the SSRIs paroxetine and fluoxetine have been reported. However, few case reports indicate that the combination of bupropion and fluoxetine (Prozac) may be associated with panic, delirium, or seizures. Bupropion in combination with lithium (Eskalith) may rarely cause CNS toxicity, including seizures.

Because of possibility of inducing a hypertensive crisis, bupropion should not be used concurrently with monoamine oxidase inhibitors (MAOIs). At least 14 days should pass after the discontinuation of an MAOI before initiating treatment with bupropion. In some cases, the addition of bupropion may permit persons taking antiparkinsonian medications to lower the doses of their dopaminergic drugs. However, delirium, psychotic symptoms, and dyskinetic movements may be associated with the coadministration of bupropion and dopaminergic agents such as levodopa (Larodopa), pergolide (Permax), ropinirole (Requip), pramipexole (Mirapex), amantadine (Symmetrel), and bromocriptine (Parlodel). Sinus bradycardia may occur when bupropion is combined with metoprolol.

Carbamazepine (Tegretol) may decrease plasma concentrations of bupropion, and bupropion may increase plasma concentrations of valproic acid (Depakene).

In vitro biotransformation studies of bupropion have found that formation of a major active metabolite, hydroxybupropion, is mediated by CYP2B6. Bupropion has a significant inhibitory effect on CYP2D6.

LABORATORY INTERFERENCES

A report has appeared indicating that bupropion may give a false-positive result on urinary amphetamine screens. No other reports have appeared of laboratory interferences clearly associated with bupropion treatment. Clinically nonsignificant changes in the electrocardiogram (premature beats and nonspecific ST-T changes) and decreases in the white blood cell count (by about 10%) have been reported in a small number of persons.

DOSAGE AND CLINICAL GUIDELINES

Immediate-release bupropion is available in 75-, 100-, and 150-mg tablets. Sustained-release bupropion is available in 100-, 150-, 200-, and 300-mg tablets. Extended-release bupropion comes in 150- and 300-mg strengths.

There have been problems associated with one of the extended-release generic versions called Budeprion XL 300-mg tablets, which was found not to be therapeutically equivalent to Wellbutrin XL 300 mg and was removed from the market.

Initiation of immediate-release bupropion in the average adult person should be 75 mg orally twice a day. On the fourth day of treatment, the dosage can be increased to 100 mg three times a day. Because 300 mg is the recommended dose, the person should be maintained on this dose for several weeks before increasing it further. The maximum dosage, 450 mg a day, should be given as 150 mg three times a day. Because of the risk of seizures, increases in dose should never exceed 100 mg in a 3-day period; a single dose of immediate-release bupropion should never exceed 150 mg, and the total daily dosage should not exceed 450 mg. The maximum of 400 mg of the sustained-release version should be used as a twice-a-day regimen of either 200 mg twice daily or 300 mg in the morning and 100 mg in the afternoon. A starting dosage of the sustained-release version, 100 mg once a day, can be increased to 100 mg twice a day after 4 days. Then, 150 mg twice a day may be used. A single dose of sustained-release bupropion should never exceed 300 mg. The maximum dosage is 200 mg twice a day of the immediate-release or extended-release formulations. An advantage of the extended-release preparation is that, after appropriate titration, a total of 450 mg can be given all at once in the morning.

For smoking cessation, the patient should start taking 150 mg a day of sustained-release bupropion 10 to 14 days before quitting smoking. On the fourth day, the dosage should be increased to 150 mg twice daily. Treatment generally lasts 7 to 12 weeks.

10
Buspirone

INTRODUCTION

Buspirone hydrochloride (BuSpar), an azapirone, is chemically distinct from other psychotropic agents. It has high affinity for the 5-HT$_{1A}$ serotonin receptor, acting as an agonist or partial agonist, and moderate affinity for the D$_2$ dopamine receptor, acting as both an agonist and an antagonist. The approved indication for buspirone is for the treatment of generalized anxiety disorder (GAD). It does not possess anti-convulsant and muscle relaxant effects. Buspirone was initially anticipated to be a better alternative to the benzodiazepines since buspirone is not sedating, does not possess potential for dependence and abuse, and does not have adverse cognitive and psychomotor effects. However, while it has these safety and tolerability advantages, combined evidence reveals that it is not more effective than benzodiazepines. Reports and studies continue to appear of some patients who benefit from the addition of buspirone to their antidepressant regimen. Its use in this adjunctive role probably is more common than its use as an anxiolytic. Interestingly, the antidepressant drug vilazodone (Viibryd) inhibits 5-HT reuptake and acts as a 5-HT$_{1A}$ receptor partial agonist.

PHARMACOLOGIC ACTIONS

Buspirone is well absorbed from the gastrointestinal tract, but absorption is delayed by food ingestion. Peak plasma levels are achieved 40 to 90 minutes after oral administration. At doses of 10 to 40 mg, single-dose linear pharmacokinetics are observed. Nonlinear pharmacokinetics are observed after multiple doses. Because of its short half-life (2 to 11 hours), buspirone is dosed three times daily. An active metabolite of buspirone, 1-pyrimidinylpiperazine (1-PP), is about 20% less potent than buspirone but is up to 30% more concentrated in the brain than the parent compound. The elimination half-life of 1-PP is 6 hours.

Buspirone has no effect on the γ-aminobutyric acid (GABA)–associated chloride ion channel or the serotonin reuptake transporter, targets of other drugs that are effective in GAD. Buspirone also has activity at 5-HT$_2$ and dopamine type 2 (D$_2$) receptors, although the significance of the effects at these receptors is unknown. At D$_2$ receptors, it has properties of both an agonist and an antagonist.

THERAPEUTIC INDICATIONS
Generalized Anxiety Disorder

Buspirone is a narrow-spectrum antianxiety agent with demonstrated efficacy only in the treatment of GAD. In contrast to the SSRIs or venlafaxine, buspirone is not effective in the treatment of panic disorder, obsessive-compulsive disorder (OCD), or social phobia. Buspirone, however, has an advantage over these agents in that it does not typically cause sexual dysfunction or weight gain.

Some evidence suggests that compared with benzodiazepines, buspirone is generally more effective for symptoms of anger and hostility, equally effective for psychic symptoms of anxiety, and less effective for somatic symptoms of anxiety. The full benefit of buspirone is evident only at dosages above 30 mg a day. Compared with the benzodiazepines, buspirone has a delayed onset of action and lacks any euphoric effect. Unlike benzodiazepines, buspirone has no immediate effects, and patients should be told that a full clinical response may take 2 to 4 weeks. If an immediate response is needed, patients can be started on a benzodiazepine and then withdrawn from the drug after buspirone's effects begin. Sometimes the sedative effects of benzodiazepines, which are not found with buspirone, are desirable; however, these sedative effects may cause impaired motor performance and cognitive deficits.

Other Disorders

Many other clinical uses of buspirone have been reported, but most have not been confirmed in controlled trials. Evidence of the efficacy of high-dosage buspirone (30 to 90 mg a day) for depressive disorders is mixed. Buspirone appears to have weak antidepressant activity, which has led to its use as an augmenting agent in patients who have failed standard antidepressant therapy. In a large study, buspirone augmentation of SSRIs worked as well as other commonly used strategies. Buspirone is sometimes used to augment SSRIs in the treatment of OCD. There are reports that buspirone may be beneficial against the increased arousal and flashbacks associated with posttraumatic stress disorder.

Because buspirone does not act on the GABA–chloride ion channel complex, the drug is not recommended for the treatment of withdrawal from benzodiazepines, alcohol, or sedative-hypnotic drugs, except as treatment of comorbid anxiety symptoms.

Scattered trials suggest that buspirone reduces aggression and anxiety in persons with organic brain disease or traumatic brain injury. It is also used for SSRI-induced bruxism and sexual dysfunction, nicotine craving, and attention-deficit/hyperactivity disorder.

PRECAUTIONS AND ADVERSE REACTIONS

Buspirone does not cause weight gain, sexual dysfunction, discontinuation symptoms, or significant sleep disturbance. It does not produce sedation or cognitive and psychomotor impairment. The most common adverse effects of buspirone are headache, nausea, dizziness, and (rarely) insomnia. No sedation is associated with buspirone. Some persons may report a minor feeling of restlessness, although that symptom may reflect an incompletely treated anxiety disorder. No deaths have been reported from overdoses of buspirone, and the median lethal dose is estimated to be 160 to 550 times the recommended daily dose. Buspirone should be used with caution by persons with hepatic and renal impairment. Buspirone can be used safely by the elderly.

USE IN PREGNANCY AND LACTATION

There is no evidence that pregnant women and nursing mothers taking buspirone have an increased risk of adverse effects on the newborn.

DRUG INTERACTIONS

The coadministration of buspirone and haloperidol (Haldol) results in increased blood concentrations of haloperidol. Buspirone should not be used with monoamine oxidase inhibitors (MAOIs) to avoid hypertensive episodes, and a 2-week washout period should pass between the discontinuation of MAOI use and the initiation of treatment with buspirone. Drugs or foods that inhibit CYP3A4, for example, erythromycin (E-mycin), itraconazole (Sporanox), nefazodone (Serzone), and grapefruit juice increase buspirone plasma concentrations.

LABORATORY INTERFERENCES

Single doses of buspirone can cause transient elevations in growth hormone, prolactin, and cortisol concentrations, although the effects are not clinically significant.

DOSAGE AND CLINICAL GUIDELINES

Buspirone is available in single-scored 5- and 10-mg tablets and triple-scored 15- and 30-mg tablets; treatment is usually initiated with either 5 mg orally three times daily or 7.5 mg orally twice daily. The dosage can be raised by 5 mg every 2 to 4 days to the usual dosage range of 15 to 60 mg a day.

Buspirone should not be used in patients with past hypersensitivity to buspirone, in cases of diabetes-associated metabolic acidosis, or in patients with severely compromised liver and/or renal function.

Switching From a Benzodiazepine to Buspirone

Buspirone is not cross-tolerant with benzodiazepines, barbiturates, or alcohol. A common clinical problem, therefore, is how to initiate buspirone therapy in a person who is currently taking benzodiazepines. There are two alternatives. First, the clinician can start buspirone treatment gradually while the benzodiazepine is being withdrawn. Second, the clinician can start buspirone treatment and bring the person up to a therapeutic dosage for 2 to 3 weeks while the person is still receiving the regular dosage of the benzodiazepine and then slowly taper the benzodiazepine dosage. Patients who have received benzodiazepines in the past, especially in recent months, may find that buspirone is not as effective as the benzodiazepines in the treatment of their anxiety. This might be explained by the absence of the immediate mildly euphoric and sedative effects of the benzodiazepines. The coadministration of buspirone and benzodiazepines may be effective in the treatment of persons with anxiety disorders who have not responded to treatment with either drug alone.

11

Calcium Channel Inhibitors

INTRODUCTION

Findings of elevated intracellular calcium ion activity in mania and bipolar depression that is attenuated by established mood-stabilizing medications may explain the effectiveness of calcium channel inhibitors, also called calcium channel blockers (CCBs), which act primarily on intracellular calcium ion, in the treatment of mood disorders. The intracellular calcium ion regulates activity of multiple neurotransmitters such as serotonin and dopamine, and that action may account for its role as a treatment in mood disorders. CCBs are used in psychiatry as antimanic agents for persons who are refractory to, or cannot tolerate, treatment with first-line mood-stabilizing agents such as lithium (Eskalith), carbamazepine (Tegretol), and divalproex (Depakote). Calcium channel inhibitors include nifedipine (Procardia, Adalat), nimodipine (Nimotop), isradipine (DynaCirc), amlodipine (Norvasc, Lotrel), nicardipine (Cardene), nisoldipine (Sular), nitrendipine (Baypress), and verapamil (Calan). They are used for control of mania and ultradian bipolar disorder (mood cycling in less than 24 hours).

The results of a large genetic study have rekindled interest in the potential clinical uses of CCBs. Two genome-wide findings implicated genes encoding L-type voltage-gated calcium channel subunits as susceptibility genes for bipolar disorder, schizophrenia, major depressive disorder, attention-deficit/hyperactivity disorder, and autism. Nimodipine probably has greater potential for psychiatric applications, because it crosses the blood–brain barrier more readily than verapamil and it acts on T- as well as L-type channels.

PHARMACOLOGIC ACTIONS

The calcium channel inhibitors are nearly completely absorbed after oral use, with significant first-pass hepatic metabolism. Considerable intra- and interindividual variations are seen in the plasma concentrations of the drugs after a single dose. Peak plasma levels of most of these agents are achieved within 30 minutes. Amlodipine does not reach peak plasma levels for about 6 hours. The half-life of verapamil after the first dose is 2 to 8 hours; the half-life increases from 5 to 12 hours after the first few days of therapy. The half-lives of the other CCBs range from 1 to 2 hours for nimodipine and isradipine from 30 to 50 hours for amlodipine (Table 11–1).

The primary mechanism of action of CCBs in bipolar illness is not known. The calcium channel inhibitors discussed in this section inhibit the influx of calcium into neurons through L-type (long-acting) voltage-dependent calcium channels.

Table 11–1
Half-Lives, Dosages, and Effectiveness of Selected Calcium Channel Inhibitors in Psychiatric Disorders

	Verapamil (Calan, Isoptin)	Nimodipine (Nimotop)	Isradipine (DynaCirc)	Amlodipine (Norvasc)
Half-life	Short (5–12 hours)	Short (1–2 hours)	Short (1–2 hours)	Long (30–50 hours)
Starting dosage	40 mg TID	30 mg TID	2.5 mg BID	5 mg HS
Peak daily dosage	360 mg	240–450 mg	20 mg	10–15 mg
Antimanic	++	++	++	a
Antidepressant	±	+	+	a
Antiultradian[b]	±	++	++	a

[a]No systematic studies, only case reports.
[b]Rapid cycling bipolar disorder.
BID, twice a day; HS, half strength; TID, three times a day.
Table adapted from Robert M. Post, MD.

THERAPEUTIC INDICATIONS

Bipolar Disorder

Nimodipine and verapamil have been demonstrated to be effective as maintenance therapy in persons with bipolar illness. Patients who respond to lithium appear to also respond to treatment with verapamil. Nimodipine may be useful for ultradian cycling and recurrent brief depression. The clinician should begin treatment with a short-acting drug such as nimodipine or isradipine, beginning with a low dosage and increasing the dosage every 4 to 5 days until a clinical response is seen or adverse effects appear. When symptoms are controlled, a longer-acting drug, such as amlodipine, can be substituted as maintenance therapy. Failure to respond to verapamil does not exclude a favorable response to one of the other drugs. Verapamil has been shown to prevent antidepressant-induced mania. The CCBs can be combined with other agents, such as carbamazepine, in patients who are partial responders to monotherapy.

Depression

None of the CCBs are effective as treatment for depression and may in fact prevent response to antidepressants.

Other Psychiatric Indications

Nifedipine is used to treat hypertensive crises associated with the use of monoamine oxidase inhibitors. Isradipine may reduce the subjective response to methamphetamine. Calcium channel inhibitors may be beneficial in Tourette's disorder, Huntington's disease, panic disorder, intermittent explosive disorder, and tardive dyskinesia.

Other Medical Uses

These drugs have been used to treat medical conditions such as angina, hypertension, migraine headaches, Raynaud's phenomenon, esophageal spasm, premature labor, and headache. Verapamil has antiarrhythmic activity and has been used to treat supraventricular arrhythmias.

PRECAUTIONS AND ADVERSE REACTIONS

The most common adverse effects associated with calcium channel inhibitors are those attributable to vasodilation: dizziness, headache, tachycardia, nausea, dysesthesias, and peripheral edema. Verapamil and diltiazem (Cardizem) in particular can cause hypotension, bradycardia, and atrioventricular heart block, which necessitate close monitoring and sometimes discontinuation of the drugs. In all patients with cardiovascular disease, the drugs should be used with caution. Other common adverse effects include constipation, fatigue, rash, coughing, and wheezing. Adverse effects noted with diltiazem include hyperactivity, akathisia, and parkinsonism; with verapamil, delirium, hyperprolactinemia, and galactorrhea; with nimodipine, subjective sense of chest tightness and skin flushing; and with nifedipine, depression.

USE IN PREGNANCY AND LACTATION

The drugs are commonly used during pregnancy and lactation to treat hypertension, arrhythmias, and preeclampsia.

DRUG INTERACTIONS

All CCBs have a potential for drug–drug interactions. The types and risks of these interactions vary by compound. Verapamil raises serum levels of carbamazepine, digoxin, and other CYP3A4 substrates. Verapamil and diltiazem, but not nifedipine, have been reported to precipitate carbamazepine-induced neurotoxicity. Calcium channel inhibitors should not be used by persons taking β-adrenergic receptor antagonists, hypotensives (e.g., diuretics, vasodilators, and angiotensin-converting enzyme inhibitors), or antiarrhythmic drugs (e.g., quinidine and digoxin) without consultation with an internist or cardiologist. Cimetidine (Tagamet) has been reported to increase plasma concentrations of nifedipine and diltiazem. Some patients who are treated with lithium and calcium channel inhibitors concurrently may be at increased risk for the signs and symptoms of neurotoxicity, and deaths have occurred.

LABORATORY INTERFERENCES

No known laboratory interferences are associated with the use of calcium channel inhibitors.

DOSAGE AND CLINICAL GUIDELINES

Verapamil is available in 40-, 80-, and 120-mg tablets; 120-, 180-, and 240-mg sustained-release tablets; and 100-, 120-, 180-, 200-, 240-, 300-, and 360-mg sustained-release capsules. The starting dosage is 40 mg orally three times a day and can be increased in increments every 4 to 5 days up to 80 to 120 mg three times a day. The patient's blood pressure, pulse, and electrocardiogram (in patients older than 40 years old or with a history of cardiac illness) should be routinely monitored.

Nifedipine is available in 10- and 20-mg capsules and 30-, 60-, and 90-mg extended-release tablets. Administration should be started at 10 mg orally three or four times a day and can be increased up to a maximum dosage of 120 mg a day.

Nimodipine is available in 30-mg capsules. It has been used at 60 mg every 4 hours for ultra–rapid-cycling bipolar disorder and sometimes briefly at up to 630 mg/day.

Isradipine is available in 2.5- and 5-mg capsules, with a maximum of 20 mg/day. An extended-release formulation of isradipine has been discontinued.

Amlodipine is available in 2.5-, 5-, and 10-mg tablets. Administration should start at 5 mg once at night and can be increased to a maximum dosage of 10 to 15 mg a day.

Diltiazem is available in 30-, 60-, 90-, and 120-mg tablets; 60-, 90-, 120-, 180-, 240-, 300-, and 360-mg extended-release capsules; and 60-, 90-, 120-, 180-, 240-, 300-, and 360-mg extended-release tablets. Administration should start with 30 mg orally four times a day and can be increased up to a maximum of 360 mg a day.

Elderly persons are more sensitive to the calcium channel inhibitors than are younger adults. No specific information is available regarding the use of the agents for children.

Carbamazepine and Oxcarbazepine

INTRODUCTION

Carbamazepine (Tegretol) is structurally similar to the tricyclic antidepressant imipramine (Tofranil), but having a very different clinical spectrum of efficacy.

It is now recognized in most guidelines as a first- or second-line mood stabilizer useful in the treatment and prevention of both phases of bipolar affective disorder. A long-acting sustained release formulation (Equetro) was approved by the FDA for the treatment of acute mania in 2002. The structure and chemistry of carbamazepine are closely related to the anticonvulsant oxcarbazepine (Trileptal). Because of its similarity to carbamazepine, many clinicians use it as a treatment for patients with bipolar disorder. Oxcarbazepine is not FDA approved for acute mania, although one study suggested better efficacy of oxcarbazepine in less severe mania compared with more severe mania, while carbamazepine is effective in severe forms of mania.

CARBAMAZEPINE

Pharmacologic Actions

Absorption of carbamazepine is slow and unpredictable. Food enhances absorption. Peak plasma concentrations are reached 2 to 8 hours after a single dose, and steady-state levels are reached after 2 to 4 days on a steady dosage. It is 70% to 80% protein bound. The half-life of carbamazepine ranges from 18 to 54 hours, with an average of 26 hours. However, with chronic administration, the half-life of carbamazepine decreases to an average of 12 hours. This results from induction of hepatic CYP450 enzymes by carbamazepine, specifically autoinduction of carbamazepine metabolism. The induction of hepatic enzymes reaches its maximum level after about 3 to 5 weeks of therapy.

The pharmacokinetics of carbamazepine are different for two long-acting preparations of carbamazepine, each of which uses slightly different technology. One formulation, Tegretol XR, requires food to ensure normal gastrointestinal (GI) transit time. The other preparation, Carbatrol, relies on a combination of intermediate, extended-release, and very slow–release beads, making it suitable for bedtime administration.

Carbamazepine is metabolized in the liver, and the 10,11-epoxide metabolite is active as an anticonvulsant. Its activity in the treatment of bipolar disorders is unknown. Long-term use of carbamazepine is associated with an increased ratio of the epoxide to the parent molecule.

The anticonvulsant effects of carbamazepine are thought to be mediated mainly by binding to voltage-dependent sodium channels in the inactive state and prolonging their inactivation. This secondarily reduces voltage-dependent calcium channel activation and, thus, synaptic transmission. Additional effects include reduction of currents through N-methyl-D-aspartate (NMDA) glutamate-receptor channels, competitive antagonism of adenosine A_1-receptors, and potentiation of central nervous system (CNS) catecholamine neurotransmission. Whether any or all of these mechanisms also result in mood stabilization is not known.

Therapeutic Indications

Bipolar Disorder

Acute Mania. The acute antimanic effects of carbamazepine are typically evident within the first several days of treatment. About 50% to 70% of all persons respond within 2 to 3 weeks of initiation. Studies suggest that carbamazepine may be especially effective in persons who are not responsive to lithium, such as persons with dysphoric mania, rapid cycling, or a negative family history of mood disorders. The antimanic effects of carbamazepine can be, and often are, augmented by concomitant administration of lithium (Eskalith), valproic acid (Depakene), thyroid hormones, dopamine receptor antagonists (DRAs), or serotonin–dopamine antagonists (SDAs). Some persons may respond to carbamazepine but not lithium or valproic acid and vice versa.

Prophylaxis. Carbamazepine is effective in preventing relapses, particularly among patients with bipolar II disorder and schizoaffective disorder, and dysphoric mania.

Acute Depression. A subgroup of treatment-refractory patients with acute depression responds well to carbamazepine. Patients with more severe episodic and less chronic depression seem to be better responders to carbamazepine. Nevertheless, carbamazepine remains an alternative drug for depressed persons who have not responded to conventional treatments, including electroconvulsive therapy (ECT).

Other Disorders. Carbamazepine helps to control symptoms associated with acute alcohol withdrawal, although benzodiazepines are more effective in this population. Carbamazepine has been suggested as a treatment for the paroxysmal recurrent component of posttraumatic stress disorder (PTSD). Uncontrolled studies suggest that carbamazepine is effective in controlling impulsive, aggressive behavior in nonpsychotic persons of all ages, including children and elderly persons. Carbamazepine is also effective in controlling nonacute agitation and aggressive behavior in patients with schizophrenia and schizoaffective disorder. Persons with prominent positive symptoms (e.g., hallucinations) may be likely to respond, as are persons who display impulsive aggressive outbursts.

Precautions and Adverse Reactions

Carbamazepine is relatively well tolerated. Mild GI (nausea, vomiting, gastric distress, constipation, diarrhea, and anorexia) and CNS (ataxia, drowsiness) side effects are the most common. The severity of these adverse effects is reduced if the dosage of carbamazepine is increased slowly and kept at the minimal effective plasma concentration. In contrast to lithium and valproate (other drugs used to manage bipolar disorder), carbamazepine does not appear to cause weight gain. Because of the phenomena of autoinduction, with consequent reductions in carbamazepine concentrations, side-effect tolerability may improve over time. Most of the adverse effects of carbamazepine are correlated with plasma concentrations above 9 μg/mL. The rarest

Table 12–1
Adverse Events Associated With Carbamazepine

Dosage-related Adverse Effects	Idiosyncratic Adverse Effects
Double or blurred vision	Agranulocytosis
Vertigo	Stevens–Johnson syndrome
GI disturbances	Aplastic anemia
Task performance impairment	Hepatic failure
Hematologic effects	Rash
	Pancreatitis
GI, gastrointestinal.	

but most serious adverse effects of carbamazepine are blood dyscrasias, hepatitis, and serious skin reactions (Table 12–1).

Blood Dyscrasias.   The drug's hematologic effects are not dose related. Severe blood dyscrasias (aplastic anemia, agranulocytosis) occur in about 1 in 125,000 persons treated with carbamazepine. There does not appear to be a correlation between the degree of benign white blood cell (WBC) suppression (leukopenia), which is seen in 1% to 2% of persons, and the emergence of life-threatening blood dyscrasias. Persons should be warned that the emergence of such symptoms as fever, sore throat, rash, petechiae, bruising, and easy bleeding can potentially herald a serious dyscrasia, and the person should seek medical evaluation immediately. Routine hematologic monitoring in carbamazepine-treated persons is recommended at 3, 6, 9, and 12 months. If there is no significant evidence of bone marrow suppression by that time, many experts would reduce the interval of monitoring. However, even assiduous monitoring may fail to detect severe blood dyscrasias before they cause symptoms.

Hepatitis.   Within the first few weeks of therapy, carbamazepine can cause both hepatitis associated with increases in liver enzymes, particularly transaminases, and cholestasis associated with elevated bilirubin and alkaline phosphatase. Mild transaminase elevations warrant observation only, but persistent elevations more than three times the upper limit of normal indicate the need to discontinue the drug. Hepatitis can recur if the drug is reintroduced to the person and can result in death.

Dermatologic Effects.   About 10% to 15% of persons treated with carbamazepine develop a benign maculopapular rash within the first 3 weeks of treatment. Stopping the medication usually leads to resolution of the rash. Some patients may experience life-threatening dermatologic syndromes, including exfoliative dermatitis, erythema multiforme, Stevens–Johnson syndrome, and toxic epidermal necrolysis. The possible emergence of these serious dermatologic problems causes most clinicians to discontinue carbamazepine use in people who develop any type of rash. The risk of drug rash is about equal between valproic acid and carbamazepine in the first 2 months of use but is subsequently much higher for carbamazepine. If carbamazepine seems to be the only effective drug for a person who has a benign rash with carbamazepine treatment, a retrial of the drug can be undertaken. Many patients can be rechallenged without reemergence of the rash. Pretreatment with prednisone (40 mg a day) may suppress the rash, although other symptoms of an allergic reaction (e.g., fever and pneumonitis) may develop even with steroid pretreatment.

Renal Effects.   Carbamazepine is occasionally used to treat diabetes insipidus not associated with lithium use. This activity results from direct or indirect effects at the vasopressin receptor. It may also lead to the development of hyponatremia and water intoxication in some patients, particularly elderly persons, or when used in high doses.

Other Adverse Effects.   Carbamazepine decreases cardiac conduction (although less than the tricyclic drugs do) and can thus exacerbate pre-existing cardiac disease. Carbamazepine should be used with caution in persons with glaucoma, prostatic hypertrophy, diabetes, or a history of alcohol abuse. Carbamazepine occasionally activates vasopressin receptor function, which results in a condition resembling the syndrome of secretion of inappropriate antidiuretic hormone, characterized by hyponatremia and, rarely, water intoxication. This is the opposite of the renal effects of lithium (i.e., nephrogenic diabetes insipidus). Augmentation of lithium with carbamazepine does not reverse the lithium effect, however. Emergence of confusion, severe weakness, or headache in a person taking carbamazepine should prompt measurement of serum electrolytes.

Carbamazepine use rarely elicits an immune hypersensitivity response consisting of fever, rash, eosinophilia, and possibly fatal myocarditis.

Use in Pregnancy and Lactation
Cleft palate, fingernail hypoplasia, microcephaly, and spina bifida in infants may be associated with the maternal use of carbamazepine during pregnancy. Pregnant women should not use carbamazepine unless absolutely necessary. All women with childbearing potential should take 1 to 4 mg of folic acid daily even if they are not trying to conceive. Carbamazepine is secreted in breast milk.

Drug Interactions
Carbamazepine decreases serum concentrations of numerous drugs as a result of prominent induction of hepatic CYP3A4 (Table 12–2). Monitoring for a decrease in clinical effects is frequently indicated. Carbamazepine can decrease the blood concentrations of oral contraceptives, resulting in breakthrough bleeding and uncertain prophylaxis against pregnancy. Carbamazepine should not be administered with monoamine oxidase inhibitors (MAOIs), which should be discontinued at least 2 weeks before initiating treatment with carbamazepine. Grapefruit juice inhibits the hepatic metabolism of carbamazepine. When carbamazepine and valproate are used in combination, the dosage of carbamazepine should be decreased because valproate displaces carbamazepine binding on proteins, and the dosage of valproate may need to be increased.

Laboratory Interferences
Circulating levels of thyroxine and triiodothyronine are associated with a decrease in thyroid-stimulating hormone and may be associated with treatment. Carbamazepine

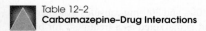

Table 12-2
Carbamazepine–Drug Interactions

Effect of Carbamazepine on Plasma Concentrations of Concomitant Agents	Agents That May Affect Carbamazepine Plasma Concentrations
Carbamazepine may decrease drug plasma concentration of	*Agents that may increase carbamazepine plasma concentration*
Acetaminophen	Allopurinol
Alprazolam	Cimetidine
Amitriptyline	Clarithromycin
Bupropion	Danazol
Clomipramine	Diltiazem
Clonazepam	Erythromycin
Clozapine	Fluoxetine
Cyclosporine	Fluvoxamine
Desipramine	Gemfibrozil
Dicumarol	Itraconazole
Doxepine	Ketoconazole
Doxycycline	Isoniazid[a]
Ethosuximide	Itraconazole
Felbamate	Lamotrigine
Fentonyl	Loratadine
Fluphenazine	Macrolides
Haloperidol	Nefazadone
Hormonal contraceptives	Nicotinamide
Imipramine	Propoxyphene
Lamotrigine	Terfenadine
Methadone	Troleandomycin
Methsuximide	Valproate[a]
Methylprednisolone	Verapamil
Nimodipino	Viloxazine
Pancuronium	*Drugs that may decrease carbamazepine plasma concentrations*
Phensuximide	Carbamazepine (autoinduction)
Phenytoin	Cisplatin
Primidone	Doxorubicin HCl
Theophylline	Felbamate
Valproate	Phenobarbital
Warfarin	Phenytoin
Carbamazepine may increase drug plasma concentrations of	Primidone
Clomipramine	Rifampin[b]
Phenytoin	Theophylline
Primidone	Valproate

[a]Increased concentrations of the active 10,11-epoxide.
[b]Decreased concentrations of carbamazepine and increased concentrations of the 10,11-epoxide.
Table by Carlos A. Zarate, Jr., MD and Mauricio Tohen, MD.

is also associated with an increase in total serum cholesterol, primarily by increasing high-density lipoproteins. The thyroid and cholesterol effects are not clinically significant. Carbamazepine may interfere with the dexamethasone suppression test and may also cause false-positive pregnancy test results.

Dosing and Administration
The target dose for antimanic activity is 1,200 mg a day, although this varies considerably. Immediate-release carbamazepine needs to be taken three or four times a day, which leads to lapses in compliance. Extended-release formulations are thus preferred because they can be taken once or twice a day. One form of extended-release

carbamazepine, Carbatrol, comes as 100-, 200-, and 300-mg capsules. Another form called Equetro is identical to Carbetrol and is marketed as a treatment for bipolar disorder. These capsules contain tiny beads with three different types of coatings so they dissolve at different times. Capsules should not be crushed or chewed. The contents can be sprinkled over food, however, without affecting the extended-release qualities. This formulation can be taken either with or without meals. The entire daily dose can be given at bedtime. The rate of absorption is faster when it is given with a high-fat meal. Another extended-release form of carbamazepine, Tegretol XR, uses a different drug-delivery system than Carbatrol. It is available in 100-, 200-, and 300-mg tablets.

Pre-existing hematologic, hepatic, and cardiac diseases can be relative contrain-dications for carbamazepine treatment. Persons with hepatic disease require only one-third to one-half the usual dosage; the clinician should be cautious about raising the dosage in such persons and should do so only slowly and gradually. The labora-tory examination should include a complete blood count with platelet count, liver function tests, serum electrolytes, and an electrocardiogram in persons older than 40 years of age or with a pre-existing cardiac disease. An electroencephalogram is not necessary before the initiation of treatment, but it may be helpful in some cases for the documentation of objective changes correlated with clinical improvement. See Table 12–3 for a brief user's guide to carbamazepine in bipolar disorder.

Routine Laboratory Monitoring.   Serum levels for antimanic efficacy have not been established. The anticonvulsant blood concentration range for carbamaz-epine is 4 to 12 μg/mL, and this range should be reached before determining that carbamazepine is not effective in the treatment of a mood disorder. A clinically

Table 12–3
Carbamazepine in Bipolar Illness: A Brief User's Guide

1. Start with low (200 mg) bedtime dose in depression or euthymia; higher doses (600–800 mg per day in divided doses) in manic inpatients.
2. All-bedtime dosing is reasonable with carbamazepine extended-release preparation.
3. Titrate slowly to the individual's response or side-effect threshold.
4. Hepatic enzyme CYP450 (3A4) induction and autoinduction occurring 2 to 3 weeks; slightly higher doses may be needed or tolerated at that time.
5. Warn regarding benign rash, which occurs in 5–10% of those taking the drug; progression to rare, severe rash is unpredictable, so the drug should be discontinued if any rash develops.
6. Benign white blood cell count decreases occur regularly (usually inconsequential).
7. Rarely, agranulocytosis and aplastic anemia may develop (several per million new exposures); warn regarding appearance of fever, sore throat, petechiae, and bleeding gums and to check with physician to obtain an immediate complete blood cell count.
8. Use adequate birth control methods, including higher dosage forms of estrogen (as carbamazepine lowers estrogen levels).
9. Avoid carbamazepine in pregnancy (spina bifida occurs in 0.5%; other severe adverse outcomes occur about 8%).
10. Some people will respond well to carbamazepine and not other mood stabilizers (lithium) or anticonvulsants (valproic acid).
11. Combination treatment often required to maintain remission and prevent loss of effect via tolerance.
12. Major drug interactions associated with increases in carbamazepine and potential toxicity from 3A4 enzyme inhibition include calcium channel blockers (isradipine and verapamil); erythromycin and related macrolide antibiotics; and valproate.

Table 12-4
Laboratory Monitoring of Carbamazepine for Adult Psychiatric Disorders

	Baseline	Weekly to Stability	Monthly for 6 Months	6-12 Months
CBC	+	+	+	+
Bilirubin	+		+	+
Alanine aminotransferase	+		+	+
Aspartate aminotransferase	+		+	+
Alkaline phosphatase	+		+	+
Carbamazepine level	+	+		+

CBC, complete blood count.

insignificant suppression of the WBC count commonly occurs during carbamazepine treatment. This benign decrease can be reversed by adding lithium, which enhances colony-stimulating factor. Potential serious hematologic effects of carbamazepine, such as pancytopenia, agranulocytosis, and aplastic anemia, occur in about one in 125,000 patients. Complete laboratory blood assessments may be performed every 2 weeks for the first 2 months of treatment and quarterly thereafter, but the FDA has revised the package insert for carbamazepine to suggest that blood monitoring be performed at the discretion of the physician. Patients should be informed that fever, sore throat, rash, petechiae, bruising, or unusual bleeding may indicate a hematologic problem and should prompt immediate notification of a physician. This approach is probably more effective than is frequent blood monitoring during long-term treatment. It has also been suggested that liver and renal function tests be conducted quarterly, although the benefit of conducting tests this frequently has been questioned. It seems reasonable, however, to assess hematologic status, along with liver and renal functions whenever a routine examination of the person is being conducted. A monitoring protocol is listed in Table 12-4.

Carbamazepine treatment should be discontinued and a consult with a hematologist should be obtained if the following laboratory values are found: total WBC count below 3,000/mm^3, erythrocytes below 4.0 × 10^6/mm^3, neutrophils below 1,500/mm^3, hematocrit less than 32%, hemoglobin less than 11 g/100 mL, platelet count below 100,000/mm^3, reticulocyte count below 0.3%, and a serum iron concentration below 150 mg/100 mL.

OXCARBAZEPINE

Although structurally related to carbamazepine, the usefulness of oxcarbazepine as a treatment for mania has not been established in controlled trials.

Pharmacokinetics

Absorption is rapid and unaffected by food. Peak concentrations occur after about 45 minutes. The elimination half-life of the parent compound is 2 hours, which remains stable over long-term treatment. The monohydroxide has a half-life of 9 hours. Most of the drug's anticonvulsant activity is presumed to result from this monohydroxy derivative.

Side Effects

The most common side effects are sedation and nausea. Less frequent side effects are cognitive impairment, ataxia, diplopia, nystagmus, dizziness, and tremor. In contrast to carbamazepine, oxcarbazepine does not have an increased risk of serious blood dyscrasias, so hematologic monitoring is not necessary. The frequency of benign rash is lower than observed with carbamazepine, and serious rashes are extremely rare. However, about 25% to 30% of patients who develop an allergic rash while taking carbamazepine also develop a rash with oxcarbazepine. Oxcarbazepine is more likely to cause hyponatremia than carbamazepine. Approximately 3% to 5% of patients taking oxcarbazepine develop this side effect. It is advisable to obtain serum sodium concentrations early in the course of treatment because hyponatremia may be clinically silent. In severe cases, confusion and seizure may occur.

Use in Pregnancy and Lactation

There is very little information about the reproductive safety of oxcarbazepine. The drug passes into breast milk.

Dosing and Administration

Oxcarbazepine dosing for bipolar disorder has not been established. It is available in 150-, 300-, and 600-mg tablets. The dose range may vary from 150 to 2,400 mg per day given in divided doses twice a day. In clinical trials for mania, the doses typically used were from 900 to 1,200 mg per day with a starting dose of 150 or 300 mg at night. Oxcarbazepine is also available in an extended release form (Oxteller ER), taken once a day on an empty stomach. It is available as 150-, 300-, and 600-mg tablets.

Drug Interactions

Drugs such as phenobarbital and alcohol, which induce CYP34A, increase the clearance and reduce oxcarbazepine concentrations. Oxcarbazepine induces CYP3A4/5 and inhibits CYP2C19, which may affect the metabolism of drugs that use that pathway. Women taking oral contraceptives should be told to consult with their gynecologists because oxcarbazepine may reduce concentrations of their contraceptive and thus decrease its efficacy.

13
Cholinesterase Inhibitors and Memantine

INTRODUCTION

The cholinesterase inhibitors, donepezil (Aricept), rivastigmine (Exelon), galantamine (Reminyl), and memantine (Namenda) are the only medications approved by the FDA for the treatment of Alzheimer's disease (AD) and other dementias (Table 13–1). Originally, cholinesterase inhibitors were indicated only for mild to moderately ill patients with AD. Recently, their indication has expanded to include patients with moderate to severe AD and patients with dementia associated with Parkinson's disease (PD). Cholinesterase inhibitors reduce the inactivation of the neurotransmitter acetylcholine and, thus, potentiate cholinergic neurotransmission, which in turn produces a modest improvement in memory and goal-directed thought. Memantine, an N-methyl-D-aspartate (NMDA) receptor antagonist, has been approved for moderate to severe AD. It is routinely used with a cholinesterase inhibitor in clinical practice and recent studies have shown that this combination may provide beneficial response compared with only cholinesterase inhibitor pharmacotherapy. This combination of memantine and donepezil is available as a fixed combination with (Namzaric).

Tacrine (Cognex), the first cholinesterase inhibitor to be introduced, is no longer available because of its multiple daily dosing regimens, its potential for hepatotoxicity, and the consequent need for frequent laboratory monitoring.

PHARMACOLOGIC ACTIONS

Donepezil is absorbed completely from the gastrointestinal (GI) tract. Peak plasma concentrations are reached about 3 to 4 hours after oral dosing. The half-life of donepezil is 70 hours in elderly persons, and it is taken only once daily. Steady-state levels are achieved within about 2 weeks. The presence of stable alcoholic cirrhosis reduces clearance of donepezil by 20%. Rivastigmine (Exelon) is rapidly and completely absorbed from the GI tract and reaches peak plasma concentrations in 1 hour, but this is delayed by up to 90 minutes if rivastigmine is taken with food. The half-life of rivastigmine is 1 hour, but because it remains bound to cholinesterases, a single dose is therapeutically active for 10 hours, and it is taken twice daily. Galantamine (Reminyl) is an alkaloid similar to codeine and extracted from daffodils of the plant *Galanthus nivalis*. It is readily absorbed, with maximum concentrations reached after 30 minutes to 2 hours. Food decreases the maximum concentration by 25%. The elimination half-life of galantamine is approximately 6 hours.

The primary mechanism of action of cholinesterase inhibitors is reversible, nonacylating inhibition of acetylcholinesterase and butyrylcholinesterase; the enzymes that catabolize acetylcholine in the central nervous system (CNS). The enzyme

Table 13-1

Medications Used in Neurocognitive Disorders

Drug (Brand)	Formulation	Indications	Starting Dose	Titration	Dosage Range
Tacrine (Cognex)	10-, 20-, 30-, 40-mg capsules	Mild to moderate AD dementia	10 mg 4 times a day	Increase by 10 mg 4 times a day (40 mg total daily) every 4 weeks	40-160 mg daily with 4 times a day dosing
Donepezil (Aricept)	5-, 10-, 23-mg tablets 5-, 10-mg disintegrated tablets	Mild to moderate and severe AD dementia	5 mg daily	Increase to 10 mg after 4 weeks. Increase to 23 mg daily after 3 months	10-23 mg daily
Rivastigmine (Exelon, Exelon Patch)	1.5-, 3-, 4.5-, 6-mg oral solution 4.6-, 9.5-, 13.3-mg transdermal patch	Mild to moderate AD dementia Major neurocognitive disorder due to Parkinson's disease	4 mg twice a day 8 mg daily extended release	By 1.5 mg twice a day every 4 weeks. Increase to 9.5 mg in 4 weeks and then to 13.3 mg after 4 weeks for transdermal patch	3-6 mg daily for oral preparation. 4.6-13.3 mg daily for transdermal patch
Galantamine (Razadyne, Razadyne ER)	4-, 8-, 12-mg tablets 8-, 16-, 24-mg extended-release capsules 4-mg/mL oral solution	Mild to moderate AD dementia	1.5 mg twice a day 4.6-mg transdermal patch	Increase by 4 mg twice a day every 4 weeks. Increase by 8 mg every 4 weeks for extended release	4-12 mg in divided doses for oral preparation. 8-24 mg daily for extended release
Memantine (Namenda, Namenda XR)	5-, 10-mg tablets 7-, 14-, 21-, 28-mg extended-release capsules 10-mg/5-mL oral solution	Moderate to severe AD dementia	5 mg daily 7-mg extended-release formula	By 5 mg daily in weekly intervals. Increase by 7 mg daily extended-release formula	10-20 mg daily in divided dose for oral preparation. 7-28 mg daily for extended release
Memantine XR and donepezil combination (Namzaric)	14-mg memantine ER/10-mg donepezil capsules 28-mg memantine ER/10-mg donepezil capsules	Moderate to severe Alzheimer's disease when patient already stabilized on memantine ER and donepezil	14-mg memantine ER/10-mg donepezil daily 28-mg memantine ER/10-mg donepezil daily in severe renal impairment		

Borrowed from Sadock BJ, Sadock VA, Kaplan HI, eds. *Kaplan & Sadock's Comprehensive Textbook of Psychiatry*. 10th ed. Philadelphia, PA: Lippincott Williams & Wilkins; 2017.

inhibition increases synaptic concentrations of acetylcholine, especially in the hippocampus and cerebral cortex. Donepezil's favorable side-effect profile appears to correlate with its lack of inhibition of cholinesterases in the GI tract. Rivastigmine appears to have somewhat more peripheral activity than donepezil and is thus more likely to cause GI adverse effects than is donepezil.

THERAPEUTIC INDICATIONS

Cholinesterase inhibitors are effective for the treatment of mild to moderate cognitive impairment in dementia of the Alzheimer's type. In long-term use, they slow the progression of memory loss and diminish apathy, depression, hallucinations, anxiety, euphoria, and purposeless motor behaviors. Functional autonomy is less well preserved. Some persons note immediate improvement in memory, mood, psychotic symptoms, and interpersonal skills. Others note little initial benefit but are able to retain their cognitive and adaptive faculties at a relatively stable level for many months. A practical benefit of cholinesterase inhibitor use is a delay or reduction of the need for nursing home placement.

Donepezil and rivastigmine may be beneficial for patients with Parkinson's disease and Lewy body disease and for treatment of cognitive deficits caused by traumatic brain injury. Donepezil is under study for treatment of mild cognitive impairment that is less severe than that caused by AD. People with vascular dementia may respond to acetylcholinesterase inhibitors. Occasionally, cholinesterase inhibitors elicit an idiosyncratic catastrophic reaction, with signs of grief and agitation, which is self-limited after the drug is discontinued. Use of cholinesterase inhibitors to improve cognition by nondemented individuals should be discouraged.

PRECAUTIONS AND ADVERSE REACTIONS
Donepezil

Donepezil is generally well tolerated at recommended dosages. Fewer than 3% of persons taking donepezil experience nausea, diarrhea, and vomiting. These mild symptoms are more common with a 10-mg dose than with a 5-mg dose, and when present, they tend to resolve after 3 weeks of continued use. Donepezil may cause weight loss. Donepezil treatment has been infrequently associated with bradyarrhythmias, especially in persons with underlying cardiac disease. A small number of persons experience syncope.

Rivastigmine

Rivastigmine is generally well tolerated, but recommended dosages may need to be scaled back in the initial period of treatment to limit GI and CNS adverse effects. These mild symptoms are more common at dosages above 6 mg a day, and when present, they tend to resolve after the dosage is lowered. The most common adverse effects associated with rivastigmine are nausea, vomiting, dizziness, headache, diarrhea, abdominal pain, anorexia, fatigue, and somnolence. Rivastigmine may cause weight loss, but it does not appear to cause hepatic, renal, hematologic, or electrolyte abnormalities.

Galantamine

The most common side effects of galantamine are dizziness, headache, nausea, vomiting, diarrhea, and anorexia. These side effects tend to be mild and transient.

Table 13–2
Incidence (%) of Major Adverse Side Effects with Cholinesterase Inhibitors

Drug	Dose (mg/day)	Nausea	Vomiting	Diarrhea	Dizziness	Muscle Cramps	Insomnia
Donepezil	5	4	3	9	15	9	7
Donepezil	10	17	10	17	13	12	8
Rivastigmine	1–4	14	7	10	15	NR	NR
Rivastigmine	6–12	48	27	17	24	NR	NR
Galantamine	8	5.7	3.6	5	NR	NR	NR
Galantamine	16	13.3	6.1	12.2	NR	NR	NR
Galantamine	24	16.5	9.9	5.5	NR	NR	NR

NR, not reported from clinical trial data; incidence less than 5%.

Since the users of these drugs are not women of child-bearing age, their off-label use in that population should be avoided. Data about use in this population are not available.

Table 13–2 summarizes the incidence of major adverse side effects associated with each of the cholinesterase inhibitors.

Drug Interactions

All cholinesterase inhibitors should be used cautiously with drugs that also possess cholinomimetic activity, such as succinylcholine (Anectine) and bethanechol (Urecholine). The coadministration of cholinesterase inhibitors and drugs that have cholinergic antagonist activity (e.g., tricyclic drugs) is probably counterproductive. Paroxetine (Paxil) has the most marked anticholinergic effects of any of the newer antidepressant and anxiolytic drugs and should be avoided for that reason, as well as its inhibiting effect on the metabolism of some of the cholinesterase inhibitors.

Donepezil undergoes extensive metabolism via both CYP2D6 and 3A4 isozymes. The metabolism of donepezil may be increased by phenytoin (Dilantin), carbamazepine (Tegretol), dexamethasone (Decadron), rifampin (Rifadin), and phenobarbital (Solfoton). Commonly used agents such as paroxetine, ketoconazole (Nizoral), and erythromycin can significantly increase donepezil concentrations. Donepezil is highly protein bound, but it does not displace other protein-bound drugs, such as furosemide (Lasix), digoxin (Lanoxin), or warfarin (Coumadin). Rivastigmine circulates mostly unbound to serum proteins and has no significant drug interactions.

Similar to donepezil, galantamine is metabolized by both CYP2D6 and 3A4 isozymes and thus may interact with drugs that inhibit these pathways. Paroxetine and ketoconazole should be used with great caution.

LABORATORY INTERFERENCES

No laboratory interferences have been associated with the use of cholinesterase inhibitors.

DOSAGE AND CLINICAL GUIDELINES

Before initiation of cholinesterase inhibitor therapy, potentially treatable causes of dementia should be ruled out and the diagnosis of dementia of the Alzheimer's type established.

Donepezil is available in 5- and 10-mg tablets. Treatment should be initiated at 5 mg each night. If well tolerated and of some discernible benefit after 4 weeks, the dosage should be increased to a maintenance dosage of 10-mg each night. Donepezil absorption is unaffected by meals.

Rivastigmine is available in 1.5-, 3-, 4.5-, and 6-mg capsules. The recommended initial dosage is 1.5 mg twice daily for a minimum of 2 weeks, after which increases of 1.5 mg a day can be made at intervals of at least 2 weeks to a target dosage of 6 mg a day, taken in two equal dosages. If tolerated, the dosage may be further titrated upward to a maximum of 6 mg twice daily. The risk of adverse GI events can be reduced by administration of rivastigmine with food.

Galantamine is available in 4-, 8-, and 16-mg tablets. The suggested dose range is 16 to 32 mg per day given twice a day. The higher dose is actually better tolerated than the lower dose. The initial dosage is 8 mg per day, and after a minimum of 4 weeks, the dose can be raised. All subsequent dosage increases should occur at 4-week intervals and should be based on tolerability.

MEMANTINE

Pharmacologic Actions

Memantine is well absorbed after oral administration with peak concentrations reached in about 3 to 7 hours. Food has no effect on the absorption of memantine. Memantine has linear pharmacokinetics over the therapeutic dose range and has a terminal elimination half-life of about 60 to 80 hours. Plasma protein binding is 45%.

Memantine undergoes little metabolism, with the majority (57% to 82%) of an administered dose excreted unchanged in urine; the remainder is converted primarily to three polar metabolites, the N-gludantan conjugate, 6-hydroxy memantine, and 1-nitroso-deaminated memantine. These metabolites possess minimal NMDA receptor antagonist activity. Memantine is a low- to moderate-affinity NMDA receptor antagonist. It is thought that overexcitation of NMDA receptors by the neurotransmitter glutamate may play a role in AD because glutamate plays an integral role in the neural pathways associated with learning and memory. Excess glutamate overstimulates NMDA receptors to allow too much calcium into nerve cells, leading to the eventual cell death observed in AD. Memantine may protect cells against excess glutamate by partially blocking NMDA receptors associated with abnormal transmission of glutamate while allowing for physiologic transmission associated with normal cell functioning.

Therapeutic Indications

Memantine is the only approved therapy in the United States for moderate to severe AD.

Precautions and Adverse Reactions

Memantine is safe and well tolerated. The most common adverse effects are dizziness, headache, constipation, and confusion. The use of memantine in patients with severe renal impairment is not recommended. In a documented case of an overdose with up to 400 mg of memantine, the patient experienced restlessness, psychosis, visual hallucinations, somnolence, stupor, and loss of consciousness. The patient recovered without permanent sequelae.

Drug Interactions

In vitro studies conducted with marker substrates of CYP450 enzymes (CYP1A2, 2A6, 2C9, 2D6, 2E1, and 3A4) showed minimal inhibition of these enzymes by memantine. No pharmacokinetic interactions with drugs metabolized by these enzymes are expected.

Because memantine is eliminated in part by tubular secretion, coadministration of drugs that use the same renal cationic system, including hydrochlorothiazide triamterene (Dyrenium), cimetidine (Tagamet), ranitidine (Zantac), quinidine, and nicotine, could potentially result in altered plasma levels of both agents. Coadministration of memantine and a combination of hydrochlorothiazide and triamterene did not affect the bioavailability of either memantine or triamterene, and the bioavailability of hydrochlorothiazide decreased by 20%.

Urine pH is altered by diet, drugs (e.g., carbonic anhydrase inhibitors, topiramate [Topamax], sodium bicarbonate), and the clinical state of the patient (e.g., renal tubular acidosis or severe infections of the urinary tract). The clearance of memantine is reduced by about 80% under alkaline urine conditions at pH 8. Therefore, alterations of urine pH toward the alkaline condition may lead to an accumulation of the drug with a possible increase in adverse effects. Hence, memantine should be used with caution under these conditions.

Laboratory Interferences

No laboratory interferences have been associated with the use of memantine.

Dosage and Clinical Guidelines

Memantine is available in 5- and 10-mg tablets, with a recommended starting dose of 5 mg daily. The recommended target dose is 20 mg per day. The drug is administered twice daily in separate doses with 5-mg increment increases weekly depending on tolerability. It is also available as 5- and 10-mg extended-release tablets and as 7-, 14-, 21- and 28-mg extended-release capsules.

The combination of donepezil and extended-release memantine is available of in fixed doses of 8-mg donepezil/10-mg memantine and 28-mg donepezil/10-mg memantine.

14

Disulfiram and Acamprosate

INTRODUCTION

The drugs disulfiram (Antabuse) and acamprosate (Campral) are used to treat alcohol dependence. Disulfiram has suffered from a reputation as a dangerous medication only suitable for highly motivated and strictly supervised drinkers because of the severe physical reactions the drug causes after drinking. In fact, disulfiram's main therapeutic effect is its ability to produce unpleasant or dangerous symptoms after alcohol intake (also known as disulfiram–alcohol reaction). In the most severe cases, when disulfiram is combined with alcohol, patients may experience respiratory depression, cardiovascular collapse, acute heart failure, convulsions, loss of consciousness. Death may occur in rare cases. Experience has shown, however, that at recommended doses it is an acceptable and safe medication for dependent drinkers seeking to sustain abstinence.

These potential complications as well as the development of alternative antialcohol medications have limited wider use of disulfiram. Unlike disulfiram, acamprosate, the other drug discussed in this section, does not produce aversive side effects. Acamprosate is now prescribed more commonly than disulfiram in outpatient settings, but disulfiram is prescribed more often in inpatient settings because it helps facilitate initial abstinence.

Other drugs that are useful in reducing alcohol consumption include naltrexone (ReVia, Trexan), nalmefene (Revex), topiramate (Topamax), and gabapentin (Neurontin). These agents are discussed in their respective chapters.

DISULFIRAM

Pharmacologic Actions

Disulfiram is almost completely absorbed from the gastrointestinal (GI) tract after oral administration. Its half-life is estimated to be 60 to 120 hours. Therefore, 1 or 2 weeks may be needed before disulfiram is totally eliminated from the body after the last dose has been taken.

The metabolism of ethanol proceeds through oxidation via alcohol dehydrogenase to the formation of acetaldehyde, which is further metabolized to acetylcoenzyme A (acetyl-CoA) by aldehyde dehydrogenase. Disulfiram is an aldehyde dehydrogenase inhibitor that interferes with the metabolism of alcohol by producing a marked increase in blood acetaldehyde concentration. The accumulation of acetaldehyde (to a level up to 10 times higher than occurs in the normal metabolism of alcohol) produces a wide array of unpleasant reactions, called the *disulfiram–alcohol reaction,* characterized by nausea, throbbing headache, vomiting, hypertension, flushing, sweating, thirst, dyspnea, tachycardia, chest pain, vertigo, and blurred vision. The reaction occurs almost immediately after the ingestion of one alcoholic drink and may last from 30 minutes to 2 hours.

Blood Concentrations in Relation to Action. Plasma concentrations of disulfiram may vary among individuals because of a number of factors, most notably age and hepatic function. In general, the severity of disulfiram–alcohol reaction has been shown to be proportional to the amount of the ingested disulfiram and alcohol. Nevertheless, disulfiram plasma levels are rarely obtained in clinical practice. The positive correlation between plasma concentrations of alcohol and the intensity of the reaction is described as follows: in sensitive individuals, as little as 5 to 10 mg per 100 mL increase of the plasma alcohol level may produce mild symptoms; fully developed symptoms occur at alcohol levels of 50 mg per 100 mL; and levels as high as 125 to 150 mg per 100 mL result in loss of consciousness and coma.

Therapeutic Indications

The primary indication for disulfiram use is as an aversive conditioning treatment for alcohol dependence. Either the fear of having a disulfiram–alcohol reaction or the memory of having had one is meant to condition the person not to use alcohol. Usually, describing the severity and the unpleasantness of the disulfiram–alcohol reaction graphically enough discourages the person from imbibing alcohol. Disulfiram treatment should be combined with such treatments as psychotherapy, group therapy, and support groups such as Alcoholics Anonymous (AA). Treatment with disulfiram requires careful monitoring because a person can simply decide not to take the medication.

Precautions and Adverse Reactions

With Alcohol Consumption. The intensity of the disulfiram–alcohol reaction varies with each person. In extreme cases, it is marked by respiratory depression, cardiovascular collapse, myocardial infarction, convulsions, and death. Therefore, disulfiram is contraindicated for persons with significant pulmonary or cardiovascular disease. In addition, disulfiram should be used with caution, if at all, by persons with nephritis, brain damage, hypothyroidism, diabetes, hepatic disease, seizures, polydrug dependence, or an abnormal electroencephalogram. Most fatal reactions occur in persons who take more than 500 mg a day of disulfiram and who consume more than 3 oz of alcohol. The treatment of a severe disulfiram–alcohol reaction is primarily supportive to prevent shock. The use of oxygen, intravenous vitamin C, ephedrine, and antihistamines has been reported to aid in recovery.

Without Alcohol Consumption. The adverse effects of disulfiram in the absence of alcohol consumption include fatigue, dermatitis, impotence, optic neuritis, a variety of mental changes, and hepatic damage. A metabolite of disulfiram inhibits dopamine-β-hydroxylase, the enzyme that metabolizes dopamine into norepinephrine and epinephrine, and thus may exacerbate psychosis in persons with psychotic disorders. Catatonic reactions may also occur.

Use in Pregnancy and Lactation

There are no well-controlled studies of disulfiram effects on the fetus or newborn, or whether it crosses into breast milk.

Drug Interactions

Disulfiram increases the blood concentration of diazepam (Valium), paraldehyde, phenytoin (Dilantin), caffeine, tetrahydrocannabinol (the active ingredient in marijuana), barbiturates, anticoagulants, isoniazid (Nydrazid), and tricyclic drugs. Disulfiram should not be administered concomitantly with paraldehyde because paraldehyde is metabolized to acetaldehyde in the liver.

Laboratory Interferences

In rare instances, disulfiram has been reported to interfere with the incorporation of iodine-131 into protein-bound iodine. Disulfiram may reduce urinary concentrations of homovanillic acid, the major metabolite of dopamine, because of its inhibition of dopamine hydroxylase.

Dosage and Clinical Guidelines

Disulfiram is supplied in 250- and 500-mg tablets. The usual initial dosage is 500 mg a day taken by mouth for the first 1 or 2 weeks followed by a maintenance dosage of 250 mg a day. The dosage should not exceed 500 mg a day. The maintenance dosage range is 125 to 500 mg a day.

Persons taking disulfiram must be instructed that the ingestion of even the smallest amount of alcohol will bring on a disulfiram–alcohol reaction, with all of its unpleasant effects. In addition, persons should be warned against ingesting any alcohol-containing preparations, such as cough drops, tonics of any kind, and alcohol-containing foods and sauces. Some reactions have occurred in patients who used alcohol-based lotions, toilet water, colognes, or perfumes and inhaled the fumes; therefore, precautions must be explicit and should include any topically applied preparations containing alcohol, such as perfume.

Disulfiram should not be administered until the person has abstained from alcohol for at least 12 hours. Persons should be warned that the disulfiram–alcohol reaction may occur as long as 1 or 2 weeks after the last dose of disulfiram. Persons taking disulfiram should carry identification cards describing the disulfiram–alcohol reaction and listing the name and telephone number of the physician to be called.

ACAMPROSATE

Pharmacologic Actions

Acamprosate's mechanism of action is not fully understood, but it is thought to antagonize neuronal overactivity related to the actions of the excitatory neurotransmitter glutamate. In part, this may result from antagonism of N-methyl-D-aspartate (NMDA) receptors.

Indications

Acamprosate is used for treating alcohol-dependent individuals seeking to continue to remain alcohol free after they have stopped drinking. Its efficacy in promoting abstinence has not been demonstrated in persons who have not undergone detoxification and who have not achieved alcohol abstinence before beginning treatment.

Precautions and Adverse Effects

Side effects are mostly seen early in treatment and are usually mild and transient in nature. The most common side effects are headache, diarrhea, flatulence, abdominal pain, paresthesias, and various skin reactions. No adverse events occur after abrupt withdrawal of acamprosate, even after long-term use. There is no evidence of addiction to the drug. Patients with severe renal impairment (creatinine clearance of less than 30 mL/min) should not be given acamprosate.

Drug Interactions

The concomitant intake of alcohol and acamprosate does not affect the pharmacokinetics of either alcohol or acamprosate. Administration of disulfiram or diazepam does not affect the pharmacokinetics of acamprosate. Coadministration of naltrexone with acamprosate produces an increase in concentrations of acamprosate. No adjustment of dosage is recommended in such patients. The pharmacokinetics of naltrexone and its major metabolite 6-β-naltrexol were unaffected after coadministration with acamprosate. During clinical trials, patients taking acamprosate concomitantly with antidepressants more commonly reported both weight gain and weight loss compared with patients taking either medication alone.

Use in Pregnancy and Lactation

There are no well-controlled studies of acamprosate effects on the fetus or newborn.

Laboratory Interferences

Acamprosate has not been shown to interfere with commonly done laboratory tests.

Dosage and Clinical Guidelines

It is important to remember that acamprosate should not be used to treat alcohol withdrawal symptoms. It should only be started after the individual has been successfully weaned off alcohol. Patients should show a commitment to remaining abstinent, and treatment should be part of a comprehensive management program that includes counseling or support group attendance.

Each tablet contains acamprosate calcium 333 mg, which is equivalent to 300 mg of acamprosate. The dose of acamprosate is different for different patients. The recommended dosage is two 333-mg tablets (each dose should total 666 mg) taken three times daily. Although dosing may be done without regard to meals, dosing with meals was used during clinical trials and is suggested as an aid to compliance in patients who regularly eat three meals daily. A lower dose may be effective in some patients. A missed dose should be taken as soon as possible. However, if it is almost time for the next dose, the missed dose should be skipped, and then the regular dosing schedule should be resumed. Doses should not be doubled up. For patients with moderate renal impairment (creatinine clearance of 30 to 50 mL/min), a starting dosage of one 333-mg tablet taken three times daily is recommended. People with severe renal insufficiency should not take acamprosate.

15

Dopamine Receptor Agonists and Precursors

INTRODUCTION

Dopamine receptor agonists (DAs) bind to and activate dopamine receptors to reproduce the activity of the endogenous neurotransmitter. These drugs were initially developed during the 1970s to treat advanced Parkinson's disease (PD). They are typically classified into nonergot and ergot derivatives. Nonergot DAs include apomorphine (Apokyn), pramipexole (Mirapex), and ropinirole (Requip). Pramipexole and ropinirole are FDA approved for use in PD and restless legs syndrome (RLS), and have been studied as an adjunctive treatment for unipolar and bipolar depression. Amantadine (Symmetrel), an adamantane derivative, is FDA approved to treat PD, drug-induced extrapyramidal symptoms (EPS), and influenza A infection. It is also used off-label to treat neuroleptic malignant syndrome (NMS) and Cotard's syndrome, a psychiatric condition that involves a delusional belief that one is dead. The ergot class includes bromocriptine (Parlodel), cabergoline (Dostinex, Caberlin), and pergolide (Permax). Bromocriptine is FDA approved for use in PD, galactorrhea (due to hyperprolactin conditions), and acromegaly, and is used off-label to treat RLS and NMS. Cabergoline is FDA approved for the treatment of hyperprolactinemic disorders, either idiopathic or due to pituitary adenomas.

Other classes of drugs may also exert agonist effects at the dopamine receptor. The wakefulness-promoting agents, modafinil (Provigil) and armodafinil (Nuvigil), have complex prodopaminergic activity, including dopamine transporter inhibition and may also have dopamine (D2) receptor partial agonist effects. These drugs have been FDA approved to improve wakefulness in adult patients with excessive sleepiness associated with narcolepsy, obstructive sleep apnea (OSA), or shift work disorder (SWD). They have been studied as an adjunctive treatment for unipolar and bipolar depression, and attention-deficit/hyperactivity disorder (ADHD). Modafinil and armodafinil are discussed in Chapter 29.

Dopamine agonists activate dopamine receptors in the absence of endogenous dopamine and have been widely used to treat idiopathic PD, hyperprolactinemia, and certain pituitary tumors (prolactinoma) and RLS. Because dopamine stimulates the heart and increases blood flow to the liver, kidneys, and other organs, low levels of dopamine are associated with low blood pressure and low cardiac input. Dopamine agonist drugs are also administered to treat shock and congestive heart failure.

PHARMACOLOGIC ACTIONS

L-Dopa is rapidly absorbed after oral administration, and peak plasma levels are reached after 30 to 120 minutes. The half-life of L-Dopa is 90 minutes. Absorption of L-Dopa can be significantly reduced by changes in gastric pH and by ingestion with meals. Bromocriptine and ropinirole are rapidly absorbed but undergo first-pass metabolism such that only about 30% to 55% of the dose is bioavailable. Peak concentrations are achieved 1.5 to 3 hours after oral administration. The half-life of ropinirole is 6 hours. Pramipexole is rapidly absorbed with little first-pass metabolism and reaches peak concentrations in 2 hours. Its half-life is 8 hours. Oral forms of apomorphine have been studied but are not available in the United States. Subcutaneous apomorphine injection results in rapid and controlled systemic delivery, with linear pharmacokinetics over a dose ranging from 2 to 8 mg.

After L-Dopa enters the dopaminergic neurons of the central nervous system (CNS), it is converted into the neurotransmitter dopamine. Apomorphine, bromocriptine, ropinirole, and pramipexole act directly on dopamine receptors. L-Dopa, pramipexole, and ropinirole bind about 20 times more selectively to dopamine D_3 than D_2 receptors; the corresponding ratio for bromocriptine is less than 2:1. Apomorphine binds selectively to D_1 and D_2 receptors, with little affinity for D_3 and D_4 receptors. L-Dopa, pramipexole, and ropinirole have no significant activity at nondopaminergic receptors, but bromocriptine binds to serotonin 5-HT$_1$ and 5-HT$_2$ and α_1-, α_2-, and β-adrenergic receptors.

THERAPEUTIC INDICATIONS
Medication-Induced Movement Disorders
In present-day clinical psychiatry, DAs are used for the treatment of medication-induced parkinsonism, EPS, akinesia, and focal perioral tremors. Their use has diminished sharply, however, because the incidence of medication-induced movement disorders is much lower with the use of the newer, atypical antipsychotics (serotonin–dopamine antagonists). DAs are effective in treating idiopathic RLS and may also be helpful when this is a medication side effect. Ropinirole has an indication for RLS.

For the treatment of medication-induced movement disorders, most clinicians rely on anticholinergics, amantadine, and antihistamines because they are equally effective and have few adverse effects. Bromocriptine remains in use in the treatment of NMS; however, the incidence of this disorder is diminishing with the decreasing use of dopamine receptor antagonists (DRAs).

DAs are also used to counteract the hyperprolactinemic effects of DRAs, which result in the side effects of amenorrhea and galactorrhea.

Mood Disorders
Bromocriptine has long been used to enhance response to antidepressant drugs in refractory patients. Ropinirole has been reported to be useful as augmentation to antidepressant therapy and as a treatment for medication-resistant bipolar II depression. Ropinirole may also be helpful in the treatment of antidepressant-induced sexual dysfunction. Pramipexole is often used in the augmentation of antidepressants in treatment-resistant depression. Some studies have found pramipexole to be superior to sertraline (Zoloft) in the treatment of depression in PD, as well as reducing anhedonia in Parkinson's patients.

Sexual Dysfunction
DAs improve erectile dysfunction in some patients. However, they are rarely used because they frequently cause adverse effects at therapeutic dosages. Phosphodiesterase-5 inhibitor agents are better tolerated and more effective (see Chapter 25).

PRECAUTIONS AND ADVERSE REACTIONS

Adverse effects are common with DAs, thus limiting the usefulness of these drugs. Adverse effects are dosage dependent and include nausea, vomiting, orthostatic hypotension, headache, dizziness, and cardiac arrhythmias. To reduce the risk of orthostatic hypotension, the initial dosage of all DAs should be quite low, with incremental increases at intervals of at least 1 week. These drugs should be used with caution in persons with hypertension, cardiovascular disease, and hepatic disease. After long-term use, persons, particularly elderly persons, may experience choreiform and dystonic movements and psychiatric disturbances—including hallucinations, delusions, confusion, depression, and mania—and other behavioral changes.

Long-term use of bromocriptine can produce retroperitoneal and pulmonary fibrosis, pleural effusions, and pleural thickening.

In general, ropinirole and pramipexole have a similar but milder adverse-effect profile than L-Dopa and bromocriptine. Pramipexole and ropinirole may cause irresistible sleep attacks that occur suddenly without warning and have caused motor vehicle accidents.

The most common adverse effects of apomorphine are yawning, dizziness, nausea, vomiting, drowsiness, bradycardia, syncope, and perspiration. Hallucinations have also been reported. Apomorphine's sedative effects are exacerbated with concurrent use of alcohol or other CNS depressants.

USE IN PREGNANCY AND LACTATION

DAs are contraindicated during pregnancy, especially for nursing mothers because they inhibit lactation.

DRUG INTERACTIONS

DRAs are capable of reversing the effects of DAs, but this is not usually clinically significant. The concurrent use of tricyclic drugs and DAs has been reported to cause symptoms of neurotoxicity, such as rigidity, agitation, and tremor. They may also potentiate the hypotensive effects of diuretics and other antihypertensive medications. DAs should not be used in conjunction with monoamine oxidase inhibitors (MAOIs), including selegiline (Eldepryl), and MAOIs should be discontinued at least 2 weeks before the initiation of dopamine receptor agonist therapy.

Benzodiazepines, phenytoin (Dilantin), and pyridoxine may interfere with the therapeutic effects of DAs. Ergot alkaloids and bromocriptine should not be used concurrently because they may cause hypertension and myocardial infarction. Progestins, estrogens, and oral contraceptives may interfere with the effects of bromocriptine and may raise plasma concentrations of ropinirole. Ciprofloxacin (Cipro) can raise plasma concentrations of ropinirole, and cimetidine (Tagamet) can raise plasma concentrations of pramipexole.

LABORATORY INTERFERENCES

L-Dopa administration has been associated with false reports of elevated serum and urinary uric acid concentrations, urinary glucose test results, urinary ketone test results, and urinary catecholamine concentrations. No laboratory interferences have been associated with the administration of the other DAs.

Table 15-1
Available Preparations of Dopamine Receptor Agonists and Carbidopa

Generic Name	Trade Name	Preparations
Amantadine	Symmetrel	100-mg capsule, 50-mg/5-mL syrup (teaspoon)
Bromocriptine	Parlodel	2.5-, 5-mg tablets
Carbidopa	Lodosyn	25 mg^a
Levodopa (L-Dopa)	Larodopa	100-, 250-, 500-mg tablets
Levodopa-carbidopa (Co-careldopa)	Sinemet, Atamet	100/10-mg, 100/25-mg, 250/25-mg tablets; 100/25-, 200/50-mg extended-release tablets
Pramipexole	Mirapex	0.125-, 0.375-, 0.75-, 1.5-, 3-, 4-mg extended-release tablets
Ropinirole	Requip	0.25-, 0.5-, 1-, 2-, 5-mg tablets

^aDrug only available directly through the manufacturer.

DOSAGE AND CLINICAL GUIDELINES

Table 15-1 lists the various DAs and their formulations. For the treatment of antipsychotic-induced parkinsonism, the clinician should start with a 100-mg dose of levodopa three times a day, which may be increased until the person is functionally improved. The maximum dosage of L-Dopa is 2,000 mg a day, but most persons respond to dosages below 1,000 mg per day. The dosage of the carbidopa component of the L-Dopa-carbidopa formulation should total at least 75 mg a day.

The dosage of bromocriptine for mental disorders is uncertain, although it seems prudent to begin with low dosages (1.25 mg twice daily) and to increase the dosage gradually. Bromocriptine is usually taken with meals to help reduce the likelihood of nausea.

The starting dosage of pramipexole is 0.125 mg three times daily, which is increased to 0.25 mg three times daily in the second week and is increased by 0.25 mg per dose each week until therapeutic benefit or adverse effects emerge. Persons with idiopathic PD usually experience benefits at total daily doses of 1.5 mg, and the maximum daily dose is 4.5 mg.

For ropinirole, the starting dosage is 0.25 mg three times daily and is increased by 0.25 mg per dose each week to a total daily dose of 3 mg, then by 0.5 mg per dose each week to a total daily dose of 9 mg, and then by 1 mg per dose each week to a maximum dosage of 24 mg a day until therapeutic benefit or adverse effects emerge. The average daily dose for persons with idiopathic PD is about 16 mg.

The recommended subcutaneous dose of apomorphine in PD is 0.2 to 0.6 mL subcutaneously during acute hypomobility episodes delivered via metered injector pen. Apomorphine can be administered three times daily, with a maximum dose of 0.6 mL five times daily.

AMANTADINE

Amantadine (Symmetrel) is an antiviral drug used for the prophylaxis and treatment of influenza. It was found to have antiparkinsonian properties and is now used to treat the disorder as well as akinesias and other extrapyramidal signs, including focal perioral tremors (rabbit syndrome).

Pharmacologic Actions

Amantadine is well absorbed from the GI tract after oral administration, reaches peak plasma concentrations in approximately 2 to 3 hours, has a half-life of about 12 to 18 hours, and attains steady-state concentrations after approximately 4 to 5 days of therapy. Amantadine is excreted unmetabolized in the urine. Amantadine plasma concentrations can be twice as high in elderly persons as in younger adults. Patients with renal failure accumulate amantadine in their bodies.

Amantadine augments dopaminergic neurotransmission in the CNS; however, the precise mechanism for the effect is unknown. The mechanism may involve dopamine release from presynaptic vesicles, blocking reuptake of dopamine into presynaptic nerve terminals, or an agonist effect on postsynaptic dopamine receptors.

Therapeutic Indications

The primary indication for amantadine use in psychiatry is to treat extrapyramidal signs and symptoms, such as parkinsonism, akinesia, and the so-called rabbit syndrome (focal perioral tremor of the choreoathetoid type) caused by the administration of DRA or SDA drugs. Amantadine is as effective as the anticholinergics (e.g., benztropine [Cogentin]) for these indications and results in improvement in approximately half of all persons who take it. Amantadine, however, is not generally considered as effective as the anticholinergics for the treatment of acute dystonic reactions and is not effective in treating tardive dyskinesia and akathisia.

Amantadine is a reasonable compromise for persons with EPS who would be sensitive to additional anticholinergic effects, particularly those taking a low-potency DRA or the elderly. Elderly persons are susceptible to anticholinergic adverse effects, both in the CNS, such as anticholinergic delirium, and in the peripheral nervous system, such as urinary retention. Amantadine is associated with less memory impairment than are the anticholinergics.

Amantadine has been reported to be of benefit in treating some selective serotonin reuptake inhibitor–associated side effects, such as lethargy, fatigue, anorgasmia, and ejaculatory inhibition.

Amantadine is used in general medical practice for the treatment of parkinsonism of all causes, including idiopathic parkinsonism.

Precautions and Adverse Effects

The most common CNS effects of amantadine are mild dizziness, insomnia, and impaired concentration (dosage related), which occur in 5% to 10% of all persons. Irritability, depression, anxiety, dysarthria, and ataxia occur in 1% to 5% of persons. More severe CNS adverse effects, including seizures and psychotic symptoms, have been reported. Nausea is the most common peripheral adverse effect of amantadine. Headache, loss of appetite, and blotchy spots on the skin have also been reported.

Livedo reticularis of the legs (a purple discoloration of the skin caused by dilation of blood vessels) has been reported in up to 5% of persons who take the drug for longer than 1 month. It usually diminishes with elevation of the legs and resolves in almost all cases when drug use is terminated.

Amantadine is relatively contraindicated in persons with renal disease or a seizure disorder. Amantadine should be used with caution in persons with edema or cardiovascular disease. Some evidence indicates that amantadine is teratogenic and therefore should not be taken by pregnant women. Because amantadine is excreted in breast milk, women who are breastfeeding should not take the drug.

Suicide attempts with amantadine overdosages are life threatening. Symptoms can include toxic psychoses (confusion, hallucinations, aggressiveness) and cardiopulmonary arrest. Emergency treatment beginning with gastric lavage is indicated.

Drug Interactions

Coadministration of amantadine with phenelzine (Nardil) or other MAOIs can result in a significant increase in resting blood pressure. The coadministration of amantadine with CNS stimulants can result in insomnia, irritability, nervousness, and possibly seizures or irregular heartbeat. Amantadine should not be coadministered with anticholinergics because unwanted side effects—such as confusion, hallucinations, nightmares, dry mouth, and blurred vision—may be exacerbated.

Dosage and Clinical Guidelines

Amantadine is available in 100-mg capsules and as a 50-mg per 5-mL syrup. The usual starting dosage of amantadine is 100 mg given orally twice a day, although the dosage can be cautiously increased up to 200 mg given orally twice a day if indicated. Amantadine should be used in persons with renal impairment *only* in consultation with the physician treating the renal condition. If amantadine is successful in the treatment of the drug-induced EPS, it should be continued for 4 to 6 weeks and then discontinued to see whether the person has become tolerant to the neurologic adverse effects of the antipsychotic medication. Amantadine should be tapered over 1 to 2 weeks after a decision has been made to discontinue the drug. Persons taking amantadine should not drink alcoholic beverages.

16

Dopamine Receptor Antagonists (First-Generation Antipsychotics)

INTRODUCTION

The dopamine receptor antagonists (DRAs) represent the first group of effective agents to prove highly effective for schizophrenia and nearly all disorders that result in psychotic symptoms. These drugs are also referred to as first-generation antipsychotics (FGAs). The first of these drugs, the phenothiazine chlorpromazine (Thorazine) was introduced in the early 1950s. Other DRAs include all of the antipsychotics in the following groups: phenothiazines, butyrophenones, thioxanthenes, dibenzoxazepines, dihydroindoles, and diphenylbutylpiperidines. Because these agents are associated with extrapyramidal syndromes (EPSs) at clinically effective dosages, newer antipsychotic drugs—the serotonin–dopamine antagonists (SDAs)—have gradually replaced the older agents in the United States. The SDAs are differentiated from earlier drugs by their lower liability to cause extrapyramidal side effects. These newer drugs have other liabilities, most notably a propensity to cause weight gain, lipid elevations, and diabetes. So a reason to still consider use of the DRAs is their lower risk of causing significant metabolic abnormalities. Intermediate-potency DRAs, such as perphenazine (Trilafon), have been shown to be as effective and well tolerated as the SDAs. Manufacturing of molindone (Moban), the DRA with the lowest risk of weight gain and metabolic side effects, has been discontinued in the United States.

PHARMACOLOGIC ACTIONS

All of the DRAs are well absorbed after oral administration, with liquid preparations being absorbed more efficiently than tablets or capsules. Peak plasma concentrations are usually reached 1 to 4 hours after oral administration and 30 to 60 minutes after parenteral administration. Smoking, coffee, antacids, and food interfere with absorption of these drugs. Steady-state levels are reached in approximately 3 to 5 days. The half-lives of these drugs are approximately 24 hours. All can be given in one daily oral dose, if tolerated, after the person is in a stable condition. Most DRAs are highly protein bound. Parenteral formulation of the DRAs results in a more rapid and more reliable onset of action. Bioavailability is also up to tenfold higher with parenteral administration. Most DRAs are metabolized by CYP2D6 and 3A isozymes. However, there are differences among the specific agents.

Long-acting depot parenteral formulations of haloperidol (Haldol, Decanoate) and fluphenazine are available in the United States. They are usually administered once every 1 to 4 weeks, depending on the dose and the person. It can take up to 6 months of treatment with depot formulations to reach steady-state plasma levels, indicating that oral therapy should be continued during the first month or so of depot antipsychotic treatment.

Table 16–1
Factors Influencing the Pharmacokinetics of Antipsychotics

Age	Elderly patients may demonstrate reduced clearance rates
Medical condition	Decreased hepatic blood flow can reduce clearance
	Hepatic disease can decrease clearance
Enzyme inducers	Carbamazepine, phenytoin, ethambutol, barbiturates
Clearance inhibitors	Include SSRIs, TCAs, cimetidine, β-blockers, isoniazid, methylphenidate, erythromycin, triazolobenzodiazepines, ciprofloxacin, and ketoconazole
Changes in binding protein	Hypoalbuminemia can occur with malnutrition or hepatic failure

SSRI, selective serotonin reuptake inhibitor; TCA, tricyclic antidepressant.
Adapted from Ereshefsky L. Pharmacokinetics and drug interactions: Update for new antipsychotics. *J Clin Psychiatry.* 1996; 57(Suppl 11):12–25.

Antipsychotic activity derives from inhibition of dopaminergic neurotransmission. The DRAs are effective when approximately 72% of D_2 receptors in the brain are occupied. The DRAs also block noradrenergic, cholinergic, and histaminergic receptors, with different drugs having different effects on these receptor systems.

There are some generalizations that can be made about the DRAs based on their potency. Potency refers to the amount of drug that is required to achieve therapeutic effects. Low-potency drugs such as chlorpromazine and thioridazine (Mellaril), given in doses of several 100 mg/day, typically produce more weight gain and sedation than high-potency agents such as haloperidol and fluphenazine, usually given in doses of less than 10 mg/day. High-potency agents are also more likely to cause EPS. Some factors influencing the pharmacologic actions of DRAs are listed in Table 16–1.

THERAPEUTIC INDICATIONS

Many types of psychiatric and neurologic disorders may benefit from treatment with DRAs. Some of these indications are shown in Table 16–2.

Schizophrenia and Schizoaffective Disorder

The DRAs are effective in both the short- and long-term management of schizophrenia and schizoaffective disorder. They reduce both acute symptoms and prevent future exacerbations. The DRAs produce their most dramatic effects against the

Table 16–2
Indications for Dopamine Receptor Antagonists

Acute psychotic episodes in schizophrenia and schizoaffective disorder
Maintenance treatment in schizophrenia and schizoaffective disorders
Mania
Depression with psychotic symptoms
Delusional disorder
Borderline personality disorder
Substance-induced psychotic disorder
Delirium and dementia
Mental disorders caused by a medical condition
Childhood schizophrenia
Pervasive developmental disorder
Tourette's syndrome
Huntington's disease

positive symptoms of schizophrenia (e.g., hallucinations, delusions, and agitation). Negative symptoms (e.g., emotional withdrawal and ambivalence) are less likely to improve significantly, and they may appear to worsen because these drugs produce constriction of facial expression and akinesia, side effects that mimic negative symptoms.

Schizophrenia and schizoaffective disorder are characterized by remission and relapse. DRAs decrease the risk of reemergence of psychosis in patients who have recovered while on medication. After a first episode of psychosis, patients should be maintained on medication for 1 to 2 years; after multiple episodes, for 2 to 5 years.

Mania

DRAs are effective to treat psychotic symptoms of acute mania. Because antimanic agents (e.g., lithium) generally have a slower onset of action than do antipsychotics in the treatment of acute symptoms, it is standard practice to initially combine either a DRA or an SDA with lithium (Eskalith), divalproex (Depakote), lamotrigine (Lamictal), or carbamazepine (Tegretol) and then gradually withdraw the antipsychotic.

Depression with Psychotic Symptoms

Combination treatment with an antipsychotic and an antidepressant is one of the treatments of choice for major depressive disorder with psychotic features; the other is electroconvulsive therapy (ECT).

Delusional Disorder

Patients with delusional disorder often respond favorably to treatment with these drugs. Some persons with borderline personality disorder who may develop paranoid thinking in the course of their disorder may respond to antipsychotic drugs.

Severe Agitation and Violent Behavior

Severely agitated and violent patients, regardless of diagnosis, may be treated with DRAs. Symptoms such as extreme irritability, lack of impulse control, severe hostility, gross hyperactivity, and agitation respond to short-term treatment with these drugs. Children with mental disabilities, especially those with profound mental retardation and autistic disorder, often have associated episodes of violence, aggression, and agitation that respond to treatment with antipsychotic drugs; however, the repeated administration of antipsychotics to control disruptive behavior in children is controversial.

Tourette's Syndrome

DRAs are used to treat Tourette's syndrome, a neurobehavioral disorder marked by motor and vocal tics. Haloperidol and pimozide (Orap) are the drugs most frequently used, but other DRAs are also effective. Some clinicians prefer to use clonidine (Catapres) for this disorder because of its lower risk of neurologic side effects.

Borderline Personality Disorder

Patients with borderline personality disorder who experience transient psychotic symptoms, such as perceptual disturbances, suspiciousness, ideas of reference, and aggression, may need to be treated with a DRA. This disorder is also associated with mood instability, so patients should be evaluated for possible treatment with mood-stabilizing agents.

Dementia and Delirium

About two-thirds of agitated, elderly patients with various forms of dementia improve when given a DRA. Low doses of high-potency drugs (e.g., 0.5 to 1 mg a day of haloperidol) are recommended. DRAs are also used to treat psychotic symptoms and agitation associated with delirium. The cause of the delirium needs to be determined because toxic deliriums caused by anticholinergic agents can be exacerbated by low-potency DRAs, which often have significant antimuscarinic activity. Orthostasis, parkinsonism, and worsened cognition are the most problematic side effects in this elderly population.

Substance-Induced Psychotic Disorder

Intoxication with cocaine, amphetamines, alcohol, phencyclidine, or other drugs can cause psychotic symptoms. Because these symptoms tend to be time limited, it is preferable to avoid use of a DRA unless the patient is severely agitated and aggressive. Usually, benzodiazepines can be used to calm the patient. Benzodiazepines should be used instead of DRAs in cases of phencyclidine intoxication. When a patient is experiencing hallucinations or delusions as a result of alcohol withdrawal, DRAs may increase the risk of seizure.

Childhood Schizophrenia

Children with schizophrenia benefit from treatment with antipsychotic medication, although considerably less research has been devoted to this population. Studies are currently under way to determine if intervention with medication at the very earliest signs of disturbance in children genetically at risk for schizophrenia can prevent the emergence of more florid symptoms. Careful consideration needs to be given to side effects, especially those involving cognition and alertness.

Other Psychiatric and Nonpsychiatric Indications

The DRAs reduce the chorea in the early stages of Huntington's disease. Patients with this disease may develop hallucinations, delusions, mania, or hypomania. These and other psychiatric symptoms respond to DRAs. High-potency DRAs should be used. However, clinicians should be aware that patients with the rigid form of this disorder may experience acute EPS. The use of DRAs to treat impulse control disorders should be reserved for patients in whom other interventions have failed. Patients with pervasive developmental disorder may exhibit hyperactivity, screaming, and agitation with combativeness. Some of these symptoms respond to high-potency DRAs, but there is little research evidence supporting benefits in these patients.

The rare neurologic disorders ballismus and hemiballismus (which affect only one side of the body), characterized by propulsive movements of the limbs away from the body, also respond to treatment with antipsychotic agents. Other miscellaneous indications for the use of DRAs include the treatment of nausea, emesis, intractable hiccups, and pruritus. Endocrine disorders and temporal lobe epilepsy may be associated with psychosis that responds to antipsychotic treatment.

The most common side effects of DRAs are neurologic. As a rule, low-potency drugs cause most nonneurologic adverse effects, and the high-potency drugs cause most neurologic adverse effects.

PRECAUTIONS AND ADVERSE REACTIONS

Table 16–3 summarizes the most common adverse events associated with the use of DRAs.

Table 16–3
Dopamine Receptor Antagonists: Potency and Adverse Effects

Drug Name	Chemical Classification	Therapeutically Equivalent Oral	Sedation	Autonomic[a]	Extrapyramidal Reactions[b]
Pimozide[c]	Diphenylbutyl-piperidine	1.5	+	+	+++
Fluphenazine	Phenothiazine: piperazine compound	2	+	+	+++
Haloperidol	Butyrophenone	2	+	+	+++
Thiothixene	Thioxanthene	4	+	+	+++
Trifluoperazine	Phenothiazine: piperazine compound	5	++	+	+++
Perphenazine	Phenothiazine: piperazine compound	8	++	+	++/+++
Molindone	Dihydroindole	10	++	+	+
Loxapine	Dibenzoxazepine	10	++	+/++	++/+++
Prochlor-perazine[c]	Phenothiazine: piperazine compound	15	++	+	+++
Aceto-phenazine	Phenothiazine: piperazine compound	20	++	+	++/+++
Triflupromazine	Phenothiazine: aliphatic compound	25	+++	++/+++	++
Mesoridazine	Phenothiazine: piperidine compound	50	+++	++	+
Chlorpromazine	Phenothiazine: aliphatic compound	100	+++	+++	++
Chlorprothixene	Thioxanthene	100	+++	+++	+/++
Thioridazine	Phenothiazine: piperidine compound	100	+++	+++	+

[a]Anti-α-adrenergic and anticholinergic effects.
[b]Excluding tardive dyskinesia, which appears to be produced to the same degree and frequency by all agents with equieffective antipsychotic dosages.
[c]Pimozide is used principally in the treatment of Tourette's syndrome; prochlorperazine is used rarely, if ever, as an antipsychotic agent.
Adapted from American Medical Association. *AMA Drug Evaluations: Annual 1992.* Chicago, IL: American Medical Association, 1992.

Neuroleptic Malignant Syndrome

A potentially fatal side effect of DRA treatment, neuroleptic malignant syndrome, can occur at any time during the course of DRA treatment. Symptoms include extreme hyperthermia, severe muscular rigidity and dystonia, akinesia, mutism, confusion, agitation, and increased pulse rate and blood pressure (BP). Laboratory findings include increased white blood cell (WBC) count, creatinine phosphokinase, liver enzymes, plasma myoglobin, and myoglobinuria, occasionally associated with renal failure. The symptoms usually evolve over 24 to 72 hours, and the untreated syndrome lasts 10 to 14 days. The diagnosis is often missed in the early stages, and the withdrawal or agitation may mistakenly be considered to reflect increased psychosis. Men are affected more frequently than are women, and young persons are affected more commonly than are elderly persons. The mortality rate can reach 20% to 30% or even higher when depot medications are involved. Rates are also increased when high doses of high-potency agents are used.

If neuroleptic malignant syndrome is suspected, the DRA should be stopped immediately and the following done: medical support to cool the person; monitoring of vital signs, electrolytes, fluid balance, and renal output; and symptomatic treatment of fever. Antiparkinsonian medications may reduce some of the muscle rigidity. Dantrolene (Dantrium), a skeletal muscle relaxant (0.8 to 2.5 mg/kg every 6 hours, up to a total dosage of 10 mg a day) may be useful in the treatment of this disorder. When the person can take oral medications, dantrolene can be given in doses of 100 to 200 mg a day. Bromocriptine (20 to 30 mg a day in four divided doses) or amantadine can be added to the regimen. Treatment should usually be continued for 5 to 10 days. When drug treatment is restarted, the clinician should consider switching to a low-potency drug or an SDA, although these agents—including clozapine—may also cause neuroleptic malignant syndrome.

Seizure Threshold

DRAs may lower the seizure threshold. Chlorpromazine, thioridazine, and other low-potency drugs are thought to be more epileptogenic than are high-potency drugs. The risk of inducing a seizure by drug administration warrants consideration when the person already has a seizure disorder or brain lesion.

Sedation

Blockade of histamine H_1 receptors is the usual cause of sedation associated with DRAs. Chlorpromazine is the most sedating typical antipsychotic. The relative sedative properties of the drugs are summarized in Table 16–3. Giving the entire daily dose at bedtime usually eliminates any problems from sedation, and tolerance for this adverse effect often develops.

Central Anticholinergic Effects

The symptoms of central anticholinergic activity include severe agitation; disorientation to time, person, and place; hallucinations; seizures; high fever; and dilated pupils. Stupor and coma may ensue. The treatment of anticholinergic toxicity consists of discontinuing the causal agent or agents, close medical supervision, and physostigmine (Antilirium, Eserine), 2 mg by slow intravenous (IV) infusion, repeated within 1 hour as necessary. Too much physostigmine is dangerous, and symptoms of physostigmine toxicity include hypersalivation and sweating. Atropine sulfate (0.5 mg) can reverse the effects of physostigmine toxicity.

Cardiac Effects

The DRAs decrease cardiac contractility, disrupt enzyme contractility in cardiac cells, increase circulating levels of catecholamines, and prolong atrial and ventricular conduction time and refractory periods. Low-potency DRAs particularly the pheno-thiazines, are usually more cardiotoxic than are high-potency drugs. One exception is haloperidol, which has been linked to abnormal heart rhythm, ventricular arrhyth-mias, torsades de pointes, and sudden death when injected IV. Pimozide, sulpiride, and droperidol (a butyrophenone) also prolong the QTc interval and have clearly been associated with torsades de pointes and sudden death. In one study, thioridazine was responsible for 28 (61%) of the 46 sudden antipsychotic deaths. In 15 of these cases, it was the only drug ingested. Chlorpromazine also causes prolongation of the QT and PR intervals, blunting of the T waves, and depression of the ST segment. These drugs are thus indicated only when other agents have been ineffective.

Sudden Death

Occasional reports of sudden cardiac death during treatment with DRAs may be the result of cardiac arrhythmias. Other causes may include seizure, asphyxiation, malignant hyperthermia, heat stroke, and neuroleptic malignant syndrome. How-ever, there does not appear to be an overall increase in the incidence of sudden death linked to the use of antipsychotics.

Orthostatic (Postural) Hypotension

Orthostatic (postural) hypotension is most common with low-potency drugs, par-ticularly chlorpromazine, thioridazine, and chlorprothixene. When using intra-muscular (IM) low-potency DRAs, the clinician should measure the person's BP (lying and standing) before and after the first dose and during the first few days of treatment.

Orthostatic hypotension is mediated by adrenergic blockade and occurs most fre-quently during the first few days of treatment. Tolerance often develops for this side effect, which is why initial dosing of these drugs is lower than the usual therapeutic dose. Fainting or falls, although uncommon, may lead to injury. Patients should be warned of this side effect and instructed to rise slowly after sitting and reclining. Patients should avoid all caffeine and alcohol; should drink at least 2 L of fluid a day; and if not under treatment for hypertension, should add liberal amounts of salt to their diet. Support hose may help some persons.

Hypotension can usually be managed by having patients lie down with their feet higher than their heads and pump their legs as if bicycling. Volume expan-sion or vasopressor agents, such as norepinephrine (Levophed), may be indicated in severe cases. Because hypotension is produced by α-adrenergic blockade, the drugs also block the α-adrenergic stimulating properties of epinephrine, leaving the β-adrenergic stimulating effects untouched. Therefore, the administration of epi-nephrine results in a paradoxical worsening of hypotension and is contraindicated in cases of antipsychotic-induced hypotension. Pure α-adrenergic pressor agents, such as metaraminol (Aramine) and norepinephrine, are the drugs of choice in the treatment of the disorder.

Hematologic Effects

A temporary leukopenia with a WBC count of about 3,500 is a common but not serious problem. Agranulocytosis, a life-threatening hematologic problem, occurs in about 1 in 10,000 persons treated with DRAs. Thrombocytopenic or nonthrombocytopenic purpura, hemolytic anemias, and pancytopenia may occur rarely in persons treated with DRAs. Although routine complete blood counts (CBCs) are not indicated, if a person reports a sore throat and fever, a CBC should be done immediately to check for the possibility. If the blood indexes are low, administration of DRAs should be stopped, and the person should be transferred to a medical facility. The mortality rate for the complication may be as high as 30%.

Tardive Dyskinesia

Discussed in Chapter 31, is one of the more concerning effects of long-term treatment with DRAs. It is an important reason to monitor patients being treated with these drugs. Clinical trials showed that patients who received 80 mg/day of the active treatment had a significant decrease in tardive dyskinesia (TD) symptoms on the Abnormal Involuntary Movement Scale (AIMS) at 6 weeks compared with those who received matching placebo. The group receiving the treatment at 40 mg/day also had a reduction on the AIMS measures.

Treatment with valbenazine may cause sleepiness and QT prolongation and its use should be avoided in patients with congenital long QT syndrome or with abnormal heartbeats associated with a prolonged QT interval.

The drug reduced involuntary movements without reducing the therapeutic effects of the DRAs.

The drug is currently being investigated as a treatment for Tourette's syndrome in adults and adolescents.

Peripheral Anticholinergic Effects

Peripheral anticholinergic effects, consisting of dry mouth and nose, blurred vision, constipation, urinary retention, and mydriasis, are common, especially with low-potency DRAs; for example, chlorpromazine, thioridazine, mesoridazine (Serentil). Some persons may also have nausea and vomiting.

Constipation should be treated with the usual laxative preparations, but severe constipation can progress to paralytic ileus. A decrease in the DRA dosage or a change to a less anticholinergic drug is warranted in such cases. Pilocarpine (Salagen) may be used to treat paralytic ileus, although the relief is only transitory. Bethanechol (Urecholine) (20 to 40 mg a day) may be useful in some persons with urinary retention.

Weight gain is associated with increased mortality and morbidity and with medication noncompliance. Low-potency DRAs may cause significant weight gain but not as much as is seen with the SDAs olanzapine (Zyprexa) and clozapine (Clozaril). Molindone and perhaps loxapine (Loxitane) appear to be least likely to cause weight gain.

Endocrine Effects

Blockade of the dopamine receptors in the tuberoinfundibular tract results in the increased secretion of prolactin, which can result in breast enlargement, galactorrhea, amenorrhea, and inhibited orgasm in women and impotence in men. The SDAs, with the exception of risperidone (Risperdal), are not particularly associated with an increase in prolactin levels and may be the drugs of choice for persons experiencing disturbing side effects from increased prolactin release.

Sexual Adverse Effects

Both men and women taking DRAs can experience anorgasmia and decreased libido. As many as 50% of men taking antipsychotics report ejaculatory and erectile disturbances. Sildenafil (Viagra), vardenafil (Levitra), and tadalafil (Cialis) are often used to treat psychotropic-induced orgasmic dysfunction, but they have not been studied in combination with the DRAs. Thioridazine is particularly associated with decreased libido and retrograde ejaculation in men. Priapism and reports of painful orgasms have also been described, both possibly resulting from α_1-adrenergic antagonist activity.

Skin and Eye Effects

Allergic dermatitis and photosensitivity may occur, especially with low-potency agents. Urticarial, maculopapular, petechial, and edematous eruptions may occur early in treatment, generally in the first few weeks, and remit spontaneously. A photosensitivity reaction that resembles a severe sunburn also occurs in some persons taking chlorpromazine. Persons should be warned of this adverse effect, should spend no more than 30 to 60 minutes in the sun, and should use sunscreens. Long-term chlorpromazine use is associated with blue-gray discoloration of skin areas exposed to sunlight. The skin changes often begin with a tan or golden brown color and progress to such colors as slate gray, metallic blue, and purple. These discolorations resolve when the patient is switched to another medication.

Irreversible retinal pigmentation is associated with the use of thioridazine at dosages above 1,000 mg a day. An early symptom of the side effect can sometimes be nocturnal confusion related to difficulty with night vision. The pigmentation can progress even after thioridazine administration is stopped, finally resulting in blindness. It is for this reason that the maximum recommended dosage of thioridazine is 800 mg/day.

Patients taking chlorpromazine may develop a relatively benign pigmentation of the eyes, characterized by whitish brown granular deposits concentrated in the anterior lens and posterior cornea and visible only by slit-lens examination. The deposits can progress to opaque white and yellow-brown granules, often stellate. Occasionally, the conjunctiva is discolored by a brown pigment. No retinal damage is seen, and vision is almost never impaired. This condition gradually resolves when chlorpromazine is discontinued.

Jaundice

Elevations of liver enzymes during treatment with a DRA tend to be transient and not clinically significant. When chlorpromazine first came into use, cases of obstructive or cholestatic jaundice were reported. It usually occurred in the first month of treatment and was heralded by symptoms of upper abdominal pain, nausea, and vomiting.

This was followed by fever; rash; eosinophilia; bilirubin in the urine; and increases in serum bilirubin, alkaline phosphatase, and hepatic transaminases. Reported cases are now extremely rare, but if jaundice occurs, the medication should be discontinued.

Overdoses

Overdoses typically consist of exaggerated DRA side effects. Symptoms and signs include central nervous system (CNS) depression, EPS, mydriasis, rigidity, restlessness, decreased deep tendon reflexes, tachycardia, and hypotension. The severe symptoms of overdose include delirium, coma, respiratory depression, and seizures. Haloperidol may be among the safest typical antipsychotics in overdose. After an overdose, the electroencephalogram (EEG) shows diffuse slowing and low voltage. Extreme overdose may lead to delirium and coma, with respiratory depression and hypotension. Life-threatening overdose usually involves ingestion of other CNS depressants, such as alcohol or benzodiazepines.

Activated charcoal, if possible, and gastric lavage should be administered if the overdose is recent. Emetics are not indicated because the antiemetic actions of the DRAs inhibit their efficacy. Seizures can be treated with IV diazepam (Valium) or phenytoin (Dilantin). Hypotension can be treated with either norepinephrine or dopamine but not epinephrine.

Use in Pregnancy and Lactation

There is a low correlation between the use of antipsychotics during pregnancy and congenital malformations. Nevertheless, antipsychotics should be avoided during pregnancy, particularly in the first trimester unless the benefit outweighs the risk. High-potency drugs are preferable to low-potency drugs because the low-potency drugs are associated with hypotension.

DRAs are secreted in the breast milk, although concentrations are low. Women taking these agents should be advised against breastfeeding.

DRUG INTERACTIONS

Many pharmacokinetic and pharmacodynamic drug interactions are associated with these drugs (Table 16–4). CYP2D6 is the most common hepatic isozyme involved in DRA pharmacokinetic interactions. Other common drug interactions affect the absorption of the DRAs.

Antacids, activated charcoal, cholestyramine (Questran), kaolin, pectin, and cimetidine (Tagamet) taken within 2 hours of antipsychotic administration can reduce the absorption of these drugs. Anticholinergics may decrease the absorption of the DRAs. The additive anticholinergic activity of the DRAs, anticholinergics, and tricyclic drugs may result in anticholinergic toxicity. Digoxin (Lanoxin) and steroids, both of which decrease gastric motility, can increase DRA absorption.

Phenothiazines, especially thioridazine, may decrease the metabolism of and cause toxic concentrations of phenytoin. Barbiturates may increase the metabolism of DRAs.

Tricyclic drugs and selective serotonin reuptake inhibitors (SSRIs) that inhibit CYP2D6—paroxetine (Paxil), fluoxetine (Prozac), and fluvoxamine (Luvox)—interact with DRAs, resulting in increased plasma concentrations of both drugs. The anticholinergic, sedative, and hypotensive effects of the drugs may also be additive.

Table 16–4
Antipsychotic Drug Interactions

Interacting Medication	Mechanism	Clinical Effect
Drug interactions assessed to have major severity		
β-Adrenergic receptor antagonists	Synergistic pharmacologic effect; antipsychotic inhibits metabolism of propranolol; antipsychotic increases plasma concentrations	Severe hypotension
Anticholinergics	Pharmacodynamic effects Additive anticholinergic effect	Decreased antipsychotic effect Anticholinergic toxicity
Barbiturates	Phenobarbital induces antipsychotic metabolism	Decreased antipsychotic concentrations
Carbamazepine	Induces antipsychotic metabolism	Up to 50% reduction in antipsychotic concentrations
Charcoal	Reduces GI absorption of antipsychotic and adsorbs drug during enterohepatic circulation	May reduce antipsychotic effect or cause toxicity when used to treat overdose or for GI disturbances
Cigarette smoking	Induction of microsomal enzymes	Reduced plasma concentrations of antipsychotic agents
Epinephrine, norepinephrine	Antipsychotic antagonizes pressor effect	Hypotension
Ethanol	Additive CNS depression	Impaired psychomotor status
Fluvoxamine	Fluvoxamine inhibits metabolism of haloperidol and clozapine	Increased concentrations of haloperidol and clozapine
Guanethidine	Antipsychotic antagonizes guanethidine reuptake	Impaired antihypertensive effect
Lithium	Unknown	Rare reports of neurotoxicity
Meperidine	Additive CNS depression	Hypotension and sedation
Drug interactions assessed to have minor or moderate severity		
Amphetamines anorexiants	Decreased pharmacologic effect of amphetamine	Diminished weight loss effect; amphetamines may exacerbate psychosis
ACEIs	Additive hypotensive crisis	Hypotension, postural intolerance
Antacids containing aluminum	Insoluble complex formed in GI tract	Possible reduced antipsychotic effect
AD nonspecific	Decreased metabolism of AD through competitive inhibition	Increased AD concentration
Benzodiazepines	Increased pharmacologic effect of the benzodiazepine	Respiratory depression, stupor, hypotension
Bromocriptine	Antipsychotic antagonizes dopamine receptor stimulation	Increased prolactin
Caffeinated beverages	Form precipitate with antipsychotic solutions	Possible diminished antipsychotic effect
Cimetidine	Reduced antipsychotic absorption and clearance	Decreased antipsychotic effect
Clonidine	Antipsychotic potentiates α-adrenergic hypotensive effect	Hypotension or hypertension
Disulfiram	Impairs antipsychotic metabolism	Increased antipsychotic concentrations
Methyldopa	Unknown	BP elevations
Phenytoin	Induction of antipsychotic metabolism; decreased phenytoin metabolism	Decreased antipsychotic concentrations; increased phenytoin levels
SSRIs	Impair antipsychotic metabolism; pharmacodynamic interaction	Sudden onset of extrapyramidal symptoms
Valproic acid	Antipsychotic inhibits valproic acid metabolism	Increased valproic acid half-life and levels

ACEI, angiotensin-converting enzyme inhibitor; AD, antidepressant; BP, blood pressure; CNS, central nervous system; GI, gastrointestinal; SSRIs, selective serotonin reuptake inhibitors.
From Ereshosky L, Overman GP, Karp JK. Current psychotropic dosing and monitoring guidelines. *Prim Psychiatry.* 1996, 3:21.

Typical antipsychotics may inhibit the hypotensive effects of α-methyldopa (Aldomet). Conversely, typical antipsychotics may have an additive effect on some hypotensive drugs. Antipsychotic drugs have a variable effect on the hypotensive effects of clonidine. Propranolol (Inderal) coadministration increases the blood concentrations of both drugs.

The DRAs potentiate the CNS-depressant effects of the sedatives, antihistamines, opiates, opioids, and alcohol, particularly in persons with impaired respiratory status. When these agents are taken with alcohol, the risk for heat stroke may be increased.

Cigarette smoking may decrease the plasma levels of the typical antipsychotic drugs. Epinephrine has a paradoxical hypotensive effect in persons taking typical antipsychotics. These drugs may decrease the blood concentration of warfarin (Coumadin), resulting in decreased bleeding time. The phenothiazines, thioridazine, and pimozide should not be coadministered with other agents that prolong the QT interval. Thioridazine is contraindicated in patients taking drugs that inhibit the CYP2D6 isoenzyme or in patients with reduced levels of CYP2D6.

LABORATORY INTERFERENCES

Chlorpromazine and perphenazine (Trilafon) may cause both false-positive and false-negative results in immunologic pregnancy tests and falsely elevated bilirubin (with reagent test strips) and urobilinogen (with Ehrlich's reagent test) values. These drugs have also been associated with an abnormal shift in results of the glucose tolerance test, although that shift may reflect the effects of the drugs on the glucose-regulating system. Phenothiazines have been reported to interfere with the measurement of 17-ketosteroids and 17-hydroxycorticosteroids and produce false-positive results in tests for phenylketonuria.

DOSAGE AND CLINICAL GUIDELINES

Contraindications to the use of DRAs include: (1) a history of a serious allergic response, (2) the possible ingestion of a substance that will interact with the antipsychotic to induce CNS depression (e.g., alcohol, opioids, barbiturates, and benzodiazepines) or anticholinergic delirium (e.g., scopolamine and possibly phencyclidine [PCP]), (3) the presence of a severe cardiac abnormality, (4) a high risk for seizures, (5) the presence of narrow-angle glaucoma or prostatic hypertrophy if a drug with high anticholinergic activity is to be used, and (6) the presence or a history of TD. Antipsychotics should be administered with caution in persons with hepatic disease because impaired hepatic metabolism may result in high plasma concentrations. The usual assessment should include a CBC with WBC indexes, liver function tests, and electrocardiography (EKG), especially in women older than 40 years of age and men older than 30 years of age. Elderly persons and children are more sensitive to side effects than are young adults, so the dosage of the drug should be adjusted accordingly.

Various patients may respond to widely different dosages of antipsychotics; therefore, there is no set dosage for any given antipsychotic drug. Because of side effects, it is reasonable clinical practice to begin at a low dosage and increase it as necessary. It is important to remember that the maximal effects of a particular dosage may not be evident for 4 to 6 weeks. Available preparations and dosages of the DRAs are given in Table 16–5.

Table 16-5
Dopamine Receptor Antagonists

Generic or Chemical	Trade	Trade (mg)	Capsules (mg)	Solution	Parenteral	Rectal Suppositories (mg)	Adult Dose Range (mg/day) Acute	Adult Dose Range (mg/day) Maintenance
Chlorpromazine	Thorazine	10, 25, 50, 100, 200	30, 75, 150, 200, 300	10 mg/5 mL, 30 mg/mL, 100 mg/mL	25 mg/mL	25, 100	100–1,600 PO 25–400 IM	50–400 PO
Prochlorperazine	Compazine	5, 10, 25	10, 15, 30	5 mg/5 mL	5 mg/mL	2.5, 5, 25	15–200 PO 40–80 IM	15–60 PO
Perphenazine	Trilafon	2, 4, 8, 16	—	16 mg/5 mL	5 mg/mL	—	12–64 PO 15–30 IM	8–24 PO
Trifluoperazine	Stelazine	1, 2, 5, 10	—	10 mg/mL	2 mg/mL	—	4–40 PO 4–10 IM	5–20 PO
Fluphenazine	Prolixin	1, 2.5, 5, 10	—	2.5 mg/5 mL 5 mg/mL	2.5 mg/mL (IM only)	—	2.5–40.0 PO 5–20 IM	1.0–15.0 PO 12.5–50.0 IM (decanoate or enanthate, weekly or biweekly)
Fluphenazine decanoate	—	—	—	—	2.5 mg/mL	—	—	—
Fluphenazine enanthate	—	—	—	2.5 mg/mL	—	—	—	—
Thioridazine	Mellaril	10, 15, 25, 50, 100, 150, 200	—	25 mg/5 mL, 100 mg/5 mL, 30 mg/mL, 100 mg/mL	—	—	200–800 PO	100–300 PO
Mesoridazine	Serentil	10, 25, 50, 100	—	25 mg/mL	25 mg/mL	—	100–400 PO 25–200 IM	30–150 PO
Haloperidol	Haldol	0.5, 1, 2, 5, 10, 20	—	2 mg/5 mL	5 mg/mL (IM only)	—	5–20 PO 12.5–25 IM	1–10 PO
Haloperidol decanoate	—	—	—	—	50 mg/mL 100 mg/mL (IM only)	—	—	25–200 IM (decanoate, monthly)
Chlorprothixene	Taractan	10, 25, 50, 100	—	100 mg/5 mL (suspension)	12.5 mg/mL	—	75–600 PO 75–200 IM	50–400
Thiothixene	Navane	—	1, 2, 5, 10, 20	5 mg/mL	5 mg/mL (IM only), 20 mg/mL	—	6–100 PO 8–30 IM	6–30
Loxapine	Loxitane	—	5, 10, 25, 50	25 mg/5 mL	50 mg/mL	—	20–250 20–75 IM	20–100
Molindone	Moban	5, 10, 25, 50, 100	—	20 mg/mL	—	—	50–225	5–150
Pimozide	Orap	2	—	—	—	—	0.5–20	0.5–5.0

IM, intramuscular; PO, oral.

Short-Term Treatment

The equivalent of 5 to 20 mg of haloperidol is a reasonable dose for an adult in an acute state. A geriatric person may benefit from as little as 1 mg of haloperidol. The administration of more than 25 mg of chlorpromazine in one injection may result in serious hypotension. IM administration results in peak plasma levels in about 30 minutes versus 90 minutes using the oral route. Doses of drugs for IM administration are about half those given by the oral route. In a short-term treatment setting, the person should be observed for 1 hour after the first dose of medication. After that time, most clinicians administer a second dose or a sedative agent (e.g., a benzodiazepine) to achieve effective behavioral control. Possible sedatives include lorazepam (Ativan) (2 mg IM) and amobarbital (50 to 250 mg IM).

Rapid Neuroleptization

Rapid neuroleptization (also called psychotolysis) is the practice of administering hourly IM doses of antipsychotic medications until marked sedation of the person is achieved. However, several research studies have shown that merely waiting several more hours after one dose yields the same clinical improvement as is seen with repeated doses. Nevertheless, clinicians must be careful to keep persons from becoming violent while they are psychotic. Clinicians can help prevent violent episodes by using adjuvant sedatives or by temporarily using physical restraints until the persons can control their behavior.

Early Treatment

A full 6 weeks may be necessary to evaluate the extent of the improvement in psychotic symptoms. However, agitation and excitement usually improve quickly with antipsychotic treatment. About 75% of persons with a short history of illness show significant improvement in their psychosis. Psychotic symptoms, both positive and negative, usually continue to improve 3 to 12 months after the initiation of treatment.

About 5 mg of haloperidol or 300 mg of chlorpromazine is a usual effective daily dose. In the past, much higher doses were used, but evidence suggests that it resulted in more side effects without additional benefits. A single daily dose is usually given at bedtime to help induce sleep and to reduce the incidence of adverse effects. However, bedtime dosing for elderly persons may increase their risk of falling if they get out of bed during the night. The sedative effects of typical antipsychotics last only a few hours in contrast to the antipsychotic effects, which last for 1 to 3 days.

Intermittent Medications

It is common clinical practice to order medications to be given intermittently as needed (PRN). Although this practice may be reasonable during the first few days that a person is hospitalized, the amount of time the person takes antipsychotic drugs, rather than an increase in dosage, is what produces therapeutic improvement. Clinicians on inpatient services may feel pressured by staff members to write PRN antipsychotic orders; such orders should include specific symptoms, how often the drugs should be given, and how many doses can be given each day. Clinicians may choose to use small doses for the PRN doses (e.g., 2 mg of haloperidol) or use a benzodiazepine instead (e.g., 2 mg of lorazepam IM). If PRN doses of an antipsychotic are necessary after the first week of treatment, the clinician may want to consider increasing the standing daily dose of the drug.

Maintenance Treatment

The first 3 to 6 months after a psychotic episode is usually considered a period of stabilization. After that time, the dosage of the antipsychotic can be decreased about 20% every 6 months until the minimum effective dosage is found. A person is usually maintained on antipsychotic medications for 1 to 2 years after the first psychotic episode. Antipsychotic treatment is often continued for 5 years after a second psychotic episode, and lifetime maintenance is considered after the third psychotic episode, although attempts to reduce the daily dosage can be made every 6 to 12 months.

Antipsychotic drugs are effective in controlling psychotic symptoms, but persons may report that they prefer being off the drugs because they feel better without them. The clinician must discuss maintenance medication with patients and take into account their wishes, the severity of their illnesses, and the quality of their support systems. It is essential for the clinician to know enough about the patient's life to try to predict upcoming stressors that might require increasing the dosage or closely monitoring compliance.

Long-Acting Depot Medications

Long-acting depot preparations may be needed to overcome problems with compliance. IM preparations are typically given once every 1 to 4 weeks.

Two depot preparations, a decanoate and an enanthate, of fluphenazine and a decanoate preparation of haloperidol are available in the United States. The preparations are injected IM into an area of large muscle tissue, from which they are absorbed slowly into the blood. Decanoate preparations can be given less frequently than enanthate preparations because they are absorbed more slowly. Although stabilizing a person on the oral preparation of the specific drugs is not necessary before initiating the depot form, it is good practice to give at least one oral dose of the drug to assess the possibility of an adverse effect, such as severe EPS or an allergic reaction.

It is reasonable to begin with either 12.5 mg (0.5 mL) of fluphenazine preparation or 25 mg (0.5 mL) of haloperidol decanoate. If symptoms emerge in the next 2 to 4 weeks, the person can be treated temporarily with additional oral medications or with additional small depot injections. After 3 to 4 weeks, the depot injection can be increased to a single dose equal to the total of the doses given during the initial period.

A good reason to initiate depot treatment with low doses is that the absorption of the preparations may be faster than usual at the onset of treatment, resulting in frightening episodes of dystonia that eventually discourage compliance with the medication. Some clinicians keep persons drug free for 3 to 7 days before initiating depot treatment and give small doses of the depot preparations (3.125 mg of fluphenazine or 6.25 mg of haloperidol) every few days to avoid those initial problems.

PLASMA CONCENTRATIONS

Genetic differences among persons and pharmacokinetic interactions with other drugs influence the metabolism of the antipsychotics. If a person has not improved after 4 to 6 weeks of treatment, the plasma concentration of the drug should be determined if feasible. After a patient has been on a particular dosage for at least five times the half-life of the drug and thus approaches steady-state concentrations, blood levels may be helpful. It is standard practice to obtain plasma samples at trough levels—just before the daily dose is given, usually at least 12 hours after the previous dose and most commonly 20 to 24 hours after the previous dose. In fact, most antipsychotics have no well-defined dose–response curve. The best-studied drug is haloperidol, which may have a therapeutic window ranging from 2 to 15 ng/mL. Other therapeutic ranges that have been reasonably well documented are 30 to 100 ng/mL for chlorpromazine and 0.8 to 2.4 ng/mL for perphenazine.

Treatment-Resistant Persons

Unfortunately, 10% to 35% of persons with schizophrenia do not obtain significant benefit from the antipsychotic drugs. Treatment resistance is a failure on at least two adequate trials of antipsychotics from two pharmacologic classes. It is useful to determine plasma concentrations for such persons because it is possible that they are slow or rapid metabolizers or are not taking their medication. Clozapine has been conclusively shown to be effective when given to patients who have failed multiple trials of DRAs.

Adjunctive Medications

It is common practice to use DRAs in conjunction with other psychotropic agents, either to treat side effects or further improve symptoms. Most commonly, this involves the use of lithium or other mood-stabilizing agents, SSRIs, or benzodiazepines. It was once held that antidepressant drugs exacerbated psychosis in schizophrenic patients. In all likelihood, this observation involved patients with bipolar disorder who were misdiagnosed as being schizophrenic. Abundant evidence suggests that antidepressants in fact improve symptoms of depression in schizophrenic patients. In some cases, amphetamines can be added to DRAs if patients remain withdrawn and apathetic.

CHOICE OF DRUG

Given their proven efficacy in managing acute psychotic symptoms and the fact that prophylactic administration of antiparkinsonian medication prevents or minimizes acute motor abnormalities, DRAs are still valuable, especially for short-term therapy. There is a considerable cost advantage to a DRA antiparkinsonian regimen compared with monotherapy with a newer antipsychotic agent. Concern about the development of DRA-induced TD is the major deterrent to long-term use of these drugs, yet it is not clear that SDAs are completely free of this complication. Thus, DRAs still occupy an important role in psychiatric treatment. DRAs are not predictably interchangeable. For reasons that cannot be explained, some patients do better on one drug than another. Choice of a particular DRA should be based on the known adverse effect profile of the drugs. Other than a significant advantage in terms of medication cost, the choice currently would be an SDA. If a DRA is thought to be preferable, a high-potency antipsychotic is favored even though it may be associated with more neurologic adverse effects, mainly because there is a higher incidence of other adverse effects (e.g., cardiac, hypotensive, epileptogenic, sexual, and allergic) with the low-potency drugs. If sedation is a desired goal, either a low-potency antipsychotic can be given in divided doses or a benzodiazepine can be coadministered.

An unpleasant or dysphoric reaction (a subjective sense of restlessness, oversedation, and acute dystonia) to the first dose of an antipsychotic predicts future poor response and noncompliance. Prophylactic use of antiparkinsonian medications may prevent this reaction. In general, clinicians should be vigilant about serious side effects and adverse events (described above) regardless of which drug is used.

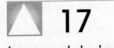

17
Lamotrigine

INTRODUCTION

After proving effectiveness in several animal models of epilepsy, lamotrigine (Lamictal) was developed as an antiepileptic drug, and was marketed for the adjunctive treatment of partial seizures in the United States in 1995. Lamotrigine later demonstrated efficacy and was approved for maintenance treatment of bipolar I disorder in 2003. However, lamotrigine has not received approval for the treatment of acute bipolar depression or rapid cycling bipolar disorder. Lamotrigine has not been shown to be effective as a main intervention in acute mania. Based on available evidence, lamotrigine is an agent that appears to "stabilize mood from below, such that it may maximally impact the depressive component of bipolar disorders and have some mood-stabilizing effects as well."

PHARMACOLOGIC ACTIONS

Lamotrigine is completely absorbed, has a bioavailability of 98%, and has a steady-state plasma half-life of 25 hours. However, the rate of lamotrigine's metabolism varies over a sixfold range, depending on which other drugs are administered concomitantly. Dosing is escalated slowly to twice-a-day maintenance dosing. Food does not affect its absorption, and it is 55% protein bound in the plasma; 94% of lamotrigine and its inactive metabolites are excreted in the urine. Among the better-delineated biochemical actions of lamotrigine are blockade of voltage-sensitive sodium channels, which in turn modulate release of glutamate and aspartate, and have the slight effect on calcium channels. Lamotrigine modestly increases plasma serotonin concentrations, possibly through inhibition of serotonin reuptake, and is a weak inhibitor of serotonin 5-HT$_3$ receptors.

THERAPEUTIC INDICATIONS

Bipolar Disorder

Lamotrigine is indicated in the treatment of bipolar disorder and may prolong the time between episodes of depression and mania. It is more effective in lengthening the intervals between depressive episodes than manic episodes. It is also effective as treatment for rapid cycling bipolar disorder.

Other Indications

There have been reports of therapeutic benefit in the treatment of borderline personality disorder and in the treatment for various pain syndromes.

PRECAUTIONS AND ADVERSE REACTIONS

Lamotrigine is remarkably well tolerated. The absence of sedation, weight gain, and other metabolic effects is noteworthy. The most common adverse effects—dizziness, ataxia, somnolence, headache, diplopia, blurred vision, and nausea—are typically mild. Anecdotal reports of cognitive impairment and joint or back pain are common.

The appearance of a rash, which is common and occasionally very severe, is a source of concern. About 8% of patients started on lamotrigine develop a benign maculopapular rash during the first 4 months of treatment, and the drug should be discontinued if a rash develops. Even though these rashes are benign, there is concern that in some cases, they may represent early manifestations of Stevens–Johnson syndrome or toxic epidermal necrolysis. Nevertheless, even if lamotrigine is discontinued immediately upon development of rash or other signs of hypersensitivity reaction, such as fever and lymphadenopathy, this may not prevent subsequent development of a life-threatening rash or permanent disfiguration.

Estimates of the rate of serious rash vary, depending on the source of the data. In some studies, the incidence of serious rashes was 0.08% in adult patients receiving lamotrigine as initial monotherapy and 0.13% in adult patients receiving lamotrigine as adjunctive therapy. German registry data, based on clinical practice, suggest that the risk of rash may be as low as 1 in 5,000 patients. If a rash occurs the patient should be told to hold the next dose and contact their physician or go to an emergency room to be evaluated. Ideally, the patient should be evaluated by a dermatologist to determine if the rash is drug related, or potentially serious. Characteristics of potentially serious rashes typically include confluent and widespread purpuric and tender lesions, with involvement of the neck or upper trunk, possible involvement of the eyes, ears and mouth, fever, pharyngitis, anorexia and lymphadenopathy. Given that this is a systemic reaction there is likely to be abnormal lab values. Patients who develop serious rashes should not be rechallenged. If on the other hand the rash is felt to be nondrug related or benign, it should be treated with a dose reduction, delay of any planned dose increases, treatment with antihistamines and or corticosteroids. Any rechallenge should be considered after a careful risk-benefit analysis. Patients who develop a serious rash should not be restarted on lamotrigine.

It is known that the likelihood of a rash increases if the recommended starting dose and speed of dose increase exceed what is recommended. Concomitant administration of valproic acid also increases risk and should be avoided if possible. If valproate is used, a more conservative dosing regimen is followed. Children and adolescents younger than age 16 years appear to be more susceptible to rash with lamotrigine. If patients miss more than 4 consecutive days of lamotrigine treatment, they need to restart therapy at the initial starting dose and titrate upward as if they had not already been on the medication.

USE IN PREGNANCY AND LACTATION

Lamotrigine has a large pregnancy registry, which supports research data that lamotrigine is not associated with congenital malformations in humans. Breastfeeding during lamotrigine treatment does not appear to adversely affect neonatal development.

LABORATORY TESTING

There is no proven correlation between lamotrigine blood concentrations and either antiseizure effects or efficacy in bipolar disorders. Laboratory tests are not useful in predicting the occurrence of adverse events.

Table 17-1
Lamotrigine Dosing (mg/day)

Treatment	Weeks 1-2	Weeks 3-4	Weeks 4-5
Lamotrigine monotherapy	25	50	100–200 (500 maximum)
Lamotrigine + carbamazepine	50	100	200–500 (700 maximum)
Lamotrigine + valproate	25 every other day	25	50–200 (200 maximum)

DRUG INTERACTIONS

Lamotrigine has significant, well-characterized drug interactions involving other anticonvulsants. The most potentially serious lamotrigine drug interaction involves concurrent use of valproic acid, which doubles serum lamotrigine concentrations. Lamotrigine decreases the plasma concentration of valproic acid by 25%. Sertraline (Zoloft) also increases plasma lamotrigine concentrations but to a lesser extent than does valproic acid. Lamotrigine concentrations are decreased by 40% to 50% with concomitant administration of carbamazepine, phenytoin, or phenobarbital. Combinations of lamotrigine and other anticonvulsants have complex effects on the time of peak plasma concentration and the plasma half-life of lamotrigine.

LABORATORY INTERFERENCES

Lamotrigine and topiramate do not interfere with any laboratory tests.

DOSAGE AND ADMINISTRATION

In the clinical trials leading to the approval of lamotrigine as a treatment for bipolar disorder, no consistent increase in efficacy was associated with doses above 200 mg per day. Most patients should take between 100 and 200 mg a day. In epilepsy, the drug is administered twice daily, but in bipolar disorder, the total dose can be taken once a day, either in the morning or night, depending on whether the patient finds the drug activating or sedating.

Lamotrigine is available as unscored 25-, 100-, 150-, and 200-mg tablets. The major determinant of lamotrigine dosing is minimization of the risk of rash. Lamotrigine should not be taken by anyone younger than the age of 16 years. Because valproic acid markedly slows the elimination of lamotrigine, concomitant administration of these two drugs necessitates a much slower titration (Table 17–1). People with renal insufficiency should aim for a lower maintenance dosage. Appearance of any type of rash necessitates immediate discontinuation of lamotrigine administration. Lamotrigine should usually be discontinued gradually over 2 weeks unless a rash emerges, in which case it should be discontinued over 1 to 2 days.

Lamotrigine orally disintegrating tablets (Lamictal ODT) are available for patients who have difficulty swallowing. It is the only antiepileptic treatment that is available in an orally disintegrating formulation. It is available in 25-, 50-, 100-, and 200-mg strengths and matches the dose of lamotrigine tablets. Chewable dispersible tablets of 2, 5, and 25 mg are also available.

18 Lithium

INTRODUCTION

John Cade, an Australian psychiatrist was the first person to treat a patient with lithium and observe its unequivocal beneficial effects in previously chronically manic patients. Clinical observations, and associated and systematic clinical trials, subsequently led to its approval by most regulatory agencies for the treatment of mania. In the United States, it was not approved for the treatment of mania until 1970, due to concerns about toxicity. The only other approved indication came in 1974, for maintenance therapy in bipolar patients with a history of mania.

Lithium use increased gradually in the late 1960s. It was not until 1970 that the Food and Drug Administration (FDA) approved its labeling for the treatment of mania. The only other approved FDA indication came in 1974 when it was accepted as maintenance therapy in patients with a history of mania. For several decades, lithium was the only drug approved for both acute and maintenance treatment. It is also used as an adjunctive medication in the treatment of major depressive disorder.

Lithium has neurotropic and neuroprotective activity that may extend its spectrum of use beyond bipolar disorder. For example, it has been shown to stimulate neurogenesis in adult rat hippocampus, and to increase total brain gray matter volume (by 3%) in 8 of 10 bipolar patients after 4 weeks of treatment.

Lithium (Li), a monovalent ion, is a member of the group IA alkali metals on the periodic table, a group that also includes sodium, potassium, rubidium, cesium, and francium. Lithium exists in nature as both ^6Li (7.42%) and ^7Li (92.58%). The latter isotope allows the imaging of lithium by magnetic resonance spectroscopy. Some 300 mg of lithium is contained in 1,597 mg of lithium carbonate (Li_2CO_3). Most lithium used in the United States is obtained from dry lake mining in Chile and Argentina.

PHARMACOLOGIC ACTIONS

Lithium is rapidly and completely absorbed after oral administration, with peak serum concentrations occurring in 1 to 1.5 hours with standard preparations and in 4 to 4.5 hours with slow- and controlled-release preparations. Lithium does not bind to plasma proteins, is not metabolized, and is excreted through the kidneys. The plasma half-life is initially 1.3 days and is 2.4 days after administration for more than 1 year. The blood–brain barrier permits only slow passage of lithium, which is why a single overdose does not necessarily cause toxicity and why long-term lithium intoxication is slow to resolve. The elimination half-life of lithium is 18 to 24 hours in young adults but is shorter in children and longer in elderly persons. Renal clearance of lithium is decreased with renal insufficiency. Equilibrium is reached after 5 to 7 days of regular intake. Obesity is associated with higher rates of lithium clearance.

The excretion of lithium is complex during pregnancy; excretion increases during pregnancy but decreases after delivery. Lithium is excreted in breast milk and in insignificant amounts in the feces and sweat. Thyroid and renal concentrations of lithium are higher than serum levels.

An explanation for the mood-stabilizing effects of lithium remains elusive. Theories include alterations of ion transport and effects on neurotransmitters and neuropeptides, signal transduction pathways, and second messenger systems.

THERAPEUTIC INDICATIONS
Bipolar I Disorder
Manic Episodes. Lithium controls acute mania and prevents relapse in about 80% of persons with bipolar I disorder and in a somewhat smaller percentage of persons with mixed (mania and depression) episodes, rapid cycling bipolar disorder, or mood changes in encephalopathy. Lithium has a relatively slow onset of action when used and exerts its antimanic effects over 1 to 3 weeks. Thus, a benzodiazepine, dopamine receptor antagonist (DRA), serotonin–dopamine antagonist (SDA), or valproic acid is usually administered for the first few weeks. Patients with mixed or dysphoric mania, rapid cycling, comorbid substance abuse, or organicity respond less well to lithium than those with classic mania.

Bipolar Depression. Lithium has been shown to be effective in the treatment of depression associated with bipolar I disorder, as well as in the role of add-on therapy for patients with severe major depressive disorder. Augmentation of lithium therapy with valproic acid (Depakene) or carbamazepine (Tegretol) is usually well tolerated, with little risk of precipitation of mania.

When a depressive episode occurs in a person taking maintenance lithium, the differential diagnosis should include lithium-induced hypothyroidism, substance abuse, and lack of compliance with the lithium therapy. Possible treatment approaches include increasing the lithium concentration (up to 1 to 1.2 mEq/L), adding supplemental thyroid hormone (e.g., 25 μg a day of liothyronine [Cytomel]) even in the presence of normal findings on thyroid function tests, augmentation with valproate or carbamazepine, the judicious use of antidepressants, or electroconvulsive therapy (ECT). After the acute depressive episode resolves, other therapies should be tapered off in favor of lithium monotherapy, if clinically tolerated.

Maintenance. Maintenance treatment with lithium markedly decreases the frequency, severity, and duration of manic and depressive episodes in persons with bipolar I disorder. Lithium provides relatively more effective prophylaxis for mania than for depression, and supplemental antidepressant strategies may be necessary either intermittently or continuously. Lithium maintenance is almost always indicated after the first episode of bipolar I disorder, depression or mania, and should be considered after the first episode for adolescents or for persons who have a family history of bipolar I disorder. Others who benefit from lithium maintenance are those who have poor support systems, had no precipitating factors for the first episode, have a high suicide risk, had a sudden onset of the first episode, or had a first episode of mania. Clinical studies have shown that lithium reduces the incidence of suicide in bipolar I disorder patients six- or sevenfold. Lithium is also an effective treatment for persons with severe cyclothymic disorder.

Initiating maintenance therapy after the first manic episode is considered a wise approach based on several observations. First, each episode of mania increases the risk of subsequent episodes. Second, among people responsive to lithium, relapses are 28 times more likely after lithium use is discontinued. Third, case reports describe persons who initially responded to lithium, discontinued taking it, and then had a relapse but no longer responded to lithium in subsequent episodes. Continued maintenance treatment with lithium is often associated with increasing efficacy and reducing mortality. Therefore, an episode of depression or mania that occurs after a relatively short time of lithium maintenance does not necessarily represent treatment failure. However, lithium treatment alone may begin to lose its effectiveness after several years of successful use. If this occurs, then supplemental treatment with carbamazepine or valproate may be useful.

Maintenance lithium dosages can often be adjusted to achieve plasma concentration somewhat lower than that needed for treatment of acute mania. If lithium use is to be discontinued, then the dosage should be slowly tapered. Abrupt discontinuation of lithium therapy is associated with an increased risk of recurrence of manic and depressive episodes.

Major Depressive Disorder

Lithium is effective in the long-term treatment of major depression but is not more effective than antidepressant drugs. The most common role for lithium in major depressive disorder is as an adjuvant to antidepressant use in persons who have failed to respond to the antidepressants alone. About 50% to 60% of antidepressant nonresponders do respond when lithium, 300 mg three times daily, is added to the antidepressant regimen. In some cases, a response may be seen within days, but most often, several weeks are required to see the efficacy of the regimen. Lithium alone may effectively treat depressed persons who have bipolar I disorder but have not yet had their first manic episode. Lithium has been reported to be effective in persons with major depressive disorder whose disorder has a particularly marked cyclicity.

Schizoaffective Disorder and Schizophrenia

Persons with prominent mood symptoms—either bipolar type or depressive type—with schizoaffective disorder are more likely to respond to lithium than those with predominant psychotic symptoms. Although SDAs and DRAs are the treatments of choice for persons with schizoaffective disorder, lithium is a useful augmentation agent. This is particularly true for persons whose symptoms are resistant to treatment with SDAs and DRAs. Lithium augmentation of an SDA or DRA treatment may be an effective treatment for persons with schizoaffective disorder even in the absence of a prominent mood disorder component. Some persons with schizophrenia who cannot take antipsychotic drugs may benefit from lithium treatment alone.

Other Indications

Over the years, reports have appeared about the use of lithium to treat a wide range of other psychiatric and nonpsychiatric conditions (Tables 18–1 and 18–2). The effectiveness and safety of lithium for most of these disorders have not been confirmed. Lithium has antiaggressive activity that is separate from its effects on mood.

Table 18–1
Psychiatric Uses of Lithium

Historical
  Gouty mania
Well established (FDA approved)
  Manic episode
  Maintenance therapy
Reasonably well established
  Bipolar I disorder
    Depressive episode
  Bipolar II disorder
    Rapid cycling bipolar I disorder
    Cyclothymic disorder
  Major depressive disorder
    Acute depression (as an augmenting agent)
    Maintenance therapy
  Schizoaffective disorder
Evidence of benefit in particular groups
  Schizophrenia
  Aggression (episodic), explosive behavior, and self-mutilation
    Conduct disorder in children and adolescents
    Mental retardation
    Cognitive disorders
    Prisoners
Anecdotal, controversial, unresolved, or doubtful
  Alcohol and other substance-related disorders
    Cocaine abuse
    Substance-induced mood disorder with manic features
Obsessive-compulsive disorder
Phobias
Posttraumatic stress disorder
ADHD
Eating disorders
Anorexia nervosa
Bulimia nervosa
Impulse-control disorders
Kleine–Levin syndrome
Mental disorders caused by a general medical condition (e.g., mood disorder caused by a
  general medical condition with manic features)
Periodic catatonia
Periodic hypersomnia
Personality disorders (e.g., antisocial, borderline, emotionally unstable, schizotypal)
Premenstrual dysphoric disorder
Sexual disorders
Transvestism
Exhibitionism
Pathologic hypersexuality

FDA, Food and Drug Administration; ADHD, attention-deficit/hyperactivity disorder.

Aggressive outbursts in persons with schizophrenia, violent prison inmates, and children with conduct disorder and aggression, or self-mutilation in persons with mental retardation can sometimes be controlled with lithium.

PRECAUTIONS AND ADVERSE EFFECTS

More than 80% of patients taking lithium experience side effects. It is important to minimize the risk of adverse events through monitoring of lithium blood

Table 18-2
Nonpsychiatric Uses of Lithium^{*a*}

Historical
  Gout and other uric acid diatheses
  Lithium bromide as anticonvulsant
Neurologic
  Epilepsy
  Headache (chronic cluster, hypnic, migraine, particularly cyclic)
  Ménière's disease (not supported by controlled studies)
  Movement disorders
  Huntington's disease
  L-Dopa–induced hyperkinesias
  On–off phenomenon in Parkinson's disease (controlled study found decreased akinesia but development of dyskinesia in a few cases)
  Spasmodic torticollis
  Tardive dyskinesia (not supported by controlled studies, and pseudoparkinsonism has been reported)
  Tourette's disorder
  Pain (facial pain syndrome, painful shoulder syndrome, fibromyalgia)
  Periodic paralysis (hypokalemic and hypermagnesic but not hyperkalemic)
Hematologic
  Aplastic anemia
  Cancer—chemotherapy induced, radiotherapy induced
  Neutropenia (one study found increased risk of sudden death in patients with pre-existing cardiovascular disorder)
  Drug-induced neutropenia (e.g., from carbamazepine, antipsychotics, immunosuppressives, and zidovudine)
  Felty's syndrome
  Leukemia
Endocrine
  Thyroid cancer as an adjunct to radioactive iodine
  Thyrotoxicosis
  Syndrome of inappropriate antidiuretic hormone secretion
Cardiovascular
  Antiarrhythmic agent (animal data only)
Dermatologic
  Genital herpes (controlled studies support topical and oral use)
  Eczematoid dermatitis
  Seborrheic dermatitis (controlled study supports)
Gastrointestinal
  Cyclic vomiting
  Gastric ulcers
  Pancreatic cholera
  Ulcerative colitis
Respiratory
  Asthma (controlled study did not support)
  Cystic fibrosis
Other
  Bovine spastic paresis

^{*a*}All the uses listed here are experimental and do not have Food and Drug Administration (FDA)-approved labeling. There are conflicting reports about many of these uses—some have negative findings in controlled studies, and a few involve reports of possible adverse effects.
L-Dopa, levodopa.

levels and to use appropriate pharmacologic interventions to counteract unwanted effects when they occur. The most common adverse effects are summarized in Table 18–3. Patient education can play an important role in reducing the incidence and severity of side effects. Patients taking lithium should be advised that changes

Table 18–3
Adverse Effects of Lithium

Neurologic
  Benign, nontoxic: dysphoria, lack of spontaneity, slowed reaction time, memory difficulties
  Tremor: postural, occasional extrapyramidal
  Toxic: coarse tremor, dysarthria, ataxia, neuromuscular irritability, seizures, coma, death
  Miscellaneous: peripheral neuropathy, benign intracranial hypertension, myasthenia gravis–like
    syndrome, altered creativity, lowered seizure threshold
Endocrine
  Thyroid: goiter, hypothyroidism, exophthalmos, hyperthyroidism (rare)
  Parathyroid: hyperparathyroidism, adenoma
Cardiovascular
  Benign T-wave changes, sinus node dysfunction
Renal
  Concentrating defect, morphologic changes, polyuria (nephrogenic diabetes insipidus), reduced
    GFR, nephrotic syndrome, renal tubular acidosis
Dermatologic
  Acne, hair loss, psoriasis, rash
Gastrointestinal
  Appetite loss, nausea, vomiting, diarrhea
Miscellaneous
  Altered carbohydrate metabolism, weight gain, fluid retention

GFR, glomerular filtration rate.

in the body's water and salt content can affect the amount of lithium excreted, resulting in either increases or decreases in lithium concentrations. Excessive sodium intake (e.g., a dramatic dietary change) lowers lithium concentrations. Conversely, too little sodium (e.g., fad diets) can lead to potentially toxic concentrations of lithium. Decreases in body fluid (e.g., excessive perspiration) can lead to dehydration and lithium intoxication. Patients should report whenever medications are prescribed by another clinician because many commonly used agents can affect lithium concentrations.

Cardiac Effects

Lithium can cause diffuse slowing, widening of frequency spectrum, potentiation and disorganization of background rhythm on electrocardiograms (EKGs). Bradycardia and cardiac arrhythmias may occur, especially in people with cardiovascular disease. Lithium infrequently reveals Brugada syndrome, an inherited, life-threatening heart problem that some people may have without knowing it. It can cause a serious abnormal heartbeat and other symptoms (such as severe dizziness, fainting, shortness of breath) that need medical attention right away. Before starting lithium treatment, clinicians should ask about known heart conditions, unexplained fainting, and family history of problems or sudden unexplained death before age 45.

Gastrointestinal Effects

Gastrointestinal (GI) symptoms—which include nausea, decreased appetite, vomiting, and diarrhea—can be diminished by dividing the dosage, administering the lithium with food, or switching to another lithium preparation. The lithium preparation least likely to cause diarrhea is lithium citrate. Some lithium preparations contain lactose, which can cause diarrhea in lactose-intolerant persons. Persons taking slow-release formulations of lithium who experience diarrhea caused by unabsorbed medication in the lower part of the GI tract may experience less diarrhea than with standard-release preparations. Diarrhea may also respond to antidiarrheal preparations such as loperamide (Imodium, Kaopectate), bismuth subsalicylate (Pepto-Bismol), or diphenoxylate with atropine (Lomotil).

Weight Gain
Weight gain results from a poorly understood effect of lithium on carbohydrate metabolism. Weight gain can also result from lithium-induced hypothyroidism, lithium-induced edema, or excessive consumption of soft drinks and juices to quench lithium-induced thirst.

Neurologic Effects
Tremor. A lithium-induced postural tremor may occur that is usually 8 to 12 Hz and is most notable in outstretched hands, especially in the fingers, and during tasks involving fine manipulations. The tremor can be reduced by dividing the daily dosage, using a sustained-release formulation, reducing caffeine intake, reassessing the concomitant use of other medicines, and treating comorbid anxiety. β-Adrenergic receptor antagonists, such as propranolol, 30 to 120 mg a day in divided doses, and primidone (Mysoline), 50 to 250 mg a day, are usually effective in reducing the tremor. In persons with hypokalemia, potassium supplementation may improve the tremor. When a person taking lithium has a severe tremor, the possibility of lithium toxicity should be suspected and evaluated.

Cognitive Effects. Lithium use has been associated with dysphoria, lack of spontaneity, slowed reaction times, and impaired memory. The presence of these symptoms should be noted carefully because they are a frequent cause of noncompliance. The differential diagnosis for such symptoms should include depressive disorders, hypothyroidism, hypercalcemia, other illnesses, and other drugs. Some, but not all, persons have reported that fatigue and mild cognitive impairment decrease with time.

Other Neurologic Effects. Uncommon neurologic adverse effects include symptoms of mild parkinsonism, ataxia, and dysarthria, although the last two symptoms may also be attributable to lithium intoxication. Lithium is rarely associated with the development of peripheral neuropathy, benign intracranial hypertension (pseudotumor cerebri), findings resembling myasthenia gravis, and increased risk of seizures.

Renal Effect
The most common adverse renal effect of lithium is polyuria with secondary polydipsia. The symptom is particularly a problem in 25% to 35% of persons taking lithium who may have a urine output of more than 3 L a day (reference range: 1 to 2 L a day). The polyuria primarily results from lithium antagonism to the effects of antidiuretic hormone, which thus causes diuresis. When polyuria is a significant problem, the person's renal function should be evaluated and followed up with 24-hour urine collections for creatinine clearance determinations. Treatment consists of fluid replacement, the use of the lowest effective dosage of lithium, and single daily dosing of lithium. Treatment can also involve the use of a thiazide or potassium-sparing

diuretic—for example, amiloride (Midamor), spironolactone (Aldactone), triamterene (Dyrenium), or amiloride–hydrochlorothiazide (Moduretic). If treatment with a diuretic is initiated, the lithium dosage should be halved, and the diuretic should not be started for 5 days because the diuretic is likely to increase lithium retention.

The most serious renal adverse effects, which are rare and associated with continuous lithium administration for 10 years or more, involve appearance of nonspecific interstitial fibrosis, associated with gradual decreases in glomerular filtration rate and increases in serum creatinine concentrations, and rarely with renal failure. Lithium is occasionally associated with nephrotic syndrome and features of distal renal tubular acidosis. Another pathologic finding in patients with lithium nephropathy is the presence of microcysts. Magnetic resonance imaging (MRI) can be used to demonstrate renal microcysts secondary to chronic lithium nephropathy and therefore avoid renal biopsy. It is prudent for persons taking lithium to check their serum creatinine concentration, urine chemistries, and 24-hour urine volume at 6-month intervals. If creatinine levels do rise, then more frequent monitoring and MRI might be considered.

Thyroid Effects

Lithium causes a generally benign and often transient diminution in the concentrations of circulating thyroid hormones. Reports have attributed goiter (5% of persons), benign reversible exophthalmos, hyperthyroidism, and hypothyroidism (7% to 10% of persons) to lithium treatment. Lithium-induced hypothyroidism is more common in women (14%) than in men (4.5%). Women are at highest risk during the first 2 years of treatment. Persons taking lithium to treat bipolar disorder are twice as likely to develop hypothyroidism if they develop rapid cycling. About 50% of persons receiving long-term lithium treatment have laboratory abnormalities, such as an abnormal thyrotropin-releasing hormone response, and about 30% have elevated concentrations of thyroid-stimulating hormone (TSH). If symptoms of hypothyroidism are present, replacement with levothyroxine (Synthroid) is indicated. Even in the absence of hypothyroid symptoms, some clinicians treat persons with significantly elevated TSH concentrations with levothyroxine. In lithium-treated persons, TSH concentrations should be measured every 6 to 12 months. Lithium-induced hypothyroidism should be considered when evaluating depressive episodes that emerge during lithium therapy.

Cardiac Effects

The cardiac effects of lithium resemble those of hypokalemia on the EKG. They are caused by the displacement of intracellular potassium by the lithium ion. The most common changes on the EKG are T-wave flattening or inversion. The changes are benign and disappear after lithium is excreted from the body.

Lithium depresses the pacemaking activity of the sinus node, sometimes resulting in sinus dysrhythmias, heart block, and episodes of syncope. Lithium treatment, therefore, is contraindicated in persons with sick sinus syndrome. In rare cases, ventricular arrhythmias and congestive heart failure have been associated with lithium therapy. Lithium cardiotoxicity is more prevalent in persons on a low-salt diet, those taking certain diuretics or angiotensin-converting enzyme inhibitors (ACEIs), and those with fluid–electrolyte imbalances or any renal insufficiency.

Dermatologic Effects

Dermatologic effects may be dose dependent. They include acneiform, follicular, and maculopapular eruptions; pretibial ulcerations; and worsening of psoriasis. Occasionally, aggravated psoriasis or acneiform eruptions may force the discontinuation of lithium treatment. Alopecia has also been reported. Persons with many of those conditions respond favorably to changing to another lithium preparation and the usual dermatologic measures. Lithium concentrations should be monitored if tetracycline is used for the treatment of acne because it can increase the retention of lithium.

Lithium Toxicity and Overdoses

The early signs and symptoms of lithium toxicity include neurologic symptoms, such as coarse tremor, dysarthria, and ataxia; GI symptoms; cardiovascular changes; and renal dysfunction. The later signs and symptoms include impaired consciousness, muscular fasciculations, myoclonus, seizures, and coma. Signs and symptoms of lithium toxicity are outlined in Table 18–4. Risk factors include exceeding the recommended dosage, renal impairment, low sodium diet, drug interaction, and dehydration. Elderly persons are more vulnerable to the effects of increased serum lithium concentrations. The greater the degree and duration of elevated lithium concentrations, the worse are the symptoms of lithium toxicity.

Table 18–4
Signs and Symptoms of Lithium Toxicity

1. Mild to moderate intoxication (lithium level, 1.5–2.0 mEq/L)	
GI	Vomiting
	Abdominal pain
	Dryness of mouth
Neurologic	Ataxia
	Dizziness
	Slurred speech
	Nystagmus
	Lethargy or excitement
	Muscle weakness
2. Moderate to severe intoxication (lithium level: 2.0–2.5 mEq/L)	
GI	Anorexia
	Persistent nausea and vomiting
Neurologic	Blurred vision
	Muscle fasciculations
	Clonic limb movements
	Hyperactive deep tendon reflexes
	Choreoathetoid movements
	Convulsions
	Delirium
	Syncope
	Electroencephalographic changes
	Stupor
	Coma
	Circulatory failure (lowered BP, cardiac arrhythmias, and conduction abnormalities)
3. Severe lithium intoxication (lithium level >2.5 mEq/L)	
Generalized convulsions	
Oliguria and renal failure	
Death	

Table 18–5
Management of Lithium Toxicity

1. Contact personal physician or go to a hospital emergency department
2. Lithium should be discontinued
3. Vital signs and a neurologic examination with complete formal mental status examination
4. Lithium level, serum electrolytes, renal function tests, and EKG
5. Emesis, gastric lavage, and absorption with activated charcoal
6. For any patient with a serum lithium level greater than 4.0 mEq/L, hemodialysis

Lithium toxicity is a medical emergency, potentially causing permanent neuronal damage and death. In cases of toxicity (Table 18–5), lithium should be stopped and dehydration treated. Unabsorbed lithium can be removed from the GI tract by ingestion of sodium polystyrene sulfonate (Kayexalate) or polyethylene glycol solution (GoLYTELY), but not activated charcoal. Ingestion of a single large dose may create clumps of medication in the stomach, which can be removed by gastric lavage with a wide-bore tube. The value of forced diuresis is still debated. In severe cases, hemodialysis rapidly removes excessive amounts of serum lithium. Postdialysis serum lithium concentrations may increase as lithium is redistributed from tissues to blood, so repeat dialysis may be needed. Neurologic improvement may lag behind clearance of serum lithium by several days because lithium crosses the blood–brain barrier slowly.

Adolescents
The serum lithium concentrations for adolescents are similar to those for adults. Weight gain and acne associated with lithium use can be particularly troublesome to adolescents.

Elderly Persons
Lithium is a safe and effective drug for elderly persons. However, the treatment of elderly persons taking lithium may be complicated by the presence of other medical illnesses, decreased renal function, special diets that affect lithium clearance, and generally increased sensitivity to lithium. Elderly persons should initially be given low dosages, their dosages should be switched less frequently than those of younger persons, and a longer time must be allowed for renal excretion to equilibrate with absorption before lithium can be assumed to have reached its steady-state concentrations.

Use in Pregnancy and Lactation
Lithium should not be administered to pregnant women in the first trimester because of the risk of birth defects. The most common malformations involve the cardiovascular system, most commonly Ebstein's anomaly of the tricuspid valves. The risk of Ebstein's malformation in lithium-exposed fetuses is 1 in 1,000, which is 20 times the risk in the general population. The possibility of fetal cardiac anomalies can be evaluated with fetal echocardiography. The teratogenic risk of lithium (4% to 12%) is higher than that for the general population (2% to 3%) but appears to be lower than that associated with the use of valproate or carbamazepine. A woman who continues to take lithium during pregnancy should use the lowest effective dosage.

The maternal lithium concentration must be monitored closely during pregnancy and especially after pregnancy because of the significant decrease in renal lithium excretion as renal function returns to normal in the first few days after delivery. Adequate hydration can reduce the risk of lithium toxicity during labor. Lithium prophylaxis is recommended for all women with bipolar disorder as they enter the postpartum period. Lithium is excreted into breast milk and should be taken by a nursing mother only after careful evaluation of potential risks and benefits. Signs of lithium toxicity in infants include lethargy, cyanosis, abnormal reflexes, and sometimes hepatomegaly.

Miscellaneous Effects

Lithium should be used with caution in diabetic persons, who should monitor their blood glucose concentrations carefully to avoid diabetic ketoacidosis. Benign, reversible leukocytosis is commonly associated with lithium treatment. Dehydrated, debilitated, and medically ill persons are most susceptible to adverse effects and toxicity.

DRUG INTERACTIONS

Lithium drug interactions are summarized in Table 18–6.

Lithium is commonly used in conjunction with DRAs. This combination is typically effective and safe. However, coadministration of higher dosages of a DRA and lithium may result in a synergistic increase in the symptoms of lithium-induced neurologic side effects and neuroleptic extrapyramidal symptoms. In rare instances, encephalopathy has been reported with this combination.

The coadministration of lithium and carbamazepine, lamotrigine, valproate, and clonazepam may increase lithium concentrations and aggravate lithium-induced neurologic adverse effects. Treatment with the combination should be initiated at slightly lower dosages than usual, and the dosages should be increased gradually. Changes from one to another treatment for mania should be made carefully, with as little temporal overlap between the drugs as possible.

Most diuretics (e.g., thiazide and potassium sparing) can increase lithium concentrations; when treatment with such diuretics is stopped, the clinician may need to increase the person's daily lithium dosage. Osmotic and loop diuretics, carbonic anhydrase inhibitors, and xanthines (including caffeine) may reduce lithium concentrations to below therapeutic concentrations. Whereas ACEIs may cause an increase in lithium concentrations, the AT_1 angiotensin II receptor inhibitors losartan (Cozaar) and irbesartan (Avapro) do not alter lithium concentrations. A wide range of nonsteroidal anti-inflammatory drugs (NSAIDs) can decrease lithium clearance, thereby increasing lithium concentrations. These drugs include indomethacin (Indocin), phenylbutazone (Azolid), diclofenac (Voltaren), ketoprofen (Orudis), oxyphenbutazone (Oxalid), ibuprofen (Motrin, Advil), piroxicam (Feldene), and naproxen (Naprosyn). Aspirin and sulindac (Clinoril) do not affect lithium concentrations.

The coadministration of lithium and quetiapine (Seroquel) may cause somnolence but is otherwise well tolerated. The coadministration of lithium and ziprasidone (Geodon) may modestly increase the incidence of tremor. The coadministration of lithium and calcium channel inhibitors should be avoided because of potentially fatal neurotoxicity.

Table 18–6
Drug Interactions With Lithium

Drug Class	Reaction
Antipsychotics	Case reports of encephalopathy, worsening of extrapyramidal adverse effects, and neuroleptic malignant syndrome; inconsistent reports of altered red blood cell and plasma concentrations of lithium, antipsychotic drug, or both
Antidepressants	Occasional reports of a serotonin-like syndrome with potent serotonin reuptake inhibitors
Anticonvulsants	No significant pharmacokinetic interactions with carbamazepine or valproate; reports of neurotoxicity with carbamazepine; combinations helpful for treatment resistance
NSAIDs	May reduce renal lithium clearance and increase serum concentration; toxicity reported (exception is aspirin)
Diuretics	
Thiazides	Well-documented reduced renal lithium clearance and increased serum concentration; toxicity reported
Potassium sparing	Limited data; may increase lithium concentration
Loop	Lithium clearance unchanged (some case reports of increased lithium concentration)
Osmotic (mannitol, urea)	Increase renal lithium clearance and decrease lithium concentration
Xanthine (aminophylline, caffeine, theophylline)	Increase renal lithium clearance and decrease lithium concentration
Carbonic anhydrase inhibitors (acetazolamide)	Increase renal lithium clearance
ACEIs	Reports of reduced lithium clearance, increased concentrations, and toxicity
Calcium channel inhibitors	Case reports of neurotoxicity; no consistent pharmacokinetic interactions
Miscellaneous	
Succinylcholine, pancuronium	Reports of prolonged neuromuscular blockade
Metronidazole	Increased lithium concentration
Methyldopa	Few reports of neurotoxicity
Sodium bicarbonate	Increased renal lithium clearance
Iodides	Additive antithyroid effects
Propranolol	Used for lithium tremor; possible slight increase in lithium concentration

NSAID, nonsteroidal anti-inflammatory drug; ACEI, angiotensin-converting enzyme inhibitor.

A person taking lithium who is about to undergo ECT should discontinue taking lithium 2 days before beginning ECT to reduce the risk of delirium.

LABORATORY INTERFERENCES

Lithium does not interfere with any laboratory tests, but lithium-induced alterations include an increased white blood cell count, decreased serum thyroxine, and increased serum calcium. Blood collected in a lithium–heparin anticoagulant tube will produce falsely elevated lithium concentrations.

DOSAGE AND CLINICAL GUIDELINES

Initial Medical Workup

All patients should have a routine laboratory workup and physical examination before being started on lithium. The laboratory tests should include serum creatinine concentration (or a 24-hour urine creatinine if the clinician has any reason to be concerned about renal function), electrolytes, thyroid function (TSH, T_3 [triiodothyronine], and T_4 [thyroxine]), a complete blood count (CBC), EKG, and a pregnancy test in women of childbearing age.

Dosage Recommendations

Lithium formulations include immediate-release 150-, 300-, and 600-mg lithium carbonate capsules (Eskalith and generic), 300-mg lithium carbonate tablets (Lithotabs), 450-mg controlled-release lithium carbonate capsules (Eskalith CR and Lithonate), and 8 mEq/5 mL of lithium citrate syrup.

The starting dosage for most adults is 300 mg of the regular-release formulation three times daily. The starting dosage for elderly persons or persons with renal impairment should be 300 mg once or twice daily. After stabilization, dosages between 900 and 1,200 mg a day usually produce a therapeutic plasma concentration of 0.6 to 1 mEq/L, and a daily dose of 1,200 to 1,800 mg usually produces a therapeutic concentration of 0.8 to 1.2 mEq/L. Maintenance dosing can be given either in two or three divided doses of the regular-release formulation or in a single dosage of the sustained-release formulation equivalent to the combined daily dosage of the regular-release formulation. The use of divided doses reduces gastric upset and avoids single high-peak lithium concentrations. Discontinuation of lithium should be gradual to minimize the risk of early recurrence of mania and to permit recognition of early signs of recurrence.

Laboratory Monitoring

The periodic measurement of serum lithium concentration is an essential aspect of patient care, but it should always be combined with sound clinical judgment. A laboratory report listing the therapeutic range as 0.5 to 1.5 mEq/L may lull a clinician into disregarding early signs of lithium intoxication in patients whose levels are less than 1.5 mEq/L. Clinical toxicity, especially in elderly persons, has been well documented within this so-called therapeutic range.

Regular monitoring of serum lithium concentrations is essential. Lithium levels should be obtained every 2 to 6 months except when there are signs of toxicity, during dosage adjustments, and in persons suspected to be noncompliant with the prescribed dosages. Under these circumstances, levels may be done weekly. Baseline EKGs are essential and should be repeated annually.

When obtaining blood for lithium levels, patients should be at steady-state lithium dosing (usually after 5 days of constant dosing), preferably using a twice- or thrice-daily dosing regimen, and the blood sample must be drawn 12 hours (±30 minutes) after a given dose. Lithium concentrations 12 hours postdose in persons treated with sustained-release preparations are generally about 30% higher than the corresponding concentrations obtained from those taking the regular-release preparations. Because available data are based on a sample population following a multiple-dosage regimen, regular-release formulations given at least twice daily should be used for initial determination of the appropriate dosages. Factors that may cause fluctuations in lithium measurements include dietary sodium intake, mood state, activity level, body position, and use of an improper blood sample tube.

Laboratory values that do not seem to correspond to clinical status may result from the collection of blood in a tube with a lithium–heparin anticoagulant (which can give results falsely elevated by as much as 1 mEq/L) or aging of the lithium ion–selective electrode (which can cause inaccuracies of up to 0.5 mEq/L). After the daily dose has been set, it is reasonable to change to the sustained-release formulation given once daily.

Effective serum concentrations for mania are 1.0 to 1.5 mEq/L, a level associated with 1,800 mg a day. The recommended range for maintenance treatment is 0.4 to 0.8 mEq/L, which is usually achieved with a daily dose of 900 to 1,200 mg. A small number of persons will not achieve therapeutic benefit with a lithium concentration of 1.5 mEq/L, yet will have no signs of toxicity. For such persons, titration of the lithium dosage to achieve a concentration above 1.5 mEq/L may be warranted. Some patients can be maintained at concentrations below 0.4 mEq/L. There may be considerable variation from patient to patient, so it is best to follow the maxim "treat the patient, not the laboratory results." The only way to establish an optimal dose for a patient may be through trial and error.

Table 18–7
Instructions to Patients Taking Lithium

Lithium can be remarkably effective in treating your disorder. If not used appropriately and not monitored closely, it can be ineffective and potentially harmful. It is important to keep the following instructions in mind.

Dosing

Take lithium exactly as directed by your doctor—never take more or less than the prescribed dose. Do not stop taking without speaking to your doctor.

If you miss a dose, take it as soon as possible. If it is within 4 hours of the next dose, skip the missed dose (about 6 hours in the case of extended- or slow-release preparations). Never double up doses.

Blood Tests

Comply with the schedule of recommended regular blood tests.

Despite their inconvenience and discomfort, your lithium blood levels, thyroid function, and kidney status need to be monitored as long as you take lithium.

When going to have lithium levels checked, you should have taken your last lithium dose 12 hours earlier.

Use of Other Medications

Do not start any prescription or over-the-counter medications without telling your doctor.

Even drugs such as ibuprofen (Advil, Motrin) and naproxen (Aleve) can significantly increase lithium levels.

Diet and Fluid Intake

Avoid sudden changes in your diet or fluid intake. If you do go on a diet, your doctor may need to increase the frequency of blood tests.

Caffeine and alcohol act as diuretics and can lower your lithium concentrations.

During treatment with lithium, it is recommended that you drink about 2 or 3 quarts of fluid daily and use normal amounts of salt.

Inform your doctor if you start or stop a low-salt diet.

Recognizing Potential Problems

If you engage in vigorous exercise or have an illness that causes sweating, vomiting, or diarrhea, consult your doctor because these might affect lithium levels.

Nausea, constipation, shakiness, increased thirst, frequency of urination, weight gain, or swelling of the extremities should be reported to your doctor.

Blurred vision, confusion, loss of appetite, diarrhea, vomiting, muscle weakness, lethargy, shakiness, slurred speech, dizziness, loss of balance, inability to urinate, or seizures could indicate severe toxicity and should prompt immediate medical attention.

US package inserts for lithium products list effective serum concentrations for mania between 1.0 and 1.5 mEq/L (usually achieved with 1,800 mg of lithium carbonate daily) and for long-term maintenance between 0.6 and 1.2 mEq/L (usually achieved with 900 to 1,200 mg of lithium carbonate daily). The dose–blood level relationship may vary considerably from patient to patient. The likelihood of achieving a response at levels above 1.5 mEq/L is usually outweighed greatly by the increased risk of toxicity, although rarely a patient may both require and tolerate a higher-than-usual blood concentration.

What constitutes the lower end of the therapeutic range remains a matter of debate. A prospective 3-year study found patients who maintained a concentration between 0.4 and 0.6 mEq/L (mean: 0.54) were 2.6 times more likely to relapse than those who maintained between 0.8 and 1.0 mEq/L (mean: 0.83). However, the higher blood concentrations produced more adverse effects and were less well tolerated.

If there is no response after 2 weeks at a concentration that is beginning to cause adverse effects, then the person should taper off lithium over 1 to 2 weeks and other mood-stabilizing drugs should be tried.

Patient Education

Lithium has a narrow therapeutic index, and many factors can upset the balance between lithium concentrations that are well tolerated and therapeutic, and those that produce side effects or toxicity. It is thus imperative that persons taking lithium be educated about signs and symptoms of toxicity, factors that affect lithium levels, how and when to obtain laboratory testing, and the importance of regular communication with the prescribing physician. Lithium concentrations can be disrupted by common factors such as excessive sweating from ambient heat or exercise or use of widely prescribed agents such as ACEIs or NSAIDs. Patients may stop taking their lithium because they are feeling well or because they are experiencing side effects. They should be advised against discontinuing or modifying their lithium regimen. Table 18–7 lists some important instructions for patients.

19

Melatonin Agonists: Ramelteon, Melatonin, and Suvorexant

INTRODUCTION

Increased attention has been focused upon melatonergic dysfunction as a pathophysiologic mechanism underlying disruptions in the circadian sleep–wake cycle associated with insomnia, depression, and other disorders, and upon melatonergic ligands as pharmacologic agents to not only promote sleep but to normalize circadian rhythmicity.

Ramelteon and melatonin are the only melatonin receptor agonists commercially available in the United States. Melatonin is available as a dietary supplement in various preparations in health food stores, and not under Food and Drug Administration (FDA) regulations. Ramelteon (Rozerem) is an FDA-approved drug for the treatment of insomnia characterized by difficulties with sleep onset.

Also included in this chapter is suvorexant (Belsomra), another drug with a unique mechanism of action that is used to treat insomnia. Suvorexant is a highly selective antagonist for orexin receptors. Orexin is a neuropeptide that promotes wakefulness.

RAMELTEON

Ramelteon (Rozerem) is a melatonin receptor agonist used to treat sleep-onset insomnia. Unlike the benzodiazepines, ramelteon has no appreciable affinity for the γ-aminobutyric acid (GABA) receptor complex.

Pharmacologic Actions

Ramelteon essentially mimics melatonin's sleep-promoting properties and has high affinity for melatonin MT1 and MT2 receptors in the brain. These receptors are believed to be critical in the regulation of the body's sleep–wake cycle.

Ramelteon is rapidly absorbed and eliminated over a dose range of 4 to 64 mg. Maximum plasma concentration (C_{max}) is reached approximately 45 minutes after administration, and the elimination half-life is 1 to 2.6 hours. The total absorption of ramelteon is at least 84%, but extensive first-pass metabolism results in a bioavailability of approximately 2%. Ramelteon is primarily metabolized via the CYP1A2 pathway and principally eliminated in urine. Repeated once-daily dosing does not appear to result in accumulation, likely because of the compound's short half-life.

Therapeutic Indications

Ramelteon was approved by the FDA for the treatment of insomnia characterized by difficulty with sleep onset. Potential off-label usage is centered on use in circadian rhythm disorders, predominantly jet lag, delayed sleep phase syndrome, and shift work sleep disorder.

Clinical trials and animal studies failed to find evidence of rebound insomnia of withdrawal effects.

Precautions and Adverse Events

Headache is the most common side effect of ramelteon. Other adverse effects may include somnolence, fatigue, dizziness, worsening insomnia, depression, nausea, and diarrhea. The drug should not be used in patients with severe hepatic impairment. It is also not recommended in patients with severe sleep apnea or severe chronic obstructive pulmonary disease. Prolactin levels may be increased in women.

Ramelteon has been found to sometimes decrease blood cortisol and testosterone and to increase prolactin. Female patients should be monitored for cessation of menses and of galactorrhea, decreased libido, and fertility problems. The safety and effectiveness of ramelteon in children has not been established.

Use in Pregnancy and Lactation

This drug should only be used in pregnancy if the potential benefit justifies the possible risk to the fetus. It is not known if ramelteon is excreted in human breast milk.

Drug Interactions

CYP1A2 is the major isozyme involved in the hepatic metabolism of ramelteon. Accordingly, fluvoxamine (Luvox) and other CYP1A2 inhibitors may increase side effects of ramelteon.

Ramelteon should be administered with caution in patients taking CYP1A2 inhibitors, strong CYP3A4 inhibitors such as ketoconazole, and strong CYP2C inhibitors such as fluconazole (Diflucan). No clinically meaningful interactions were found when ramelteon was coadministered with omeprazole, theophylline, dextromethorphan, midazolam, digoxin, and warfarin.

Dosing and Clinical Guidelines

The usual dose of ramelteon is 8 mg within 30 minutes of going to bed. It should not be taken with or immediately after high-fat meals.

MELATONIN

Melatonin (*N*-acetyl-5-methoxytryptamine) is a hormone mainly produced at night in the pineal gland. Ingested melatonin has been shown to be capable of reaching and binding to melatonin-binding sites in the brains of mammals and to produce somnolence when used at high doses. Melatonin is available as a dietary supplement and is not a medication. Few well-controlled clinical trials have been conducted to determine its effectiveness in treating such conditions as insomnia, jet lag, and sleep disturbances related to shift work.

Pharmacologic Actions

Melatonin's secretion is stimulated by the dark and inhibited by the light. It is naturally synthesized from the amino acid tryptophan. Tryptophan is converted to serotonin and finally converted to melatonin. The suprachiasmatic nuclei (SCN) of the hypothalamus have melatonin receptors, and melatonin may have a direct action on SCN to influence circadian rhythms. These include jet lag and sleep disturbances.

In addition to the pineal gland, melatonin is also produced in the retina and gastrointestinal tract.

Melatonin has a very short half-life of 0.5 to 6 minutes. Plasma concentrations are a function of the dose administered and the endogenous rhythm. Approximately 90% of melatonin is cleared through first-pass metabolism via the CYP1A1 and CYP1A2 pathways. Elimination occurs principally in urine.

Exogenous melatonin interacts with the melatonin receptors that suppress neuronal firing and promote sleep. There does not appear to be a dose–response relationship between exogenous melatonin administrations and sleep effects.

Therapeutic Indications

Melatonin is not regulated by the FDA. Individuals have used exogenous melatonin to address sleep difficulties (insomnia, circadian rhythm disorders), cancer (breast, prostate, colorectal), seizures, depression, anxiety, and seasonal affective disorder. Some studies suggest that exogenous melatonin may have some antioxidant effects and antiaging properties.

Precautions and Adverse Reactions

Adverse events associated with melatonin include fatigue, dizziness, headache, irritability, and somnolence. Disorientation, confusion, sleepwalking, vivid dreams, and nightmares have also been observed, often with effects resolving after melatonin administration was suspended.

Melatonin may reduce fertility in both men and women. In men, exogenous melatonin reduces sperm motility, and long-term administration has been shown to inhibit testicular aromatase levels. In women, exogenous melatonin may inhibit ovarian function and for that reason has been evaluated as a contraceptive, but with inconclusive results.

Use in Pregnancy and Lactation

Melatonin occurs naturally in the body, so it is considered safe to take during pregnancy. However, there is no good scientific evidence of either its safety or risks. Doses above 3 mg/day should not be used.

Drug Interactions

As a dietary supplement preparation, exogenous melatonin is not regulated by the FDA and has not been subjected to the same type of drug interaction studies that were performed for ramelteon. Caution is suggested in coadministering melatonin with blood thinners (e.g., warfarin [Coumadin], aspirin, and heparin), antiseizure medications, and medications that lower blood pressure.

Laboratory Interference

Melatonin is not known to interfere with any commonly used clinical laboratory tests.

Dosage and Administration

Over-the-counter melatonin is available in the following formulations: 1-, 2.5-, 3-, and 5-mg capsules; 1-mg/4-mL liquid; 0.5- and 3-mg lozenges; 2.5-mg sublingual tablets; and 1-, 2-, and 3-mg timed-release tablets.

Standard recommendations are to take the desired melatonin dose at bedtime, but some evidence from clinical trials suggests that dosing up to 2 hours before habitual bedtime may produce greater improvement in sleep onset.

Agomelatine (Valdoxan)

Agomelatine is structurally related to melatonin and is used in Europe as a treatment of major depressive disorder. It acts as an agonist at melatonin (MT1 and MT2) receptors. It also acts as a serotonin antagonist. Analysis of agomelatine clinical trial data raised serious questions about the efficacy and safety of the drug. The drug is not being marketed in the United States.

SUVOREXANT

The FDA has approved suvorexant to treat insomnia in adults.

Pharmacologic Actions

It is the only available orexin receptor antagonist. It has no effects on the GABAergic system. Although the FDA has determined that suvorexant is effective, it cautions that it may not be safe at the higher doses. The drug is primarily eliminated through the feces, with approximately 66% of the drug recovered in the feces compared to 23% in the urine. The systemic pharmacokinetics of suvorexant are linear with an accumulation of one- to twofold with once-daily dosing. Steady state is achieved by 3 days.

Interactions

There are no serious interactions, but coadministration with strong CYP3A4 inhibitors, including grapefruit juice, is not recommended. Blood levels are increased in obese compared with nonobese patients, and in women compared with men. Particularly in obese women, the increased risk of exposure-related adverse effects should be considered before increasing the dose. Suvorexant will begin to work faster if taken on an empty stomach.

Precautions and Adverse Events

More common side effects include drowsiness, dizziness, headache, unusual dreams, dry mouth, cough, and diarrhea. Some serious side effects include temporary inability to move or speak for up to several minutes while going to sleep or waking up, and temporary leg weakness during the day or at night. Symptoms of overdose typically include extreme drowsiness.

Use in Pregnancy and Lactation

The safety and effectiveness of suvorexant and during pregnancy has not been established.

It is not known if suvorexant is excreted in human breast milk.

Dosing

The recommended starting dose is 10 mg at night within 30 minutes of going to bed, with at least 7 hours of planned sleep time before awakening. The lower doses studied were found to have similar efficacy and better safety. The lowest dose developed,

15 mg, may not be low enough for safe use in some patients. Data suggest that 10 mg may be effective. Less than 10 mg was not studied, but can be tried if the 10 mg dose is effective, but not well tolerated. If the 10 mg dose is well tolerated but not effective, the dose can be increased to 20 mg. Dosage should not exceed 20 mg once a day. No dosage adjustment is required in patients with renal impairment or in patients with mild to moderate hepatic impairment. But the drug is not recommended if hepatic impairment is severe. Suvorexant is available as 5-, 10-, 15- and 20-mg tablets.

INTRODUCTION

Mirtazapine (Remeron) is a drug used to treat major depression that increases both norepinephrine and serotonin without having a significant effect on monoamine uptake (as in the case of tricyclic agents or selective serotonin reuptake inhibitors [SSRIs]) or monoamine oxidase inhibition (as in the case of phenelzine or tranyl-cypromine). Its effects are the result of inhibition of α_2-adrenergic receptors and blockade of postsynaptic serotonin type 2 (5-HT$_2$) and type 3 (5-HT$_3$) receptors.

Mirtazapine is more likely to reduce rather than cause nausea and diarrhea, the result of its effects on the serotonin 5-HT$_3$ receptors. Characteristic side effects include increased appetite and sedation. Its potent antagonist of histamine H$_1$ receptors accounts for its sedative and appetite-enhancing properties. Fifteen to 25% of patients gain an unwanted amount of weight during mirtazapine therapy.

PHARMACOLOGIC ACTIONS

Mirtazapine is administered orally and is rapidly and completely absorbed. It has a half-life of about 30 hours. Peak concentration is achieved within 2 hours of ingestion, and steady state is reached after 6 days. Plasma clearance may be slowed up to 30% in persons with impaired hepatic function, up to 50% in those with impaired renal function, up to 40% slower in elderly men, and up to 10% slower in elderly women.

The mechanism of action of mirtazapine is antagonism of central presynaptic α_2-adrenergic receptors and blockade of postsynaptic serotonin 5-HT$_2$ and 5-HT$_3$ receptors. The α_2-adrenergic receptor antagonism causes increased firing of norepinephrine and serotonin neurons. The potent antagonist of serotonin 5-HT$_2$ and 5-HT$_3$ receptors serves to decrease anxiety, relieve insomnia, and stimulate appetite. Mirtazapine is a potent antagonist of histamine H$_1$ receptors and is a moderately potent antagonist at α_1-adrenergic and muscarinic-cholinergic receptors.

THERAPEUTIC INDICATIONS

Mirtazapine is effective for the treatment of depression. It is highly sedating, making it a reasonable choice for use in depressed patients with severe or long-standing insomnia. Some patients find the residual daytime sedation associated with initiation of treatment to be quite pronounced. However, the more extreme sedating properties of the drug generally lessen over the first week of treatment. Combined with the tendency to cause sometimes a ravenous appetite, mirtazapine is well suited for depressed patients with melancholic features such as insomnia, weight loss, and agitation. Elderly depressed patients in particular are good candidates for mirtazapine; young adults are more likely to object to this side-effect profile.

Mirtazapine's blockade of 5-HT$_3$ receptors, a mechanism associated with medications used to combat the severe gastrointestinal side effects of cancer chemotherapy agents, has led to the use of the drug in a similar role. In this population, sedation and stimulation of appetite clearly could be seen as being beneficial instead of unwelcome side effects.

Mirtazapine is often combined with SSRIs or venlafaxine to augment antidepressant response or counteract serotonergic side effects of those drugs, particularly nausea, agitation, and insomnia. Mirtazapine has no significant pharmacokinetic interactions with other antidepressants.

PRECAUTIONS AND ADVERSE REACTIONS

Somnolence, the most common adverse effect of mirtazapine, occurs in more than 50% of persons (Table 20–1). Persons starting mirtazapine should thus exercise caution when driving or operating dangerous machinery and even when getting out of bed at night. This adverse effect is why mirtazapine is almost always given before sleep. Mirtazapine potentiates the sedative effects of other central nervous system depressants, so potentially sedating prescription or over-the-counter drugs and alcohol should be avoided during use of mirtazapine. Mirtazapine also causes dizziness in 7% of persons. It does not appear to increase the risk for seizures. Mania or hypomania occurred in clinical trials at a rate similar to that of other antidepressant drugs.

Mirtazapine increases appetite and may also increase serum cholesterol concentration to 20% or more above the upper limit of normal in 15% of persons and increase triglycerides to 500 mg/dL or more in 6% of persons. Elevations of alanine transaminase levels to more than three times the upper limit of normal were seen in 2% of mirtazapine-treated persons, as opposed to 0.3% of placebo-controlled subjects.

In limited premarketing experience, the absolute neutrophil count dropped to 500/mm^3 or less within 2 months of the onset of use in 0.3% of persons, some of whom developed symptomatic infections. This hematologic condition was reversible in all cases and was more likely to occur when other risk factors for neutropenia were present. Increases in the frequency of neutropenia have not, however, been reported during the extensive postmarketing period. Persons who develop fever, chills, sore throat, mucous membrane ulceration, or other signs of infection should nevertheless be evaluated medically. If a low white blood cell count is found,

Table 20–1
Adverse Reactions Reported With Mirtazapine Clinical Trials

Event	Percentage (%)
Somnolence	54
Dry mouth	25
Increased appetite	17
Constipation	13
Weight gain	12
Dizziness	7
Myalgias	5
Disturbing dreams	4

mirtazapine should be immediately discontinued, and the infectious disease status should be followed closely.

A small number of persons experience orthostatic hypotension while taking mirtazapine.

USE IN PREGNANCY AND LACTATION

Mirtazapine use by pregnant women has not been studied, so no data exist regarding the effects on fetal development and mirtazapine should be used with caution during pregnancy. Since the drug may be excreted in breast milk, it should not be taken by nursing mothers.

Because of the risk of agranulocytosis associated with mirtazapine use, persons should be attuned to signs of infection. Because of the sedating effects of mirtazapine, persons should determine the degree to which they are affected before engaging in driving or other potentially dangerous activities.

DRUG INTERACTIONS

Mirtazapine can potentiate the sedation of alcohol and benzodiazepines. Mirtazapine should not be used within 14 days of use of a monoamine oxidase inhibitor.

LABORATORY INTERFERENCES

No laboratory interferences have yet been described for mirtazapine.

DOSAGE AND ADMINISTRATION

Mirtazapine is available in 15-, 30-, and 45-mg scored tablets. Mirtazapine is also available in 15-, 30- and 45-mg orally disintegrating tablets for persons who have difficulty swallowing pills. If persons fail to respond to the initial dose of 15 mg of mirtazapine before sleep, the dose may be increased in 15-mg increments every 5 days to a maximum of 45 mg before sleep. Lower dosages may be necessary in elderly persons or persons with renal or hepatic insufficiency.

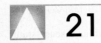

21
Monoamine Oxidase Inhibitors

INTRODUCTION

Monoamine oxidase inhibitors (MAOIs) were the first class of approved antidepressant drugs. Their antidepressant properties were discovered by chance while the drug isoniazid (Marsilid) was being investigated as a treatment for tuberculosis. Some patients treated for tuberculosis experienced elevation of mood during treatment. A subsequent study of psychotically depressed patients showed substantial improvement of symptoms in 70% of those taking the drug. In 1961 isoniazid was withdrawn from the US market because it caused jaundice and hepatotoxicity. Other MAOIs without these side effects were synthesized.

The currently available MAOIs include phenelzine (Nardil), isocarboxazid (Marplan), and tranylcypromine (Parnate). These drugs are irreversible inhibitors of MAO, and are nonselective, inactivating the MAO-A and MAO-B isoforms. Another MAOI, selegiline (Eldepryl), is an irreversible and selective inhibitor of the MAO-B isoform. In its oral form, it is used for the treatment of Parkinson's disease. In a transdermal delivery form (Emsam), it is approved as an antidepressant.

Two other MAOIs should be mentioned. Rasagiline (Azilect), an irreversible MAO-B inhibitor, is used in Parkinson's disease. It has no approved psychiatric indications. Moclobemide (Manerix), a selective reversible inhibitor of MAO-A (RIMA), is approved as an antidepressant in many countries, but not the United States.

Despite the proven effectiveness of phenelzine, isocarboxazid and tranylcypromine, prescription of these drugs as first-line agents has always been limited by concern about the development of potentially lethal hypertension and the consequent need for a restrictive diet. Use of MAOIs declined further after the introduction of the selective serotonin reuptake inhibitors (SSRIs) and other new agents. They are now mainly relegated to use in treatment-resistant cases. Thus, the second-line status of MAOIs has less to do with considerations of efficacy than with concerns for safety.

PHARMACOLOGIC ACTIONS

Phenelzine, tranylcypromine, and isocarboxazid are readily absorbed after oral administration and reach peak plasma concentrations within 2 hours. Whereas their plasma half-lives are in the range of 2 to 3 hours, their tissue half-lives are considerably longer. Because they irreversibly inactivate MAOs, the therapeutic effect of a single dose of irreversible MAOIs may persist for as long as 2 weeks. The RIMA moclobemide is rapidly absorbed and has a half-life of 0.5 to 3.5 hours. Because it is a reversible inhibitor, moclobemide has a much briefer clinical effect after a single dose than do irreversible MAOIs.

The MAO enzymes are found on the outer membranes of mitochondria, where they degrade cytoplasmic and extraneuronal monoamine neurotransmitters such as norepinephrine, serotonin, dopamine, epinephrine, and tyramine. MAOIs act in the central nervous system (CNS), the sympathetic nervous system, the liver, and the gastrointestinal (GI) tract. There are two types of MAOs, MAO_A and MAO_B. MAO_A primarily metabolizes norepinephrine, serotonin, and epinephrine; dopamine and tyramine are metabolized by both MAO_A and MAO_B.

The structures of phenelzine and tranylcypromine are similar to those of amphetamine and have similar pharmacologic effects in that they increase the release of dopamine and norepinephrine with attendant-stimulant effects on the brain.

THERAPEUTIC INDICATIONS

MAOIs are used for treatment of depression. Some research indicates that phenelzine is more effective than tricyclic antidepressants (TCAs) in depressed patients with mood reactivity, extreme sensitivity to interpersonal loss or rejection, prominent anergia, hyperphagia, and hypersomnia—a constellation of symptoms conceptualized as atypical depression. Evidence also suggests that MAOIs are more effective than TCAs as a treatment for bipolar depression.

Patients with panic disorder and social phobia respond well to MAOIs. MAOIs have also been used to treat bulimia nervosa, posttraumatic stress disorder, anginal pain, atypical facial pain, migraine, attention-deficit disorder, idiopathic orthostatic hypotension, and depression associated with traumatic brain injury.

PRECAUTIONS AND ADVERSE REACTIONS

The most frequent adverse effects of MAOIs are orthostatic hypotension, insomnia, weight gain, edema, and sexual dysfunction. Orthostatic hypotension can lead to dizziness and falls. Thus, cautious upward tapering of the dosage should be used to determine the maximum tolerable dosage. Treatment for orthostatic hypotension includes avoidance of caffeine; intake of 2 L of fluid per day; addition of dietary salt or adjustment of antihypertensive drugs (if applicable); support stockings; and in severe cases, treatment with fludrocortisone (Florinef), a mineralocorticoid, 0.1 to 0.2 mg a day. Orthostatic hypotension associated with tranylcypromine use can usually be relieved by dividing the daily dosage.

Insomnia can be treated by dividing the dose, not giving the medication after dinner, and using trazodone (Desyrel) or a benzodiazepine hypnotic if necessary. Weight gain, edema, and sexual dysfunction often do not respond to any treatment and may warrant switching to another agent. When switching from one MAOI to another, the clinician should taper and stop use of the first drug for 10 to 14 days before beginning use of the second drug.

Paresthesias, myoclonus, and muscle pains are occasionally seen in persons treated with MAOIs. Paresthesias may be secondary to MAOI-induced pyridoxine deficiency, which may respond to supplementation with pyridoxine, 50 to 150 mg orally each day. Occasionally, persons complain of feeling drunk or confused, perhaps indicating that the dosage should be reduced and then increased gradually. Reports that the hydrazine MAOIs are associated with hepatotoxic effects are relatively uncommon. MAOIs are less cardiotoxic and less epileptogenic than are the tricyclic and tetracyclic drugs.

The most common adverse effects of the RIMA moclobemide are dizziness, nausea, and insomnia or sleep disturbance. RIMAs cause fewer GI adverse effects than do SSRIs. Moclobemide does not have adverse anticholinergic or cardiovascular effects, and it has not been reported to interfere with sexual function.

MAOIs should be used with caution by persons with renal disease, cardiovascular disease, or hyperthyroidism. MAOIs may alter the dosage of a hypoglycemic agent required by diabetic persons. MAOIs have been particularly associated with induction of mania in persons in the depressed phase of bipolar I disorder and triggering of a psychotic decompensation in persons with schizophrenia.

Use in Pregnancy and Lactation
Little is known about the MAOIs during pregnancy. Data on their teratogenic risk are minimal. MAOIs should not be taken by nursing women because the drugs can pass into the breast milk.

Tyramine-Induced Hypertensive Crisis
The most worrisome side effect of MAOIs is the tyramine-induced hypertensive crisis. The amino acid tyramine is normally transformed via GI metabolism. However, MAOIs inactivate GI metabolism of dietary tyramine, thus allowing intact tyramine to enter the circulation. A hypertensive crisis may subsequently occur as a result of a powerful pressor effect of the amino acid. Tyramine-containing foods should be avoided for 2 weeks after the last dose of an irreversible MAOI to allow resynthesis of adequate concentrations of MAO enzymes.

Accordingly, foods rich in tyramine (Table 21–1) or other sympathomimetic amines, such as ephedrine, pseudoephedrine (Sudafed), or dextromethorphan (Trocal), should be avoided by persons who are taking irreversible MAOIs. Patients should be advised to continue the dietary restrictions for 2 weeks after they stop MAOI treatment to allow the body to resynthesize the enzyme. Bee stings may cause a hypertensive crisis. In addition to severe hypertension, other symptoms may include headache, stiff neck, diaphoresis, nausea, and vomiting. A patient with these symptoms should seek immediate medical treatment.

An MAOI-induced hypertensive crisis should be treated with α-adrenergic antagonists, for example, phentolamine (Regitine) or chlorpromazine (Thorazine). These drugs lower blood pressure within 5 minutes. Intravenous furosemide (Lasix) can be used to reduce fluid load, and a β-adrenergic receptor antagonist can control tachycardia. A sublingual 10-mg dose of nifedipine (Procardia) can be given and repeated after 20 minutes. MAOIs should not be used by persons with thyrotoxicosis or pheochromocytoma.

The risk of tyramine-induced hypertensive crises is relatively low for persons who are taking RIMAs, such as moclobemide and befloxatone. These drugs have relatively little inhibitory activity for MAO_B, and because they are reversible, normal activity of existing MAO_A returns within 16 to 48 hours of the last dose of a RIMA. Therefore, the dietary restrictions are less stringent for RIMAs, applying only to foods containing high concentrations of tyramine, which need be avoided for 3 days

Table 21-1
Tyramine-Rich Foods to Be Avoided in Planning MAOI Diets

High tyramine content[a] (≥2 mg of tyramine a serving)
   Cheese: English Stilton, blue cheese, white (3 years old), extra old, old cheddar, Danish blue,
     mozzarella, cheese snack spreads
   Fish, cured meats, sausage; pâtés and organs: salami: mortadella: air-dried sausage
   Alcoholic beverages[b]: Liqueurs and concentrated after-dinner drinks
   Marmite (concentrated yeast extract)
   Sauerkraut (Krakus)
Moderate tyramine content[a] (0.5–1.99 mg of tyramine a serving)
   Cheese: Swiss Gruyere, muenster, feta, parmesan, gorgonzola, blue cheese dressing, Black
     Diamond
   Fish, cured meats, sausage, pâtés and organs: chicken liver (5 days old): bologna; aged sausage,
     smoked meat; salmon mousse
   Alcoholic beverages: Beer and ale (12 oz per bottle)—Amstel, Export Draft, Blue Light, Guinness
     Extra Stout, Old Vienna, Canadian, Miller Light, Export, Heineken, Blue Wines (per 4-oz glass)—
     Rioja (red wine)
Low tyramine content[a] (0.01 to >0.49 mg of tyramine a serving)
   Cheese: Brie, Camembert, Cambozola with or without rind
   Fish, cured meat, sausage, organs, and pâtés; pickled herring; smoked fish; kielbasa sausage;
     chicken liver; liverwurst (<2 days old)
   Alcoholic beverages: Red wines, sherry, scotch[c]
   Others: Banana or avocado (ripe or not), banana peel

[a]Any food left out to age or spoil can spontaneously develop tyramine through fermentation.
[b]Alcohol can produce profound orthostasis interacting with MAOIs but cannot produce direct hypotensive reactions.
[c]White wines, gin, and vodka have no tyramine content.
Table by Jonathan M. Himmelhoch, MD.
MAOI, monoamine oxidase inhibitor.

after the last dose of a RIMA. A reasonable dietary recommendation for persons taking RIMAs is to avoid eating tyramine-containing foods 1 hour before and 2 hours after taking a RIMA.

Spontaneous, nontyramine-induced hypertensive crisis is a rare occurrence, usually shortly after the first exposure of an MAOI. Persons experiencing such a crisis should avoid MAOIs altogether.

Withdrawal

Abrupt cessation of regular doses of MAOIs may cause a self-limited discontinuation syndrome consisting of arousal, mood disturbances, and somatic symptoms. To avoid these symptoms when discontinuing use of an MAOI, dosages should be gradually tapered over several weeks.

Overdose

There is often an asymptomatic period of 1 to 6 hours after an MAOI overdose before the occurrence of the symptoms of toxicity. MAOI overdose is characterized by agitation that can progress to coma with hyperthermia, hypertension, tachypnea, tachycardia, dilated pupils, and hyperactive deep tendon reflexes. Involuntary movements may be present, particularly in the face and the jaw. Acidification of the urine markedly hastens the excretion of MAOIs, and dialysis can be of some use. Phentolamine or chlorpromazine may be useful if hypertension is a problem. Moclobemide alone in overdosage causes relatively mild and reversible symptoms.

DRUG INTERACTIONS

The major drug–drug and food–drug interactions involving MAOIs are listed in Table 21–2. Most antidepressants as well as precursor agents should be avoided. Persons should be instructed to tell any other physicians or dentists who are treating them that they are taking an MAOI. MAOIs may potentiate the action of CNS depressants, including alcohol and barbiturates. MAOIs should not be coadministered with serotonergic drugs, such as SSRIs and clomipramine (Anafranil), because this combination can trigger a serotonin syndrome. Use of lithium or tryptophan with an irreversible MAOI may also induce a serotonin syndrome. Initial symptoms of a serotonin syndrome can include tremor, hypertonicity, myoclonus, and autonomic signs, which can then progress to hallucinosis, hyperthermia, and even death. Fatal reactions have occurred when MAOIs were combined with meperidine (Demerol) or fentanyl (Sublimaze).

When switching from an irreversible MAOI to any other type of antidepressant drug, persons should wait at least 14 days after the last dose of the MAOI before beginning use of the next drug to allow replenishment of the body's MAOs. When switching from an antidepressant to an irreversible MAOI, persons should wait 10 to 14 days (or 5 weeks for fluoxetine [Prozac]) before starting use of the MAOI to avoid drug–drug interactions. In contrast, MAO activity recovers completely 24 to 48 hours after the last dose of a RIMA.

The effects of the MAOIs on hepatic enzymes are poorly studied. Tranylcypromine inhibits CYP2C19. Moclobemide inhibits CYP2D6, CYP2C19, and CYP1A2 and is a substrate for 2C19.

Cimetidine (Tagamet) and fluoxetine significantly reduce the elimination of moclobemide. Modest doses of fluoxetine and moclobemide administered

Table 21–2
Drugs to Be Avoided During Monoamine Oxidase Inhibitor Treatment (Part of Listing)

Never use
Antiasthmatics
Antihypertensives (methyldopa, guanethidine, reserpine)
Buspirone
Levodopa
Opioids (especially meperidine, dextromethorphan, propoxyphene, tramadol; morphine or codeine may be less dangerous.)
Cold, allergy, or sinus medications containing dextromethorphan or sympathomimetics
SSRIs, clomipramine, venlafaxine, sibutramine
Sympathomimetics (amphetamines, cocaine, methylphenidate, dopamine, epinephrine, norepinephrine, isoproterenol, ephedrine, pseudoephedrine, phenylpropanolamine)
L-Tryptophan
Use carefully
Anticholinergics
Antihistamines
Disulfiram
Bromocriptine
Hydralazine
Sedative-hypnotics
Terpin hydrate with codeine
Tricyclics and tetracyclics (avoid clomipramine)

SSRI, selective serotonin reuptake inhibitor.

concurrently may be well tolerated, with no significant pharmacodynamic or pharmacokinetic interactions.

LABORATORY INTERFERENCES

MAOIs may lower blood glucose concentrations. MAOIs artificially raise urinary metanephrine concentrations and may cause a false-positive test result for pheochromocytoma or neuroblastoma. MAOIs have been reported to be associated with a minimal false elevation in thyroid function test results.

DOSAGE AND CLINICAL GUIDELINES

There is no definitive rationale for choosing one irreversible MAOI over another. Table 21–3 lists MAOI preparations and typical dosages. Phenelzine use should begin with a test dose of 15 mg on the first day. The dosage can be increased to 15 mg three times daily during the first week and increased by 15 mg a day each week thereafter until the dosage of 90 mg a day, in divided doses, is reached by the end of the fourth week. Tranylcypromine and isocarboxazid use should begin with a test dosage of 10 mg and may be increased to 10 mg three times daily by the end of the first week. Many clinicians and researchers have recommended upper limits of 50 mg a day for isocarboxazid and 40 mg a day for tranylcypromine. Administration of tranylcypromine in multiple small daily doses may reduce its hypotensive effects.

Even though coadministration of MAOIs with TCAs, SSRIs, or lithium is generally contraindicated, these combinations have been used successfully and safely to treat patients with refractory depression. However, they should be used with extreme caution.

Hepatic transaminase serum concentrations should be monitored periodically because of the potential for hepatotoxicity, especially with phenelzine and isocarboxazid. Elderly persons may be more sensitive to MAOI adverse effects than are younger adults. MAO activity increases with age, so MAOI dosages for elderly persons are the same as those required for younger adults. The use of MAOIs for children has had minimal study.

Table 21–3
Selectivity, Reversibility, Typical Dosage Forms, and Recommended Dosages for Currently Available Monoamine Oxidase Inhibitors

Drug	Selectivity/ Reversibility	Usual Dose (mg/day)	Maximum Dose (mg/day)	Dosage (Oral) Formulation
Isocarboxazid (Marplan)	MAO-A and MAO-B/ Irreversible	20–40	60	10-mg tablets
Phenelzine (Nardil)	MAO-A and MAO-B/Irreversible	30–60	90	15-mg tablets
Tranylcypromine (Parnate)	MAO-A and MAO-B/Irreversible	20–60	60	10-mg tablets
Rasagiline (Azilect)[a]	MAO-B/Irreversible	0.5–1.0	1.0	0.5- or 1.0-mg tablets
Selegiline (Eldepryl)	MAO-B/Irreversible	10	30	5-mg tablets
Moclobemide (Manerix)[b]	MAO-A/Reversible	300–600	600	100- or 150-mg tablets

[a]Indicated for Parkinson's disease.
[b]Not available in the United States, but indicated for depression in countries where it is available.

Table 21-4
Classification of Monoamine Oxidase Inhibitors

Drug	Reversibility	Selectivity	Indication
Iproniazid[a] (Marsilid)	Irreversible	MAO-A MAO-B	Depression
Isocarboxazid (Marplan)	Irreversible	MAO-A MAO-B	Depression
Phenelzine (Nardil)	Irreversible	MAO-A MAO-B	Depression
Tranylcypromine (Parnate)	Irreversible	MAO-A MAO-B	Depression
Isoniazid (Nydrazid)	Irreversible	MAO-A MAO-B	Antituberculosis
Nialamide[a] (Niamid)	Irreversible	MAO-A MAO-B	Depression
Procarbazine (Matulane)	Weak irreversible	MAO-A MAO-B	Antineoplastic
Clorgyline[b]	Irreversible	MAO-A only	Depression
Selegiline (Deprenyl)	Irreversible	MAO-B only	Depression, Parkinson's disease
Rasagiline (Azilect)	Irreversible	MAO-B only	Parkinson's disease
Pargyline[a] (Eutonyl)	Irreversible	MAO-B only	Antihypertensive
Linezolid	Reversible	MAO-A MAO-B	Antibiotic
Lazabemide[c] (Pakio)	Reversible	MAO-B only	Parkinson's disease
Moclobemide[c] (Aurorix/Manerix)	Reversible	MAO-A only	Depression
Brofaromine[c] (Consonar)	Reversible	MAO-A only	Depression
Befloxatone[c] (Synthelabo)	Reversible	MAO-A only	Depression
Pirlindole[c] (Pirazidol)	Reversible	MAO-A only	Depression
Toloxatone[c] (Humoryl)	Reversible	MAO-A only	Depression

[a]Discontinued.
[b]Used in research only.
[c]Available outside the United States only.
Borrowed from Sadock BJ, Sadock VA, Kaplan HI, eds. *Kaplan & Sadock's Comprehensive Textbook of Psychiatry.* 10th ed. Philadelphia, PA: Lippincott Williams & Wilkins; 2017.

There have been studies that suggest transdermal selegiline has antidepressant properties. Although selegiline is a type B inhibitor at low doses, as the dose is increased, it becomes less selective.

Table 21–4 summarizes the reversibility, selectivity, and indications for MAOIs.

Nefazodone and Trazodone

INTRODUCTION

Mechanistically and structurally related, the drugs nefazodone (Serzone) and trazodone (Desyrel, Oleptro) are approved as treatments for depression. These drugs have differing pharmacologic properties, but they share one clinical activity is presumed to account for their antidepressant effects: antagonism of the 5-hydroxytryptamine, type 2A (5-HT$_{2A}$) receptor.

Trazodone was the first of these drugs to be introduced, in 1981. Because of its generally benign side-effect profile, there were high expectations that it would replace the older drugs as a mainstay of treatment for depression. However, the extreme sedation associated with trazodone, even at subtherapeutic doses, limited the clinical effectiveness of the drug. However, its soporific properties have made trazodone a favorite alternative to standard hypnotics as a sleep-inducing agent. Unlike conventional sleeping pills, trazodone is not a controlled substance. In 2010, the FDA approved an extended-release, once-daily formulation (Oleptro) as a treatment for major depressive disorder (MDD) in adults. In the trial leading to the approval of the extended-release formulation, the most common adverse events were somnolence or sedation, dizziness, constipation, and blurred vision.

Nefazodone is an analog of trazodone. When nefazodone was introduced in 1995, there were expectations that it would become widely used because it did not cause the sexual side effects and sleep disruption associated with the selective serotonin reuptake inhibitors (SSRIs). Although it was devoid of these side effects, it was nevertheless found to produce problematic sedation, nausea, dizziness, and visual disturbances. Consequently, nefazodone was never extensively adopted in clinical practice. This fact, as well as reports of rare cases of sometimes fatal hepatotoxicity, led the original manufacturer to discontinue production of branded nefazodone in 2004. Generic nefazodone remains available in the US market though its clinical utilization continues to decline. Sales of nefazodone in Canada were discontinued in 2003.

NEFAZODONE

Pharmacologic Actions

Nefazodone is rapidly and completely absorbed but is then extensively metabolized so that the bioavailability of active compounds is about 20% of the oral dose. Its half-life is 2 to 4 hours. Steady-state concentrations of nefazodone and its principal active metabolite, hydroxynefazodone, are achieved within 4 to 5 days. Metabolism of nefazodone in elderly persons, especially women, is about half of that seen in younger persons, so lowered doses are recommended for elderly persons. An important metabolite of nefazodone is meta-chlorophenylpiperazine (mCPP), which has some serotonergic effects and may cause migraine, anxiety, and weight loss.

Although nefazodone is an inhibitor of serotonin uptake and, more weakly, of norepinephrine reuptake, its antagonism of serotonin 5-HT$_A$ receptors is thought to produce its antianxiety and antidepressant effects. Nefazodone is also a mild antagonist of the α_1-adrenergic receptors, which predisposes some persons to orthostatic hypotension but is not sufficiently potent to produce priapism.

Therapeutic Indications

Nefazodone is effective for the treatment of major depression. The usual effective dosage is 300 to 600 mg a day. In direct comparison with SSRIs, nefazodone is less likely to cause inhibition of orgasm or decreased sexual desire. Nefazodone is also effective for treatment of panic disorder and panic with comorbid depression or depressive symptoms, generalized anxiety disorder, and premenstrual dysphoric disorder and for management of chronic pain. It is not effective for the treatment of obsessive-compulsive disorder. Nefazodone increases rapid eye movement (REM) sleep and increases sleep continuity. Nefazodone is also of use in patients with post-traumatic stress disorder and chronic fatigue syndrome. It may also be effective in patients who have been treatment-resistant to other antidepressant drugs.

Precautions and Adverse Reactions

The most common reasons for discontinuing nefazodone use are sedation, nausea, dizziness, insomnia, weakness, and agitation. Many patients report no specific side effect but describe a vague sense of feeling medicated. Nefazodone also causes visual trails, in which patients see an afterimage when looking at moving objects or when moving their heads quickly.

A major safety concern with the use of nefazodone is severe elevation of hepatic enzymes, and, in some instances, liver failure. Accordingly, serial hepatic function tests need to be done when patients are treated with nefazodone. Hepatic effects can be seen early in treatment, and are more likely to develop when nefazodone is combined with other drugs metabolized in the liver.

Some patients taking nefazodone may experience a decrease in blood pressure that can cause episodes of postural hypotension. Nefazodone should therefore be used with caution by persons with underlying cardiac conditions or history of stroke or heart attack, dehydration, or hypovolemia or by persons being treated with antihypertensive medications. Patients switched from SSRIs to nefazodone may experience an increase in side effects, possibly because nefazodone does not protect against SSRI withdrawal symptoms. One of its metabolites, mCPP, may actually intensify these discontinuation symptoms. Patients have survived nefazodone overdoses in excess of 10 g, but deaths have been reported when it has been combined with alcohol. Nausea, vomiting, and somnolence are the most common signs of toxicity. The nefazodone dosage should be lowered in persons with severe hepatic disease, but no adjustment is necessary for persons with renal disease (Table 22–1).

Use in Pregnancy and Lactation

The effects of nefazodone in human mothers are not as well understood as those of the SSRIs, mainly due to the paucity of its clinical use. Nefazodone should therefore be used during pregnancy only if the potential benefit to the mother outweighs the

Table 22–1
Adverse Reactions Reported with Nefazodone (300–600 mg a Day)

Reaction	Patients (%)
Headache	36
Dry mouth	25
Somnolence	25
Nausea	22
Dizziness	17
Constipation	14
Insomnia	11
Weakness	11
Lightheadedness	10
Blurred vision	9
Dyspepsia	9
Infection	8
Confusion	7
Scotomata	7

potential risks to the fetus. It is not known whether nefazodone is excreted in human breast milk and should be used with caution by lactating mothers.

Drug Interactions and Laboratory Interferences

Nefazodone should not be given concomitantly with monoamine oxidase inhibitors (MAOIs). In addition, nefazodone has particular drug–drug interactions with the triazolobenzodiazepines, triazolam (Halcion) and alprazolam (Xanax) because of the inhibition of CYP3A4 by nefazodone. Potentially elevated levels of each of these drugs can develop after administration of nefazodone, but the levels of nefazodone are generally not affected. The dose of triazolam should be lowered by 75% and the dose of alprazolam should be lowered by 50% when given concomitantly with nefazodone.

Nefazodone may slow the metabolism of digoxin; therefore, digoxin levels should be monitored carefully in persons taking both medications. Nefazodone also slows the metabolism of haloperidol (Haldol) so that the dosage of haloperidol should be reduced in persons taking both medications. Addition of nefazodone may also exacerbate the adverse effects of lithium carbonate (Eskalith).

There are no known laboratory interferences associated with nefazodone.

Dosage and Clinical Guidelines

Nefazodone is available in 50-, 200-, and 250-mg unscored tablets and 100- and 150-mg scored tablets. The recommended starting dosage of nefazodone is 100 mg twice a day, but 50 mg twice a day may be better tolerated, especially by elderly persons. To limit the development of adverse effects, the dosage should be slowly raised in increments of 100 to 200 mg a day at intervals of no less than 1 week per increase. The optimal dosage is 300 to 600 mg daily in two divided doses. However, some studies report that nefazodone is effective when taken once a day, especially at bedtime. Geriatric persons should receive dosages about two-thirds of the usual nongeriatric dosages, with a maximum of 400 mg a day. Similar to other antidepressants, clinical benefit of nefazodone usually appears after 2 to 4 weeks of treatment. Patients with premenstrual syndrome are treated with a flexible dosage that averages about 250 mg a day.

TRAZODONE

Pharmacologic Actions

Trazodone is readily absorbed from the gastrointestinal tract and reaches peak plasma levels in about 1 hour. It has a half-life of 5 to 9 hours. Trazodone is metabolized in the liver, and 75% of its metabolites are excreted in the urine.

Trazodone is a weak inhibitor of serotonin reuptake and a potent antagonist of serotonin 5-HT$_{2A}$ and 5-HT$_{2C}$ receptors. The active metabolite of trazodone is mCPP, which is an agonist at 5-HT$_{2C}$ receptors and has a half-life of 14 hours. mCPP has been associated with migraine, anxiety, and weight loss. The adverse effects of trazodone are partially mediated by α_1-adrenergic receptor antagonism.

Therapeutic Indications

Depressive Disorders.   The main indication for the use of trazodone is MDD. There is a clear dose–response relationship, with dosages of 250 to 600 mg a day being necessary for trazodone to have therapeutic benefit. Trazodone increases total sleep time, decreases the number and the duration of nighttime awakenings, and decreases the amount of REM sleep. Unlike tricyclic drugs, trazodone does not decrease stage 4 sleep. Trazodone is thus useful for depressed persons with anxiety and insomnia.

Insomnia.   Trazodone is a first-line agent for the treatment of insomnia because of its marked sedative qualities and favorable effects on sleep architecture (see above) combined with its lack of anticholinergic effects. Trazodone is effective for insomnia caused by depression or use of drugs. When used as a hypnotic, the usual initial dosage is 25 to 100 mg at bedtime.

Erectile Disorder.   Trazodone is associated with an increased risk of priapism. Trazodone can potentiate erections resulting from sexual stimulation. It has thus been used to prolong erectile time and turgidity in some men with erectile disorder. The dosage for this indication is 150 to 200 mg a day. Trazodone-triggered priapism (an erection lasting more than 3 hours with pain) is a medical emergency. The use of trazodone for treatment of male erectile dysfunction has diminished considerably since the introduction of phosphodiesterase (PDE)-5 agents (see Chapter 25).

Other Indications.   Trazodone may be useful in low dosages (50 mg a day) for controlling severe agitation in children with developmental disabilities and elderly persons with dementia. At dosages above 250 mg a day, trazodone reduces the tension and apprehension associated with generalized anxiety disorder. It has been used to treat depression in schizophrenia patients. Trazodone may have a beneficial effect on insomnia and nightmares in persons with posttraumatic stress disorder.

Precautions and Adverse Reactions

The most common adverse effects associated with trazodone are sedation, orthostatic hypotension, dizziness, headache, and nausea. Some persons experience dry mouth or gastric irritation. The drug is not associated with anticholinergic adverse effects, such as urinary retention, weight gain, and constipation. A few case reports have noted an association between trazodone and arrhythmias in persons with pre-existing premature ventricular contractions or mitral valve prolapse. Neutropenia, usually not of clinical significance, may develop, which should be considered if persons have fever or sore throat.

Trazodone may cause significant orthostatic hypotension 4 to 6 hours after a dose is taken, especially if taken concurrently with antihypertensive agents or if a large dose is taken without food. Administration of trazodone with food slows absorption and reduces the peak plasma concentration, thus reducing the risk of orthostatic hypotension.

Because suicide attempts often involve ingestion of sleeping pills, it is important to be familiar with the symptoms and treatment of trazodone overdose. Patients have survived trazodone overdoses of more than 9 g. Symptoms of overdose include lethargy, vomiting, drowsiness, headache, orthostasis, dizziness, dyspnea, tinnitus, myalgias, tachycardia, incontinence, shivering, and coma. Treatment consists of emesis or lavage and supportive care. Forced diuresis may enhance elimination. Treat hypotension and sedation as appropriate.

Trazodone causes priapism, prolonged erection in the absence of sexual stimuli, in one of every 10,000 men. Trazodone-induced priapism usually appears in the first 4 weeks of treatment but may occur as late as 18 months into treatment. It can appear at any dose. In such cases, trazodone use should be discontinued, and another antidepressant should be used. Painful erections or erections lasting more than 1 hour are warning signs that warrant immediate discontinuation of the drug and medical evaluation. The first step in the emergency management of priapism is intracavernosal injection of an α_1-adrenergic agonist pressor agent, such as metaraminol (Aramine) or epinephrine. In about one-third of reported cases, surgical intervention was required. In some cases, permanent impairment of erectile function or impotence resulted.

Trazodone should be used with caution in persons with hepatic and renal diseases.

Use in Pregnancy and Lactation
This drug should only be used in pregnancy if the potential benefit justifies the possible risk to the fetus. Very small amounts of trazodone are excreted in human breast milk.

Drug Interactions
Trazodone potentiates the central nervous system depressant effects of other centrally acting drugs and alcohol. Concurrent use of trazodone and antihypertensives may cause hypotension. No cases of hypertensive crisis have been reported when trazodone has been used to treat MAOI-associated insomnia. Trazodone can increase levels of digoxin and phenytoin. Trazodone should be used with caution in combination with warfarin. Drugs that inhibit CYP3A4 can increase levels of trazodone's major metabolite, mCPP, leading to an increase in side effects.

Laboratory Interferences
No known laboratory interferences are associated with the administration of trazodone.

Dosage and Clinical Guidelines
Trazodone is available in 50-, 100-, 150-, and 300-mg tablets. Once-a-day dosing is as effective as divided dosing and reduces daytime sedation. The usual starting dose

is 50 mg before sleep. The dosage can be increased in increments of 50 mg every 3 days if sedation or orthostatic hypotension does not become a problem. The therapeutic range for trazodone is 200 to 600 mg a day in divided doses. Some reports indicate that dosages of 400 to 600 mg a day are required for maximal therapeutic effects; other reports indicate that 250 to 400 mg a day is sufficient. The dosage may be titrated up to 300 mg a day; then the person can be evaluated for the need for further dosage increases on the basis of the presence or the absence of signs of clinical improvement.

Once-daily trazodone is available as bisectable tablets of 150 mg or 300 mg. The starting dosage of the extended-release formulation is 150 mg once daily. It may be increased by 75 mg per day every 3 days. The maximum dosage is 375 mg per day. Dosing should be at the same time every day in the late evening, preferably at bedtime, on an empty stomach. Tablets should be swallowed whole or broken in half along the score line.

23

Opioid Receptor Agonists: Methadone and Buprenorphine

INTRODUCTION

The opioid receptor agonists are the mainstays of pain management. They are a structurally diverse group of compounds also called narcotics. While highly effective as analgesics, they often cause dependence and are frequently diverted for recreational use and rates of death from overdose of opioids has reached epidemic proportions in some parts of the United States.

Commonly used opioid agonists for pain relief include morphine, hydromorphone (Dilaudid), codeine, meperidine (Demerol), oxycodone (OxyContin), buprenorphine (Buprenex), hydrocodone (Robidone), tramadol (Ultram), and fentanyl (Durogesic). Heroin is used as a street drug. Methadone is used both for pain management and for treatment of opiate addiction. The efficacy of opioid agonist medications, such as methadone and buprenorphine, has been clearly established in the treatment of opioid dependence.

It is now recognized that the pharmacology of the opioid system is complex. There are multiple types of opioid receptors, with μ- and κ-opioid receptors representing functionally opposing endogenous systems (Table 23–1). All of the compounds above, which represent the most extensively used narcotic analgesics, are agonists at μ-opioid receptors. However, analgesic and antidepressant effects also result from antagonist effects on the κ-opioid receptor. Buprenorphine has mixed receptor effects, being primarily a μ-opioid receptor agonist as well as κ-opioid antagonist effects. This chapter focuses on the μ-opioid receptor agonists, drugs that are most likely to be used in the treatment of pain management, but κ-opioid receptor antagonism has been shown to have antidepressant activity. A drug that incorporates buprenorphine is in late stages of clinical trials as an antidepressant.

While there is growing interest in the use of some drugs that act on opioid receptors as alternative treatments for a subpopulation of patients with refractory depression, as well as treatment for cutting behavior in patients with borderline personality disorder.

Before using opioid receptor agonists with patients who have failed on multiple conventional therapeutic agents, screen carefully for history of drug abuse, document the rationale for off-label use, establish treatment ground rules, obtain written consent, consult with primary care physician, and monitor closely. Consideration of off-label use should always consider that ongoing, regular use of opioids produces dependence and tolerance and may lead to maladaptive use, functional impairment, and withdrawal symptoms. Avoid replacing "lost" prescriptions and providing early prescription renewals.

Table 23–1
μ- and κ-Opiate Receptors

Receptor	Agonist Effects	Antagonist Effects
Mu (μ)	Analgesia	Anxiety
	Euphoria	Hostility
	Antidepressant	
	Anxiety	
Kappa (κ)	Analgesia	Antidepressant
	Dysphoria	
	Depression	
	Stress-induced anxiety	

PHARMACOLOGIC ACTIONS

Methadone and buprenorphine are absorbed rapidly from the gastrointestinal (GI) tract. Hepatic first-pass metabolism significantly affects the bioavailability of each of the drugs but in markedly different ways. For methadone, hepatic enzymes reduce the bioavailability of an oral dosage by about half, an effect that is easily managed with dosage adjustments.

For buprenorphine, first-pass intestinal and hepatic metabolism eliminates oral bioavailability almost completely. When used in opioid detoxification, buprenorphine is given sublingually in either a liquid or a tablet formulation.

The peak plasma concentrations of oral methadone are reached within 2 to 6 hours, and the plasma half-life initially is 4 to 6 hours in opioid-naive persons and 24 to 36 hours after steady dosing of any type of opioid. Methadone is highly protein bound and equilibrates widely throughout the body, which ensures little postdosage variation in steady-state plasma concentrations. In opioid-naïve patients, methadone can be lethal in relatively small doses.

Elimination of a sublingual dosage of buprenorphine occurs in two phases: an initial phase with a half-life of 3 to 5 hours and a terminal phase with a half-life of more than 24 hours. Buprenorphine dissociates from its receptor binding site slowly, which permits an every-other-day dosing schedule.

Methadone acts as pure agonists at μ-opioid receptors and has negligible agonist or antagonist activity at κ- or δ-opioid receptors. Buprenorphine is a partial agonist at μ-receptors, a potent antagonist at κ-receptors, and neither an agonist nor an antagonist at δ-receptors.

THERAPEUTIC INDICATIONS

Methadone

Methadone is used for short-term detoxification (7 to 30 days), long-term detoxification (up to 180 days), and maintenance (treatment beyond 180 days) of opioid-dependent individuals. For these purposes, it is only available through designated clinics called methadone maintenance treatment programs (MMTPs) and in hospitals and prisons. Methadone is a schedule II drug, which means that its administration is tightly governed by specific federal laws and regulations.

Enrollment in a methadone program reduces the risk of death by 70%; reduces illicit use of opioids and other substances of abuse; reduces criminal activity; reduces the risk of infectious diseases of all types, most importantly HIV and hepatitis B and C infection; and in pregnant women, reduces the risk of fetal and neonatal morbidity and mortality. The use of methadone maintenance frequently requires lifelong treatment.

Some opioid-dependence treatment programs use a stepwise detoxification protocol in which a person addicted to heroin switches first to the strong agonist methadone; then to the weaker agonist buprenorphine; and finally, to maintenance on an opioid receptor antagonist, such as naltrexone (ReVia). This approach minimizes the appearance of opioid withdrawal effects, which, if they occur, are mitigated with clonidine (Catapres). However, compliance with opioid receptor antagonist treatment is poor outside of settings using intensive cognitive-behavioral techniques. In contrast, noncompliance with methadone maintenance precipitates opioid withdrawal symptoms, which serve to reinforce the use of methadone and make cognitive-behavioral therapy less than essential. Thus, some well-motivated, socially integrated former heroin addicts are able to use methadone for years without participation in a psychosocial support program.

Data pooled from many reports indicate that methadone is more effective when taken at dosages in excess of 60 mg a day. The analgesic effects of methadone are sometimes used in the management of chronic pain when less addictive agents are ineffective.

Use Pregnancy and Lactation.   Methadone maintenance, combined with effective psychosocial services and regular obstetric monitoring, significantly improves obstetric and neonatal outcomes for women addicted to heroin. Enrollment of a heroin-addicted pregnant woman in such a maintenance program reduces the risk of malnutrition, infection, preterm labor, spontaneous abortion, preeclampsia, eclampsia, abruptio placenta, and septic thrombophlebitis.

The dosage of methadone during pregnancy should be the lowest effective dosage, and no withdrawal to abstinence should be attempted during pregnancy. Methadone is metabolized more rapidly in the third trimester, which may necessitate higher dosages. To avoid potentially sedating postdose peak plasma concentrations, the daily dose can be administered in two divided doses during the third trimester. Methadone treatment has no known teratogenic effects.

Neonatal Methadone Withdrawal Symptoms.   Withdrawal symptoms in newborns frequently include tremor, a high-pitched cry, increased muscle tone and activity, poor sleep and eating, mottling, yawning, perspiration, and skin excoriation. Convulsions that require aggressive anticonvulsant therapy may also occur. Withdrawal symptoms may be delayed in onset and prolonged in neonates because of their immature hepatic metabolism. Women taking methadone are sometimes counseled to initiate breastfeeding as a means of gently weaning their infants from methadone dependence, but they should not breastfeed their babies while still taking methadone.

Buprenorphine

The analgesic effects of buprenorphine are sometimes used in the management of chronic pain when less addictive agents are ineffective. Because buprenorphine is a partial agonist rather than a full agonist at the μ-receptor and is a weak antagonist at the κ-receptor, this agent produces a milder withdrawal syndrome and has a wider margin of safety than the full μ-agonist compounds generally used in treatment. Buprenorphine has a ceiling effect beyond which dose increases prolong the duration of action of the drug without further increasing the agonist effects. Because of this, buprenorphine has a high clinical safety profile, with limited respiratory depression, therefore decreasing the likelihood of lethal overdose. Buprenorphine does have the capacity to cause typical side effects associated with opioids, including sedation, nausea and vomiting, constipation, dizziness, headache, and sweating. A relevant pharmacokinetic consideration when using buprenorphine is the fact that it requires hepatic conversion to become analgesic (N-dealkylation catalyzed by CYP3A4). This may explain why some patients do not benefit from buprenorphine. Genetics, grapefruit juice, and many medications (including fluoxetine and fluvoxamine) can reduce a person's ability to metabolize buprenorphine into its bioactive form.

To reduce the likelihood of abusing buprenorphine via the intravenous route, buprenorphine has been combined with the narcotic antagonist naloxone for sublingual administration. Because naloxone is poorly absorbed by the sublingual route, when the combination drug is taken sublingually, there is no effect of the naloxone on the efficacy of buprenorphine. If an opioid-dependent individual injects the combination medication, the naloxone precipitates a withdrawal reaction, therefore reducing the likelihood of illicit injection use of the sublingual preparation.

Inducting and stabilizing a patient on buprenorphine is analogous to inducting and stabilizing a patient on methadone except that, as a partial agonist, buprenorphine has the potential to cause precipitated withdrawal in patients who have recently taken full agonist opioids. Thus, a patient must abstain from the use of short-acting opioids for 12 to 24 hours before starting buprenorphine and from longer-acting opioids such as methadone for 24 to 48 hours or longer. The physician must assess the patient clinically and determine that the patient is in mild to moderate opioid withdrawal with objectively observable withdrawal signs before initiating buprenorphine.

In most instances, a relatively low dose of buprenorphine (2 to 4 mg) can then be administered with additional doses given in 1 to 2 hours if withdrawal signs persist. The goal for the first 24 hours is to suppress withdrawal signs and symptoms, and the total 24-hour dose to do so can range from 2 to 16 mg on the first day. In subsequent days, the dose can be adjusted upward or downward to resolve withdrawal fully and, as with methadone, to achieve an absence of craving, adequate tolerance to prevent reinforcement from the use of other opioids, and ultimately abstinence from other opioids while minimizing side effects. Dose-ranging studies have demonstrated that dosages of 6 to 16 mg per day are associated with improved treatment outcomes compared with lower doses of buprenorphine (1 to 4 mg). Sometimes patients seem to need dosages higher than 16 mg per day, although there is no evidence for any benefit of dosages beyond 32 mg per day. For the treatment of opioid dependence, a dose of approximately 4 mg of sublingual buprenorphine is the equivalent of a daily dose of 40 mg of oral methadone. It has also been demonstrated that daily, alternate-day, or three-times-per-week administration have equivalent effects in suppressing the symptoms of opioid withdrawal in dependent individuals. The combination tablet is recommended for most clinical purposes, including induction and maintenance. The buprenorphine mono should be used only for pregnant patients or for patients who have a documented anaphylactic reaction to naloxone.

Newer forms of buprenorphine delivery, including a transdermal skin patch, a long-acting depot intramuscular injection that provides therapeutic plasma levels for several weeks, and subcutaneous buprenorphine implants that may provide thera-peutic plasma levels for 6 months, are being investigated. The last two delivery sys-tems could obviate the need for taking medications daily while virtually eliminating the risk of medication nonadherence.

Tramadol

There are multiple reports of tramadol's antidepressant effects, both as monotherapy and augmentation agent in treatment-resistant depression. Clinical and experimental data suggest that tramadol has an inherent antidepressant-like activity. Tramadol has a complex pharmacology. It is a weak μ-opioid receptor agonist, a 5-HT–releasing agent, a DA-releasing agent, a 5-HT$_{2C}$ receptor antagonist, an NE reuptake inhibi-tor, an NMDA receptor antagonist, a nicotinic acetylcholine receptor antagonist, a TRPV1 receptor agonist, and M1 and M3 muscarinic acetylcholine receptor antago-nists. Consistent with the evidence of its antidepressant effects is the fact that tramadol has a close structural similarity to the antidepressant venlafaxine.

Both venlafaxine and tramadol inhibit norepinephrine/serotonin reuptake, and inhibit the reserpine-induced syndrome completely. Both compounds also have an analgesic effect on chronic pain. Venlafaxine may have an opioid component and naloxone reverses the antipain effect of venlafaxine. Nonopioid activity is demon-strated by the fact that its analgesic effect is not fully antagonized by the μ-opioid receptor antagonist naloxone. Indicative of their structural similarities, venlafaxine may cause false-positive results on liquid chromatography tests to detect urinary tramadol levels.

Other relevant properties of tramadol are its relatively long half-life, which reduces the potential for misuse. Its habituating effects are found to be much less than other opiate agonists, but abuse, withdrawal, and dependence are risks. Trama-dol requires metabolism to become analgesic: individuals who are CYP2D6 "poor metabolizers," or use drugs that are CYP2D6 inhibitors reduce the efficacy of trama-dol (same is true of codeine).

PRECAUTIONS AND ADVERSE REACTIONS

The most common adverse effects of opioid receptor agonists are lightheaded-ness, dizziness, sedation, nausea, constipation, vomiting, perspiration, weight gain, decreased libido, inhibition of orgasm, and insomnia or sleep irregularities. Opioid receptor agonists are capable of inducing tolerance as well as producing physiologic and psychological dependence. Other central nervous system (CNS) adverse effects include depression, sedation, euphoria, dysphoria, agitation, and seizures. Delirium has been reported in rare cases. Occasional non-CNS adverse effects include periph-eral edema, urinary retention, rash, arthralgia, dry mouth, anorexia, biliary tract spasm, bradycardia, hypotension, hypoventilation, syncope, antidiuretic hormone–like activity, pruritus, urticaria, and visual disturbances. Menstrual irregularities are common in women, especially in the first 6 months of use. Various abnormal endo-crine laboratory indexes of little clinical significance may also be seen.

Most persons develop tolerance to the pharmacologic adverse effects of opioid agonists during long-term maintenance, and relatively few adverse effects are expe-rienced after the induction period.

Overdosage

The acute effects of opioid receptor agonist overdosage include sedation, hypotension, bradycardia, hypothermia, respiratory suppression, miosis, and decreased GI motility. Severe effects include coma, cardiac arrest, shock, and death. The risk of overdosage is greatest in the induction stage of treatment and in persons with slow drug metabolism caused by pre-existing hepatic insufficiency. Deaths have been caused during the first week of induction by methadone dosages of only 50 to 60 mg a day.

The risk of overdosage with buprenorphine appears to be lower than with methadone. However, deaths have been caused by use of buprenorphine in combination with benzodiazepines.

Withdrawal Symptoms

Abrupt cessation of methadone use triggers withdrawal symptoms within 3 to 4 days, which usually reach peak intensity on the sixth day. Withdrawal symptoms include weakness, anxiety, anorexia, insomnia, gastric distress, headache, sweating, and hot and cold flashes. The withdrawal symptoms usually resolve after 2 weeks. However, a protracted methadone abstinence syndrome is possible that may include restlessness and insomnia.

The withdrawal symptoms associated with buprenorphine are similar to, but less marked than, those caused by methadone. In particular, buprenorphine is sometimes used to ease the transition from methadone to opioid receptor antagonists or abstinence because of the relatively mild withdrawal reaction associated with discontinuation of buprenorphine.

DRUG–DRUG INTERACTIONS

Opioid receptor agonists can potentiate the CNS-depressant effects of alcohol, barbiturates, benzodiazepines, other opioids, low-potency dopamine receptor antagonists, tricyclic and tetracyclic drugs, and monoamine oxidase inhibitors (MAOIs). Carbamazepine (Tegretol), phenytoin (Dilantin), barbiturates, rifampin (Rimactane, Rifadin), and heavy long-term consumption of alcohol may induce hepatic enzymes, which may lower the plasma concentration of methadone or buprenorphine and thereby precipitate withdrawal symptoms. In contrast, however, hepatic enzyme induction may increase the plasma concentration of active levomethadyl metabolites and cause toxicity.

Acute opioid withdrawal symptoms may be precipitated in persons on methadone maintenance therapy who take pure opioid receptor antagonists such as naltrexone, nalmefene (Revex), and naloxone (Narcan); partial agonists such as buprenorphine; or mixed agonist–antagonists such as pentazocine (Talwin). These symptoms may be mitigated by use of clonidine, a benzodiazepine, or both.

Competitive inhibition of methadone or buprenorphine metabolism after short-term use of alcohol or administration of cimetidine (Tagamet), erythromycin, ketoconazole (Nizoral), fluoxetine (Prozac), fluvoxamine (Luvox), loratadine (Claritin), quinidine (Quinidex), and alprazolam (Xanax) may lead to higher plasma concentrations or a prolonged duration of action of methadone or buprenorphine. Medications that alkalinize the urine may reduce methadone excretion.

Methadone maintenance may also increase plasma concentrations of desipramine (Norpramin, Pertofrane) and fluvoxamine. Use of methadone may increase zidovudine (Retrovir) concentrations, which increases the possibility of zidovudine toxicity at otherwise standard dosages. Moreover, in vitro human liver microsome studies demonstrate competitive inhibition of methadone demethylation by several protease inhibitors, including ritonavir (Norvir), indinavir (Crixivan), and saquinavir (Invirase). The clinical relevance of this finding is unknown.

Fatal drug–drug interactions with the MAOIs are associated with use of the opioids fentanyl (Sublimaze) and meperidine (Demerol), but not with use of methadone, levomethadyl, or buprenorphine.

Tramadol may interact with drugs that inhibit serotonin reuptake. Such combinations can trigger seizures and serotonin syndrome. These events may also develop during tramadol monotherapy, either at routine or excessive doses. Risk of interactions is increased when tramadol is combined with virtually all classes of antidepressants and with drugs that lower the seizure threshold, especially the antidepressant bupropion.

LABORATORY INTERFERENCES

Methadone and buprenorphine can be tested for separately in urine toxicology to distinguish them from other opioids. No known laboratory interferences are associated with the use of methadone or buprenorphine.

DOSAGE AND CLINICAL GUIDELINES
Methadone

Methadone is supplied in 5-, 10-, and 40-mg dispersible scored tablets; 40-mg scored wafers; 5-mg/5-mL, 10-mg/5-mL, and 10-mg/mL solutions; and a 10-mg/mL parenteral form. In maintenance programs, methadone is usually dissolved in water or juice, and dose administration is directly observed to ensure compliance. For induction of opioid detoxification, an initial methadone dose of 15 to 20 mg will usually suppress craving and withdrawal symptoms. However, some individuals may require up to 40 mg a day in single or divided doses. Higher dosages should be avoided during induction of treatment to reduce the risk of acute toxicity from overdosage.

Over several weeks, the dosage should be raised to at least 70 mg a day. The maximum dosage is usually 120 mg a day, and higher dosages require prior approval from regulatory agencies. Dosages above 60 mg a day are associated with much more complete abstinence from use of illicit opioids than are dosages less than 60 mg a day.

The duration of treatment should not be predetermined but should be based on response to treatment and assessment of psychosocial factors. All studies of methadone maintenance programs endorse long-term treatment (i.e., several years) as more effective than short-term programs (i.e., less than 1 year) for prevention of relapse into opioid abuse. In actual practice, however, a minority of programs are permitted by policy or approved by insurers to provide even 6 months of continuous maintenance treatment. Moreover, some programs actually encourage withdrawal from methadone in less than 6 months after induction. This is quite ill conceived because more than 80% of persons who terminate methadone maintenance treatment eventually return to illicit drug use within 2 years. In programs that offer both maintenance and withdrawal treatments, the overwhelming majority of participants enroll in the maintenance treatment.

Buprenorphine

Buprenorphine is supplied as a 0.3-mg/mL solution in 1-mL ampules. Sublingual tablet formulations of buprenorphine containing buprenorphine only or buprenorphine combined with naloxone in a 4:1 ratio are used for opioid maintenance treatment. Buprenorphine is not used for short-term opioid detoxification. Maintenance dosages of 8 to 16 mg thrice weekly have effectively reduced heroin use. Physicians must be trained and certified to carry out this therapy in their private offices. There are a number of approved training programs in the United States.

Tramadol

There are no controlled trials establishing the appropriate dosing schedule for tramadol when used for conditions other than pain. Tramadol is available in many formulations. These range from capsules (regular and extended release) to tablets (regular, extended release, chewable tablets) that can be taken sublingually, suppositories and injectable ampules. It also comes as tablets and capsules containing acetaminophen or aspirin. Doses reported in case reports of treatment for depression or obsessive-compulsive disorder range from 50 to 200 mg/day, and involve short-term use. The long-term use of tramadol in the treatment of psychiatric disorders has not been studied.

Opioid Receptor Antagonists: Naltrexone, Nalmefene, and Naloxone

INTRODUCTION

Competitive opioid antagonists bind to opioid receptors without causing their activation. Because these drugs induce opioid withdrawal effects in people using full opioid agonists, these drugs are classified as opioid antagonists. Naltrexone and naloxone are the most widely used of these drugs. Naltrexone is more widely used for preventing relapse to opiate use in detoxified opiate addicts because it has a relatively long half-life, is orally effective, is not associated with dysphoria, and is administered once daily.

Since its introduction, naltrexone (ReVia, Depade) has been tried for the treatment of a wide range of psychiatric disorders, but only has two FDA-approved indications. Naltrexone is approved for the treatment of opiate dependence and alcohol dependence. An extended-release, once-a-month injectable suspension (Vivitrol) is available. Some individuals may lose a considerable amount of weight from naltrexone treatment, and in 2014 the FDA-approved Contrave, which is a trade name for the combination of naltrexone hydrochloride and bupropion hydrochloride in an extended-release formulation, for treatment of obesity.

Nalmefene (Revex) is indicated for the complete or partial reversal of opioid drug effects and in the management of known or suspected opioid overdose. An oral formulation of nalmefene is available in some countries but not in the United States. Naloxone, an opiate antagonist, has been FDA approved for reversal of opioid overdose. It is an effective medication in reversing respiratory depression and preventing fatalities secondary to opioid overdose.

PHARMACOLOGIC ACTIONS

Oral opioid receptor antagonists are rapidly absorbed from the gastrointestinal (GI) tract, but because of first-pass hepatic metabolism, only 60% of a dose of naltrexone and 40% to 50% of a dose of nalmefene reach the systemic circulation unchanged. Peak concentrations of naltrexone and its active metabolite, 6β-naltrexol, are achieved within 1 hour of ingestion. The half-life of naltrexone is 1 to 3 hours and the half-life of 6β-naltrexol is 13 hours. Peak concentrations of nalmefene are achieved in about 1 to 2 hours, and the half-life is 8 to 10 hours. Clinically, a single dose of naltrexone effectively blocks the rewarding effects of opioids for 72 hours. Traces of 6β-naltrexol may linger for up to 125 hours after a single dose.

Naltrexone and nalmefene are competitive antagonists of opioid receptors. Understanding the pharmacology of opioid receptors can explain the difference in adverse effects caused by naltrexone and nalmefene. Opioid receptors in the body are typed pharmacologically as μ, κ, or δ. Whereas activation of the κ- and δ-receptors is thought to reinforce opioid and alcohol consumption centrally, activation of μ-receptors is more closely associated with central and peripheral antiemetic effects. Because naltrexone is a relatively weak antagonist of κ- and δ-receptors and a potent μ-receptor antagonist, dosages of naltrexone that effectively reduce opioid and alcohol consumption also strongly block μ-receptors and therefore may cause nausea. Nalmefene, in contrast, is an equally potent antagonist of all three opioid receptor types, and dosages of nalmefene that effectively reduce opioid and alcohol consumption have no particularly increased effect on μ-receptors. Thus, nalmefene is associated clinically with few GI adverse effects.

Naloxone has the highest affinity for the μ-receptor but is a competitive antagonist at the μ-, κ-, and δ-receptors.

Whereas the effects of opioid receptor antagonists on opioid use are easily understood in terms of competitive inhibition of opioid receptors, the effects of opioid receptor antagonists on alcohol dependence are less straightforward and probably relate to the fact that the desire for and the effects of alcohol consumption appear to be regulated by several neurotransmitter systems, both opioid and nonopioid.

THERAPEUTIC INDICATIONS

The combination of a cognitive-behavioral program plus use of opioid receptor antagonists is more successful than either the cognitive-behavioral program or use of opioid receptor antagonists alone. Naltrexone is used as a screening test to ensure that the patient is opioid-free before the induction of therapy with naltrexone (see Table 24–1).

Table 24–1
Naloxone (Narcan) Challenge Test

The naloxone challenge test should not be performed in a patient showing clinical signs or symptoms of opioid withdrawal or in a patient whose urine contains opioids. The naloxone challenge test may be administered by either the intravenous (IV) or the subcutaneous route.
IV challenge: After appropriate screening of the patient, 0.8 mg of naloxone should be drawn into a sterile syringe. If the IV route of administration is selected, 0.2 mg of naloxone should be injected, and while the needle is still in the patient's vein, the patient should be observed for 30 seconds for evidence of withdrawal signs or symptoms. If there is no evidence of withdrawal, the remaining 0.6 mg of naloxone should be injected and the patient observed for an additional 20 minutes for signs and symptoms of withdrawal.
Subcutaneous challenge: If the subcutaneous route is selected, 0.8 mg should be administered subcutaneously and the patient observed for signs and symptoms of withdrawal for 20 minutes.
Conditions and technique for observation of patient: During the appropriate period of observation, the patient's vital signs should be monitored, and the patient should be monitored for signs of withdrawal. It is also important to question the patient carefully. The signs and symptoms of opioid withdrawal include, but are not limited to, the following:
Withdrawal signs: Stuffiness or running nose, tearing, yawning, sweating, tremor, vomiting, or piloerection
Withdrawal symptoms: Feeling of temperature change, joint or bone and muscle pain, abdominal cramps, and formication (feeling of bugs crawling under skin)
Interpretation of the challenge: Warning—the elicitation of the enumerated signs or symptoms indicates a potential risk for the subject, and naltrexone should not be administered. If no signs or symptoms of withdrawal are observed, elicited, or reported, naltrexone may be administered. If there is any doubt in the observer's mind that the patient is not in an opioid-free state or is in continuing withdrawal, naltrexone should be withheld for 24 hours and the challenge repeated.

Opioid Dependence

Patients in detoxification programs are usually weaned from potent opioid agonists such as heroin over a period of days to weeks, during which emergent adrenergic withdrawal effects are treated as needed with clonidine (Catapres). A serial protocol is sometimes used in which potent agonists are gradually replaced by weaker agonists followed by mixed agonist–antagonists and then finally by pure antagonists. For example, an abuser of the potent agonist heroin would switch first to the weaker agonist methadone (Dolophine), then to the partial agonist buprenorphine (Buprenex) or levomethadyl acetate (ORLAAM)—commonly called LAAM—and finally, after a 7- to 10-day washout period, to a pure antagonist, such as naltrexone or nalmefene. However, even with gradual detoxification, some persons continue to experience mild adverse effects or opioid withdrawal symptoms for the first several weeks of treatment with naltrexone.

As the opioid receptor agonist potency diminishes, so do the adverse consequences of discontinuing the drug. Thus, because there are no pharmacologic barriers to discontinuation of pure opioid receptor antagonists, the social environment and frequent cognitive-behavioral intervention become extremely important factors supporting continued opioid abstinence. Because of poorly tolerated adverse symptoms, most persons not simultaneously enrolled in a cognitive-behavioral program stop taking opioid receptor antagonists within 3 months. Compliance with the administration of an opioid receptor antagonist regimen can also be increased with participation in a well-conceived voucher program.

Issues of medication compliance should be a central focus of treatment. If a person with a history of opioid addiction stops taking a pure opioid receptor antagonist, the person's risk of relapse into opioid abuse is exceedingly high because reintroduction of a potent opioid agonist would yield a very rewarding subjective "high." In contrast, compliant persons do not develop tolerance to the therapeutic benefits of naltrexone even if it is administered continuously for 1 year or longer. Individuals may undergo several relapses and remissions before achieving long-term abstinence.

Persons taking opioid receptor antagonists should also be warned that sufficiently high dosages of opioid agonists can overcome the receptor antagonism of naltrexone or nalmefene, which may lead to hazardous and unpredictable levels of receptor activation (see Precautions and Adverse Reactions).

Rapid Detoxification

To avoid the 7- to 10-day period of opioid abstinence generally recommended before use of opioid receptor antagonists, rapid detoxification protocols have been developed. Continuous administration of adjunct clonidine—to reduce the adrenergic withdrawal symptoms—and adjunct benzodiazepines, such as oxazepam (Serax)—to reduce muscle spasms and insomnia—can permit use of oral opioid receptor antagonists on the first day of opioid cessation. Detoxification can thus be completed within 48 to 72 hours, at which point opioid receptor antagonist maintenance is initiated. Moderately severe withdrawal symptoms may be experienced on the first day, but they tail off rapidly thereafter.

Because of the potential hypotensive effects of clonidine, the blood pressure (BP) of persons undergoing rapid detoxification must be closely monitored for the first

8 hours. Outpatient rapid detoxification settings must therefore be adequately prepared to administer emergency care.

The main advantage of rapid detoxification is that the transition from opioid abuse to maintenance treatment occurs over just 2 or 3 days. The completion of detoxification in as little time as possible minimizes the risk that the person will relapse into opioid abuse during the detoxification protocol.

Alcohol Dependence

Opioid receptor antagonists are also used as adjuncts to cognitive-behavioral programs for treatment of alcohol dependence. Opioid receptor antagonists reduce alcohol craving and alcohol consumption, and they ameliorate the severity of relapses. The risk of relapse into heavy consumption of alcohol attributable to an effective cognitive-behavioral program alone may be halved with concomitant use of opioid receptor antagonists.

The newer agent nalmefene has a number of potential pharmacologic and clinical advantages over its predecessor naltrexone for treatment of alcohol dependence. Whereas naltrexone may cause reversible transaminase elevations in persons who take dosages of 300 mg a day (which is six times the recommended dosage for treatment of alcohol and opioid dependence [50 mg a day]), nalmefene has not been associated with any hepatotoxicity. Clinically effective dosages of naltrexone are discontinued by 10% to 15% of persons because of adverse effects, most commonly nausea. In contrast, discontinuation of nalmefene because of an adverse event is rare at the clinically effective dosage of 20 mg a day and in the range of 10% at excessive dosages—that is, 80 mg a day. Because of its pharmacokinetic profile, a given dosage of nalmefene may also produce a more sustained opioid antagonist effect than does naltrexone.

The efficacy of opioid receptor antagonists in reducing alcohol craving may be augmented with a selective serotonin reuptake inhibitor, although data from large trials are needed to assess this potential synergistic effect more fully.

PRECAUTIONS AND ADVERSE REACTIONS

Because opioid receptor antagonists are used to maintain a drug-free state after opioid detoxification, great care must be taken to ensure that an adequate washout period elapses—at least 5 days for a short-acting opioid such as heroin and at least 10 days for longer-acting opioids such as methadone—after the last dose of opioids and before the first dose of an opioid receptor antagonist is taken. The opioid-free state should be determined by self-report and urine toxicology screens. If any question persists of whether opioids are in the body despite a negative urine screen result, then a *naloxone challenge test* should be performed. Naloxone challenge is used because its opioid antagonism lasts less than 1 hour, but those of naltrexone and nalmefene may persist for more than 24 hours. Thus, any withdrawal effects elicited by naloxone will be relatively short-lived (see Dosage and Clinical Guidelines). Symptoms of acute opioid withdrawal include drug craving, feeling of temperature change, musculoskeletal pain, and GI distress. Signs of opioid withdrawal include confusion, drowsiness, vomiting, and diarrhea. Naltrexone and nalmefene should not be taken if naloxone infusion causes any signs of opioid withdrawal except as part of a supervised rapid detoxification protocol.

A set of adverse effects resembling a vestigial withdrawal syndrome tends to affect up to 10% of persons who take opioid receptor antagonists. Up to 15% of persons taking naltrexone may experience abdominal pain, cramps, nausea, and vomiting, which may be limited by transiently halving the dosage or altering the time of administration. Adverse central nervous system effects of naltrexone, experienced by up to 10% of persons, include headache, low energy, insomnia, anxiety, and nervousness. Joint and muscle pains may occur in up to 10% of persons taking naltrexone, as may rash.

Naltrexone may cause dosage-related hepatic toxicity at dosages well in excess of 50 mg a day; 20% of persons taking 300 mg a day of naltrexone may experience serum aminotransferase concentrations 3 to 19 times the upper limit of normal. The hepatocellular injury of naltrexone appears to be a dose-related toxic effect rather than an idiosyncratic reaction. At the lowest dosages of naltrexone required for effective opioid antagonism, hepatocellular injury is not typically observed. However, naltrexone dosages as low as 50 mg a day may be hepatotoxic in persons with underlying liver disease, such as persons with cirrhosis of the liver caused by chronic alcohol abuse. Serum aminotransferase concentrations should be monitored monthly for the first 6 months of naltrexone therapy and thereafter on the basis of clinical suspicion. Hepatic enzyme concentrations usually return to normal after discontinuation of naltrexone therapy.

If analgesia is required while a dose of an opioid receptor antagonist is pharmacologically active, opioid agonists should be avoided in favor of benzodiazepines or other nonopioid analgesics. Persons taking opioid receptor antagonists should be instructed that low dosages of opioids will have no effect but larger dosages could overcome the receptor blockade and suddenly produce symptoms of profound opioid overdosage, with sedation possibly progressing to coma or death. Use of opioid receptor antagonists is contraindicated in persons who are taking opioid agonists, small amounts of which may be present in over-the-counter antiemetic and antitussive preparations; in persons with acute hepatitis or hepatic failure; and in persons who are hypersensitive to the drugs.

USE IN PREGNANCY AND LACTATION

Because naltrexone is transported across the placenta, it should only be taken by pregnant women if a compelling need outweighs the potential risks to the fetus. A minimal amount of naltrexone is in maternal milk. The safety of nalmefene in pregnancy and breastfeeding has not been confirmed.

Opioid receptor antagonists are relatively safe drugs, and ingestion of high doses of opioid receptor antagonists should be treated with supportive measures combined with efforts to decrease GI absorption.

Because buprenorphine has a high affinity and slow displacement from the opioid receptors, nalmefene may not completely reverse buprenorphine-induced respiratory depression.

DRUG INTERACTIONS

Many drug interactions involving opioid receptor antagonists have been discussed earlier, including those with opioid agonists associated with drug abuse as well as those involving antiemetics and antitussives. Because of its extensive hepatic metabolism, naltrexone may affect or be affected by other drugs that influence hepatic enzyme levels. However, the clinical importance of these potential interactions is not known.

One potentially hepatotoxic drug that has been used in some cases with opioid receptor antagonists is disulfiram (Antabuse). Although no adverse effects were observed, frequent laboratory monitoring is indicated when such combination therapy is contemplated. Opioid receptor antagonists have been reported to potentiate the sedation associated with use of thioridazine (Mellaril), an interaction that probably applies equally to all low-potency dopamine receptor antagonists.

Intravenous nalmefene has been administered after benzodiazepines, inhalational anesthetics, muscle relaxants, and muscle relaxant antagonists administered in conjunction with general anesthetics without any adverse reactions. Care should be taken when using flumazenil and nalmefene together because both of these agents have been shown to induce seizures in preclinical studies.

LABORATORY INTERFERENCES

The potential for a false-positive urine for opiates using less specific urine screens such as enzyme multiplied immunoassay technique (EMIT) may exist, given that naltrexone and nalmefene are derivatives of oxymorphone. Thin-layer, gas–liquid, and high-pressure liquid chromatographic methods used for the detection of opiates in the urine are not interfered with by naltrexone.

DOSAGE AND CLINICAL GUIDELINES

To avoid the possibility of precipitating an acute opioid withdrawal syndrome, several steps should be taken to ensure that the person is opioid-free. Within a supervised detoxification setting, at least 5 days should elapse after the last dose of short-acting opioids, such as heroin, hydromorphone (Dilaudid), meperidine (Demerol), or morphine, and at least 10 days should elapse after the last dose of longer-acting opioids, such as methadone, before opioid antagonists are initiated. Briefer periods off opioids have been used in rapid detoxification protocols. To confirm that opioid detoxification is complete, urine toxicologic screens should demonstrate no opioid metabolites. However, an individual may have a negative urine opioid screen result, yet still be physically dependent on opioids and thus susceptible to antagonist-induced withdrawal effects. Therefore, after the urine screen result is negative, a naloxone challenge test is recommended unless an adequate period of opioid abstinence can be reliably confirmed by observers (Table 24–1).

The initial dosage of naltrexone for treatment of opioid or alcohol dependence is 50 mg a day, which should be achieved through gradual introduction, even when the naloxone challenge test result is negative. Various authorities begin with 5, 10, 12.5, or 25 mg and titrate up to the 50-mg dosage over a period ranging from 1 hour to 2 weeks while constantly monitoring for evidence of opioid withdrawal. When a daily dose of 50 mg is well tolerated, it may be averaged over a week by giving 100 mg on alternate days or 150 mg every third day. Such schedules may increase compliance. The corresponding therapeutic dosage of nalmefene is 20 mg a day divided into two equal doses. Gradual titration of nalmefene to this daily dose is probably a wise strategy, although clinical data on dosage strategies for nalmefene are not yet available.

To maximize compliance, it is recommended that family members directly observe ingestion of each dose. Random urine tests for opioid receptor antagonists and their metabolites as well as for ethanol or opioid metabolites should also be taken. Opioid receptor antagonists should be continued until the person is no longer considered psychologically at risk for relapse into opioid or alcohol abuse. This generally requires at least 6 months but may take longer, particularly if there are external stresses.

Nalmefene is available as a sterile solution for intravenous, intramuscular, and subcutaneous administration in two concentrations, containing 100 μg or 1 mg of nalmefene free base per mL. The 100 μg/mL concentration contains 110.8 μg of nalmefene hydrochloride and the 1.0 mg/mL concentration contains 1.108 mg of nalmefene hydrochloride per mL. Both concentrations contain 9.0 mg of sodium chloride per mL and the pH is adjusted to 3.9 with hydrochloric acid. Pharmacodynamic studies have shown that nalmefene has a longer duration of action than naloxone at fully reversing opiate activity.

Rapid Detoxification

Rapid detoxification has been standardized using naltrexone, although nalmefene would be expected to be equally effective with fewer adverse effects. In rapid detoxification protocols, the addicted person stops opioid use abruptly and begins the first opioid-free day by taking clonidine, 0.2 mg, orally every 2 hours for nine doses, to a maximum dose of 1.8 mg, during which time the BP is monitored every 30 to 60 minutes for the first 8 hours. Naltrexone, 12.5 mg, is administered 1 to 3 hours after the first dose of clonidine. To reduce muscle cramps and later insomnia, a short-acting benzodiazepine, such as oxazepam, 30 to 60 mg, is administered simultaneously with the first dose of clonidine, and half of the initial dose is readministered every 4 to 6 hours as needed. The maximum daily dosage of oxazepam should not exceed 180 mg. The person undergoing rapid detoxification should be accompanied home by a reliable escort. On the second day, similar doses of clonidine and the benzodiazepine are administered but with a single dose of naltrexone, 25 mg, taken in the morning. Relatively asymptomatic persons may return home after 3 to 4 hours. Administration of the daily maintenance dose of 50 mg of naltrexone is begun on the third day, and the dosages of clonidine and the benzodiazepine are gradually tapered off over 5 to 10 days.

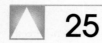

25

Phosphodiesterase-5 Inhibitors

INTRODUCTION

The phosphodiesterase (PDE)-5 inhibitors, such as sildenafil (Viagra), cause vaso-dilation in the penis, thus prolonging penile erections. They have revolutionized the treatment of the major sexual dysfunction affecting men—erectile disorder. Silde-nafil (Viagra) was the first drug of this class, with two congeners that subsequently came on the market—vardenafil (Levitra) and tadalafil (Cialis). These drugs have changed people's expectations of sexual functioning. Although indicated only for the treatment of male erectile dysfunction (ED), there is anecdotal evidence of their being effective in women. They are also being misused as recreational drugs that are believed to enhance sexual performance. These drugs have been used by more than 20 million men, if not more, around the world.

All these drugs work the same way. The development of sildenafil provided important information about the physiology of erection. Sexual stimulation causes the release of the neurotransmitter nitric oxide (NO), which increases the synthesis of cyclic guanosine monophosphate (cGMP), causing smooth muscle relaxation in the corpus cavernosum that allows blood to flow into the penis and that results in turgidity and tumescence. The concentration of cGMP is regulated by the enzyme PDE-5, which, when inhibited, allows cGMP to increase and enhance erectile func-tion. Because sexual stimulation is required to cause the release of NO, PDE-5 inhibitors have no effect in the absence of such stimulation, an important point to understand when providing information to patients about their use. The congeners vardenafil and tadalafil work in the same way, by inhibiting PDE-5, thus allowing an increase in cGMP and enhancing the vasodilatory effects of NO. For this reason, these drugs are sometimes referred to as NO enhancers.

PHARMACOLOGIC ACTIONS

All three substances are fairly rapidly absorbed from the gastrointestinal tract, with maximum plasma concentrations reached in 30 to 120 minutes (median, 60 minutes) in the fasting state. Because it is lipophilic, concomitant ingestion of a high-fat meal delays the rate of absorption by up to 60 minutes and reduces the peak concentra-tion by one-quarter. These drugs are principally metabolized by the CYP3A4 system, which may lead to clinically significant drug–drug interactions, not all of which have been documented. Excretion of 80% of the dose is via feces, and another 13% is elim-inated in the urine. Elimination is reduced in persons older than age 65 years, which results in plasma concentrations 40% higher than in persons aged 18 to 45 years. Elimination is also reduced in the presence of severe renal or hepatic insufficiency.

The mean half-lives of sildenafil and vardenafil are 3 to 4 hours, and that of tadalafil is about 18 hours. Tadalafil can be detected in the bloodstream 5 days after ingestion, and because of its long half-life, it has been marketed as effective for up to 36 hours—the so-called weekend pill. The onset of sildenafil occurs about 30 minutes after ingestion on an empty stomach; tadalafil and vardenafil act somewhat more quickly.

Clinicians need to be aware of the important clinical observation that these drugs do not by themselves create an erection. Rather, the mental state of sexual arousal brought on by erotic stimulation must first lead to activity in the penile nerves, which then release NO into the cavernosum, triggering the erectile cascade, the resulting erection being prolonged by the NO enhancers. Thus, full advantage may be taken of a sexually exciting stimulus, but the drug is not a substitute for foreplay and emotional arousal.

THERAPEUTIC INDICATIONS

EDs have traditionally been classified as organic, psychogenic, or mixed. Cialis is approved for BPH. Organic causes of ED include diabetes mellitus, hypertension, hypercholesterolemia, cigarette smoking, peripheral vascular disease, pelvic or spinal cord injury, pelvic or abdominal surgery (especially prostate surgery), multiple sclerosis, peripheral neuropathy, and Parkinson's disease; alcohol, nicotine, and other substances of abuse; and by prescription drugs. PDE-5 inhibitors are also effective in psychogenic-induced ED.

These drugs are effective regardless of the baseline severity of ED, race, or age. Among those responding to sildenafil are men with coronary artery disease, hypertension, other cardiac disease, peripheral vascular disease, diabetes mellitus, depression, coronary artery bypass graft surgery, radical prostatectomy, transurethral resection of the prostate, spina bifida, and spinal cord injury, as well as persons taking antidepressants, antipsychotics, antihypertensives, and diuretics. However, the response rate is variable.

Sildenafil has been reported to reverse selective serotonin reuptake inhibitor–induced anorgasmia in men. There are anecdotal reports of sildenafil having a therapeutic effect on sexual inhibition in women as well.

PRECAUTIONS AND ADVERSE REACTIONS

A major potential adverse effect associated with use of these drugs is myocardial infarction (MI). The Food and Drug Administration (FDA) distinguished the risk of MI caused directly by these drugs from that caused by underlying conditions such as hypertension, atherosclerotic heart disease, diabetes mellitus, and other atherogenic conditions. The FDA concluded that when used according to the approved labeling, the drugs do not by themselves confer an increased risk of death. However, there is increased oxygen demand and stress placed on the cardiac muscle by sexual intercourse. Thus, coronary perfusion may be severely compromised, and cardiac failure may occur as a result. For that reason, any person with a history of MI, stroke, renal failure, hypertension, or diabetes mellitus and any person older than the age of 70 years should discuss plans to use these drugs with an internist or a cardiologist. The cardiac evaluation should specifically address exercise tolerance and the use of nitrates.

Use of PDE-5 inhibitors is contraindicated in persons who are taking organic nitrates in any form. Also, amyl nitrate (poppers), a popular substance of abuse to enhance the intensity of orgasm, should not be used with any of the erection-enhancing drugs. The combination of organic nitrates and PDE inhibitors can cause a precipitous lowering of blood pressure and can reduce coronary perfusion to the point of causing MI and death.

Adverse effects are dose dependent, occurring at higher rates with higher dosages. The most common adverse effects are headache, flushing, and stomach pain. Other, less common adverse effects include nasal congestion, urinary tract infection, abnormal vision (colored tinge [usually blue], increased sensitivity to light, or blurred vision), diarrhea, dizziness, and rash. Supportive management is indicated in cases of overdosage. Tadalafil has been associated with back and muscle pain in about 10% of patients.

Recently, there have been 50 reports and 14 verified cases of a serious condition in men taking sildenafil called nonarteritic anterior ischemic optic neuropathy. This is an eye ailment that causes restriction of blood flow to the optic nerve and can result in permanent vision loss. The first symptoms appear within 24 hours after use of sildenafil and include blurred vision and some degree of vision loss. The incidence of this effect is very rare—1 in 1 million. In the reported cases, many patients had preexisting eye problems that may have increased their risk, and many had a history of heart disease and diabetes, which may indicate vulnerability in these men to endothelial damage.

In addition to vision problems, in 2010, a warning of possible hearing loss was reported based on 29 incidents of the problem since introduction of these drugs. Hearing loss usually occurs within hours or days of using the drug and in some cases is both unilateral and temporary.

USE IN PREGNANCY AND LACTATION

No data are available on the effects on human fetal growth and development or testicular morphologic or functional changes. However, because these drugs are not considered an essential treatment, they should not be used during pregnancy.

TREATMENT OF PRIAPISM

Phenylephrine (Neo-Synephrine, Pseudophed?) is the drug of choice and first-line treatment of priapism because the drug has almost pure α-agonist effects and minimal β-activity. In short-term priapism (less than 6 hours), especially for drug-induced priapism, intracavernosal injection of phenylephrine can be used to cause detumescence. A mixture of one ampule of phenylephrine (1 mL/1,000 μg) should be diluted with an additional 9 mL of normal saline. Using a 29-gauge needle, 0.3 to 0.5 mL should be injected into the corpora cavernosa, with 10 to 15 minutes between injections. Vital signs should be monitored, and compression should be applied to the area of injection to help prevent hematoma formation.

Phenylephrine can also be used orally, 10 to 20 mg every 4 hours as needed, but it may not be as effective or act as rapidly as the injectable route.

DRUG INTERACTIONS

The major route of PDE-5 metabolism is through CYP3A4, and the minor route is through CYP2C9. Inducers or inhibitors of these enzymes will therefore affect the plasma concentration and half-life of sildenafil. For example, 800 mg of cimetidine

(Tagamet), a nonspecific CYP inhibitor, increases plasma sildenafil concentrations by 56%, and erythromycin (E-Mycin) increases plasma sildenafil concentrations by 182%. Other, stronger inhibitors of CYP3A4 include ketoconazole (Nizoral), itraconazole (Sporanox), and mibefradil (Posicor). In contrast, rifampicin, a CYP3A4 inducer, decreases plasma concentrations of sildenafil.

LABORATORY INTERFERENCES

No laboratory interferences have been described.

DOSAGE AND CLINICAL GUIDELINES

Sildenafil is available as 25-, 50-, and 100-mg tablets. The recommended dose of sildenafil is 50 mg taken by mouth 1 hour before intercourse. However, sildenafil may take effect within 30 minutes. The duration of the effect is usually 4 hours, but in healthy young men, the effect may persist for 8 to 12 hours. Based on effectiveness and adverse effects, the dose should be titrated between 25 and 100 mg. Sildenafil is recommended for use no more than once a day. The dosing guidelines for use by women, an off-label use, are the same as those for men.

Increased plasma concentrations of sildenafil may occur in persons older than 65 years of age and those with cirrhosis or severe renal impairment or using CYP3A4 inhibitors. A starting dose of 25 mg should be used in these circumstances.

An investigational nasal spray formulation of sildenafil has been developed that acts within 5 to 15 minutes of administration. This formulation is highly water soluble, and it is rapidly absorbed directly into the bloodstream. Such a formulation would permit more ease of use.

Vardenafil is supplied in 2.5-, 5-, 10-, and 20-mg tablets. The initial dose is usually 10 mg taken with or without food about 1 hour before sexual activity. The dose can be increased to a maximum of 20 mg or decreased to 5 mg based on efficacy and side effects. The maximum dosing frequency is once per day. As with sildenafil, dosages may have to be adjusted in patients with hepatic impairment or in patients using certain CYP3A4 inhibitors. A 10-mg orally disintegrating form of vardenafil (Staxyn) is available. It is placed on the tongue approximately 60 minutes before sexual activity and should not be used more than once a day.

Tadalafil is available in 2.5-, 5-, or 20-mg tablets for oral administration. The recommended dose of tadalafil is 10 mg before sexual activity, which may be increased to 20 mg or decreased to 5 mg depending on efficacy and side effects. Once-a-day use of the 2.5- or 5-mg pill is acceptable for most patients. Similar cautions apply as mentioned earlier in patients with hepatic impairment and in those taking concomitant potent inhibitors of CYP3A4. As with other PDE-5 inhibitors, concomitant use of nitrates in any form is contraindicated.

26

Selective Serotonin–Norepinephrine Reuptake Inhibitors

INTRODUCTION

Four serotonin–norepinephrine reuptake inhibitors (SNRIs) are approved for use as antidepressants in the United States: Venlafaxine (Effexor and Effexor XR), desvenlafaxine succinate (DVS; Pristiq), duloxetine (Cymbalta), and levomilnacipran (Fetzima). A fifth SNRI, milnacipran (Savella), available in other countries as an antidepressant, has Food and Drug Administration (FDA) approval in the United States as a treatment for fibromyalgia. The term SNRI reflects the belief that the therapeutic effects of these medications are mediated by concomitant blockade of neuronal serotonin (5-HT) and norepinephrine uptake transporters. The SNRIs are also sometimes referred to as dual reuptake inhibitors, a broader functional class of antidepressant medications that includes tricyclic antidepressants (TCAs) such as clomipramine and, to a lesser extent, imipramine and amitriptyline. What distinguishes the SNRIs from TCAs is their relative lack of affinity for other receptors, especially muscarinic, histaminergic, and the families of α- and β-adrenergic receptors. This distinction is an important one because the SNRIs have a more favorable tolerability profile than the TCAs.

VENLAFAXINE AND DESVENLAFAXINE

Therapeutic Indications

Venlafaxine is approved for treatment of four therapeutic disorders: Major depressive disorder, generalized anxiety disorder, social anxiety disorder, and panic disorder. Major depressive disorder is currently the only FDA-approved indication for DVS.

Depression. The FDA does not recognize any class of antidepressant as being more effective than any other. This does not mean that differences do not exist, but no study to date has sufficiently demonstrated such superiority. It has been argued that direct modulation of serotonin and norepinephrine may convey greater antidepressant effects than are exerted by medications that selectively enhance only noradrenergic or serotoninergic neurotransmission. This greater therapeutic benefit could result from an acceleration of postsynaptic adaptation to increased neuronal signaling; simultaneous activation of two pathways for intracellular signal transduction; additive effects on the activity of relevant genes such as brain-derived neurotrophic factor; or, quite simply, broader coverage of depressive symptoms. Clinical evidence supporting this hypothesis first emerged in a pair of studies conducted by the Danish University Antidepressant Group, which found an advantage for the dual reuptake inhibitor clomipramine compared with the selective serotonin reuptake inhibitors (SSRIs) citalopram and paroxetine. Another report, which compared the results of a group of patients prospectively treated with the combination of the

TCAs, desipramine and fluoxetine, with a historical comparison group treated with desipramine alone, provided additional support. A meta-analysis of 25 inpatient studies comparing the efficacy of TCAs and SSRIs yielded the strongest evidence. Specifically, although the TCAs were found to have a modest overall advantage, superiority versus SSRIs was almost entirely explained by the studies that used the TCAs that are considered to be dual reuptake inhibitors—clomipramine, amitriptyline, and imipramine. Meta-analyses of head-to-head studies suggest that venlafaxine has a potential to induce higher rates of remission in depressed patients than do the SSRIs. This difference of the venlafaxine advantage is about 6%. DVS has not been extensively compared with other classes of antidepressants with respect to efficacy.

Generalized Anxiety Disorder.   The extended-release formulation of venlafaxine is approved for treatment of generalized anxiety disorder. In clinical trials lasting 6 months, dosages of 75 to 225 mg a day were effective in treating insomnia, poor concentration, restlessness, irritability, and excessive muscle tension related to generalized anxiety disorder.

Social Anxiety Disorder.   The extended-release formulation of venlafaxine is approved for treatment of social anxiety disorder. Its efficacy was established in 12-week studies.

Other Indications.   Case reports and uncontrolled studies have indicated that venlafaxine may be beneficial in the treatment of obsessive-compulsive disorder, panic disorder, agoraphobia, social phobia, attention-deficit/hyperactivity disorder, and patients with a dual diagnosis of depression and cocaine dependence. It has also been used in chronic pain syndromes with good effect.

Precautions and Adverse Reactions

Venlafaxine has a safety and tolerability profile similar to that of the more widely prescribed SSRI class. Nausea is the most frequently reported treatment-emergent adverse effect associated with venlafaxine and DVS therapy. Initiating therapy at lower dosages may also attenuate nausea. When extremely problematic, treatment-induced nausea can be controlled by prescribing a selective 5-HT$_3$ antagonist or mirtazapine.

Venlafaxine and DVS therapy is associated with sexual side effects, predominantly decreased libido and a delay to orgasm or ejaculation. The incidence of these side effects may exceed 30% to 40% when there is direct, detailed assessment of sexual function.

Other common side effects include headache, insomnia, somnolence, dry mouth, dizziness, constipation, asthenia, sweating, and nervousness. Although several side effects are suggestive of anticholinergic effects, these drugs have no affinity for muscarinic or nicotinic receptors. Thus, noradrenergic agonism is likely to be the culprit.

Higher-dose venlafaxine therapy is associated with an increased risk of sustained elevations of blood pressure (BP). Experience with the instant-release (IR) formulation in studies of depressed patients indicated that sustained hypertension was dose related, increasing from 3% to 7% at doses of 100 to 300 mg per day and to 13% at doses greater than 300 mg per day. In this data set, venlafaxine therapy did not adversely affect BP control of patients taking antihypertensives and actually lowered mean values of patients with elevated BP readings before therapy. In controlled studies of the extended-release formulation, venlafaxine therapy resulted in only approximately a 1% greater risk of high BP when compared to placebo. Arbitrarily capping the upper dose of venlafaxine used in these studies thus greatly attenuated concerns about elevated BP. When higher doses of the extended-release formulation are used, however, monitoring of BP is recommended.

Venlafaxine and DVS are commonly associated with a discontinuation syndrome. This syndrome is characterized by the appearance of a constellation of adverse effects during a rapid taper or abrupt cessation, including dizziness, dry mouth, insomnia, nausea, nervousness, sweating, anorexia, diarrhea, somnolence, and sensory disturbances. It is recommended that, whenever possible, a slow taper schedule should be used when longer-term treatment must be stopped. On occasion, substituting a few doses of the sustained-release formulation of fluoxetine may help to bridge this transition.

There were no overdose fatalities in premarketing trials of venlafaxine, although electrocardiographic changes (e.g., prolongation of QT interval, bundle branch block, QRS interval prolongation), tachycardia, bradycardia, hypotension, hypertension, coma, serotonin syndrome, and seizures were reported. Fatal overdoses have been documented subsequently, typically involving venlafaxine ingestion in combination with other drugs, alcohol, or both.

Use in Pregnancy and Lactation

Information concerning use of venlafaxine and desvenlafaxine by pregnant and nursing women is limited, but they appear to be safe. Venlafaxine and desvenlafaxine are excreted in human milk.

Drug Interactions

Venlafaxine is metabolized in the liver primarily by the CYP2D6 isoenzyme. Because the parent drug and principal metabolite are essentially equipotent, medications that inhibit this isoenzyme usually do not adversely affect therapy. Venlafaxine is itself a relatively weak inhibitor of CYP2D6, although it can increase levels of substrates such as desipramine or risperidone (Risperdal). In vitro and in vivo studies have shown venlafaxine to cause little or no inhibition of CYP1A2, CYP2C9, CYP2C19, and CYP3A4.

Venlafaxine is contraindicated in patients taking monoamine oxidase inhibitors (MAOIs) because of the risk of a pharmacodynamic interaction (i.e., serotonin syndrome). An MAOI should not be started for at least 7 days after stopping venlafaxine. Few data are available regarding the combination of venlafaxine with atypical neuroleptics, benzodiazepines, lithium (Eskalith), and anticonvulsants; therefore, clinical judgment should be exercised when combining medications.

Laboratory Interferences

Data are not currently available on laboratory interferences with venlafaxine.

Dosage and Administration

Venlafaxine is available in 25-, 37.5-, 50-, 75-, and 100-mg tablets and 37.5-, 75-, and 150-mg extended-release capsules. The tablets and the extended-release capsules are equally potent, and persons stabilized with one can switch to an equivalent dosage of the other. Since the immediate-release tablets are rarely used because of their tendency to cause nausea and the need for multiple daily doses, the dosage recommendations that follow refer to use the extended-release capsules.

In depressed persons, venlafaxine demonstrates a dose–response curve. The initial therapeutic dosage is 75 mg a day given once a day. However, most persons are started at a dosage of 37.5 mg for 4 to 7 days to minimize adverse effects, particularly nausea. A convenient starter kit for the drug contains a 1-week supply of both the 37.5- and 75-mg strengths. If a rapid titration is preferred, the dosage can be raised to 150 mg per day after day 4. As a rule, the dosage can be raised in increments of 75 mg a day every 4 or more days. Although the recommended upper dosage of the extended-release preparation (venlafaxine XR) is 225 mg per day, it is approved by the FDA for use at dosages up to 375 mg a day. The dosage of venlafaxine should be halved in persons with significantly diminished hepatic or renal function. If discontinued, venlafaxine use should be gradually tapered over 2 to 4 weeks to avoid withdrawal symptoms.

There are minor differences in the doses used for major depression, generalized anxiety disorder, and social anxiety disorder. In the treatment of these disorders, for example, a dose–response effect has not been found. In addition, lower mean dosages are typically used, with most patients taking 75 to 150 mg per day.

DVS is available as 50- and 100-mg extended-release tablets. The therapeutic dose for most patients is 50 mg a day. Although some patients may need higher doses, in clinical trials, no greater therapeutic benefit was noted when the dose was increased. At higher doses, adverse event and discontinuation rates were increased.

DULOXETINE

Pharmacologic Actions

Duloxetine is formulated as a delayed-release capsule to reduce the risk of severe nausea associated with the drug. It is well absorbed, but there is a 2-hour delay before absorption begins. Peak plasma concentrations occur 6 hours after ingestion. Food delays the time to achieve maximum concentrations from 6 to 10 hours and reduces the extent of absorption by about 10%. Duloxetine has an elimination half-life of about 12 hours (range: 8 to 17 hours). Steady-state plasma concentrations occur after 3 days. Elimination is mainly through the isozymes CYP2D6 and CYP1A2. Duloxetine undergoes extensive hepatic metabolism to numerous metabolites. About 70% of the drug appears in the urine as metabolites and about 20% is excreted in the feces. Duloxetine is 90% protein bound.

Therapeutic Indications

Depression. In contrast to venlafaxine, a small number of studies have compared duloxetine with the SSRIs. Although these studies are suggestive of some advantage in efficacy, their findings are limited by the use of fixed, low starting doses of paroxetine and fluoxetine, but dosages of duloxetine in some studies were as high as 120 mg per day. Any inferences on whether duloxetine is superior to the SSRIs in any aspect of treatment for depression thus await more evidence from properly designed trials.

Neuropathic Pain Associated with Diabetes and Stress Urinary Incontinence. Duloxetine is the first drug to be approved by the FDA as a treatment for neuropathic pain associated with diabetes. The drug has been studied for its effects on physical symptoms, including pain, in depressed patients, but these effects have not been compared with those seen with other widely used agents such as venlafaxine and the TCAs. Duloxetine has been studied as a treatment for stress urinary incontinence, the inability to voluntarily control bladder voiding, which is the most frequent type of incontinence in women. The action of duloxetine in the treatment of stress urinary incontinence is associated with its effects in the sacral spinal cord, which in turn increase the activity of the striated urethral sphincter. Duloxetine is marketed under the name Yentreve in the United Kingdom.

Precautions and Adverse Reactions. The most common adverse reactions are nausea, dry mouth, dizziness, constipation, fatigue, decreased appetite, anorexia, somnolence, and increased sweating. Nausea was the most common side effect leading to treatment discontinuation in clinical trials. The true incidence of sexual dysfunction is unknown; the long-term effects on body weight are also unknown. In clinical trials, treatment with duloxetine was associated with mean increases in BP averaging 2 mm Hg systolic and 0.5 mm Hg diastolic versus placebo. No studies have compared the BP effects of venlafaxine and duloxetine at equivalent therapeutic doses.

Close monitoring is suggested when using duloxetine in patients who have or are at risk for diabetes. Duloxetine has been shown to increase blood sugar and hemoglobin A1C levels during long-term treatment.

Patients with substantial alcohol use should not be treated with duloxetine because of possible hepatic effects. It also should not be prescribed for patients with hepatic insufficiency and end-stage renal disease or for patients with uncontrolled narrow-angle glaucoma.

Abrupt discontinuation of duloxetine should be avoided because it may produce a discontinuation syndrome similar to that of venlafaxine. A gradual dose reduction is recommended.

Use in Pregnancy and Lactation

Information concerning use of duloxetine by pregnant and nursing women is limited, but fetal risk appears to be low. Levels of duloxetine excreted in human milk are low.

Drug Interactions

Duloxetine is a moderate inhibitor of CYP450 enzymes.

Laboratory Interferences

Data are not currently available on laboratory interferences with duloxetine.

Dosage and Administration

Duloxetine is available in 20-, 30-, and 60-mg tablets. The recommended therapeutic, and maximum, dosage is 60 mg per day. The 20- and 30-mg doses are useful for either initial therapy or for twice-daily use as strategies to reduce side effects. In clinical trials, dosages of up to 120 mg per day were studied, but no consistent advantage in efficacy was noted at dosages higher than 60 mg per day. Duloxetine thus does not appear to demonstrate a dosage–response curve. However, there were difficulties in tolerability with single doses above 60 mg. Accordingly, when dosages of 80 and 120 mg per day were used, they were administered as 40 or 60 mg twice daily. Because of limited clinical experience with duloxetine, it remains to be seen to what extent dosages above 60 mg per day will be necessary and whether this will actually require divided doses to make the drug tolerable.

MILNACIPRAN AND LEVOMILNACIPRAN

Milnacipran is only FDA approved for the treatment of fibromyalgia. Although some countries have approved milnacipran for general use as an antidepressant, efficacy is not as well established. Unlike milnacipran, levomilnacipran is not approved for the management of fibromyalgia. Compared with venlafaxine, milnacipran is approximately five times more potent for inhibition of norepinephrine uptake than for 5-HT reuptake inhibition. Milnacipran has a half-life of approximately 8 hours and shows linear pharmacokinetics between doses of 50 and 250 mg per day. Metabolized in the liver, milnacipran has no active metabolites. Milnacipran is primarily excreted by the kidneys.

Milnacipran is available as 12.5-, 25-, 50-, and 100-mg tablets. The standard recommended milnacipran dose is as follows: Day 1, 12.5 mg once daily; days 2 and 3, 12.5 mg twice daily; days 4 to 7, 25 mg twice daily; and day 7 and beyond, 50 mg twice daily.

LEVOMILNACIPRAN (FETZIMA)

Levomilnacipran is an active enantiomer of the racemic drug milnacipran. In vitro studies have shown that it has greater potency for norepinephrine reuptake inhibition than for serotonin reuptake inhibition and does not directly affect the uptake of dopamine or other neurotransmitters. It is taken once daily as a sustained-release formulation. In clinical trials, doses of 40, 80, or 120 mg improved symptoms compared with placebo.

The most common adverse reactions in the placebo-controlled trials were nausea, constipation, hyperhidrosis, increased heart rate, erectile dysfunction, tachycardia, vomiting, and palpitations.

Adverse events associated with the use of levomilnacipran may include, but are not limited to, the following: Nausea, constipation, hyperhidrosis, heart rate increase, erectile dysfunction, tachycardia, vomiting, and palpitations. The only dose-related adverse events in clinical trials were urinary hesitation and erectile dysfunction.

The recommended dose range for levomilnacipran is 40 to 120 mg once daily, with or without food. Levomilnacipran should be initiated at 20 mg once daily for 2 days and then increased to 40 mg once daily. Based on efficacy and tolerability, the drug may then be increased in increments of 40 mg at intervals of 2 or more days. The maximum recommended dose is 120 mg once daily. Levomilnacipran should be taken at approximately the same time each day and should be swallowed whole. Capsules should not be opened, chewed, or crushed. As with most newly approved antidepressants, efficacy of levomilnacipran has not been established beyond 8 weeks.

Dose adjustment is not recommended in patients with mild renal impairment (creatinine clearance of 60 to 89 mL/min). For patients with moderate renal impairment (creatinine clearance of 30 to 59 mL/min), the maintenance dose should not exceed 80 mg once daily. For patients with severe renal impairment (creatinine clearance of 15 to 29 mL/min), the maintenance dose should not exceed 40 mg once daily. Levomilnacipran is not recommended for patients with end-stage renal disease.

The dose of levomilnacipran should not exceed 80 mg once daily when used with strong CYP3A4 inhibitors (e.g., ketoconazole, clarithromycin, ritonavir) (see Drug Interactions).

Levomilnacipran is supplied as 20-, 40-, 80-, and 120-mg extended-release capsules for oral administration. The recommended dose is 40 to 120 mg once daily with or without food. Initiate dose at 20 mg once daily for 2 days and then increase to 40 mg once daily. The dose should be increased in increments of 40 mg at intervals of 2 or more days. The maximum recommended dose is 120 mg once daily. The capsules should be swallowed whole.

Selective Serotonin Reuptake Inhibitors

INTRODUCTION

For nearly three decades, the selective serotonin reuptake inhibitors (SSRIs) have been the most widely used class of psychopharmacological agents used to treat depression and anxiety. They are considered "selective" because they have little effect on reuptake of norepinephrine or dopamine, exerting their therapeutic effects through serotonin reuptake inhibition. From a historic perspective, the most significant impact of fluoxetine, the first SSRI to be marketed in the United States, was the positive attention it generated in the popular press and the consequent reduction in the longstanding stigma and fear of taking antidepressants. Also, patients no longer experienced such side effects as dry mouth, constipation, sedation, orthostatic hypotension, and tachycardia, common side effects associated with the earlier antidepressant drugs—the tricyclic antidepressants (TCAs) and monoamine oxidase inhibitors (MAOIs). Prozac is also significantly safer when taken in overdose than previously available antidepressants.

Fluoxetine has been followed by other SSRIs. These include sertraline (Zoloft), paroxetine (Paxil), fluvoxamine (Luvox), citalopram (Celexa), escitalopram (Lexapro), and vilazodone (Viibryd). Vortioxetine (Trintellix) is unofficially considered to be an SSRI because its major pharmacologic effect is to inhibit the serotonin reuptake transporter. However, since the FDA has designated the drug a "serotonin modulator and stimulator," it is discussed separately in this chapter. Regardless of pharmacodynamics variations of these drugs, they are all equally effective in treating depression. Some are approved by the Food and Drug Administration (FDA) for multiple indications, such as major depression, obsessive-compulsive disorder (OCD), posttraumatic stress disorder (PTSD), premenstrual dysphoric disorder (PMDD), panic disorder, and social phobia (social anxiety disorder) (Table 27–1). Note that fluvoxamine is not FDA approved as an antidepressant, a fact that is due to a marketing decision. It is considered an antidepressant in other countries.

While all SSRIs are equally effective, there are meaningful differences in pharmacodynamics, pharmacokinetics, and side effects, differences that might affect clinical responses among individual patients. This would explain why some patients have better clinical responses to a particular SSRI than another. The SSRIs have proven more problematic in terms of some side effects than the original clinical trials suggested. Quality-of-life–associated adverse effects such as nausea, sexual dysfunction, and weight gain sometimes mitigate the therapeutic benefits of the SSRIs. There can also be distressing withdrawal symptoms when SSRIs are stopped abruptly. This is especially true with paroxetine but also occurs when other SSRIs with short half-lives are stopped.

Table 27-1
Currently Approved Indications of the Selective Serotonin Reuptake Inhibitors in the United States for Adult and Pediatric Populations

	Citalopram (Celexa)	Escitalopram (Lexapro)	Fluoxetine (Prozac)	Fluvoxamine (Luvox)	Paroxetine (Paxil)	Sertraline (Zoloft)	Vilazodone (Viibryd)
Major depressive disorder	Adult	Adult	Adult[a] and pediatric	—	Adult[c]	Adult	Adult
Generalized anxiety disorder	—	Adult	—	—	Adult	—	—
OCD	—	—	Adult and pediatric	Adult and pediatric	Adult	Adult and pediatric	—
Panic disorder	—	—	Adult	—	Adult[c]	Adult	—
PTSD	—	—	—	—	Adult[c]	Adult	—
Social anxiety disorder	—	—	Adult	—	Adult[c]	Adult	—
Bulimia nervosa	—	—	Adult	—	—	—	—
Premenstrual dysphoric disorder	—	—	Adult[b]	—	Adult[d]	Adult	—

[a] Weekly fluoxetine is approved for continuation and maintenance therapy in adults.
[b] Marketed as Sarafem.
[c] Paroxetine- and paroxetine-controlled release.
[d] Paroxetine-controlled release is approved for premenstrual dysphoric disorder.
OCD, obsessive-compulsive disorder; PTSD, posttraumatic stress disorder.

PHARMACOLOGIC ACTIONS

Pharmacokinetics

A significant difference among the SSRIs is their broad range of serum half-lives. Fluoxetine has the longest half-life: 4 to 6 days; its active metabolite has a half-life of 7 to 9 days. The half-life of sertraline is 26 hours, and its less active metabolite has a half-life of 3 to 5 days. The half-lives of the other three, which do not have metabolites with significant pharmacologic activity, are 35 hours for citalopram, 27 to 32 hours for escitalopram, 21 hours for paroxetine, and 15 hours for fluvoxamine. As a rule, the SSRIs are well absorbed after oral administration and have their peak effects in the range of 3 to 8 hours. Absorption of sertraline may be slightly enhanced by food.

There are also differences in plasma protein–binding percentages among the SSRIs, with sertraline, fluoxetine, and paroxetine being the most highly bound and escitalopram being the least bound.

All SSRIs are metabolized in the liver by the CYP450 enzymes. Because the SSRIs have such a wide therapeutic index, it is rare that other drugs produce problematic increases in SSRI concentrations. The most important drug–drug interactions involving the SSRIs occur as a result of the SSRIs inhibiting the metabolism of the coadministered medication. Each of the SSRIs possesses a potential for slowing or blocking the metabolism of many drugs (Table 27–2). Fluvoxamine is the most problematic of the drugs in this respect. It has a marked effect on several of the CYP enzymes. Examples of clinically significant interactions include fluvoxamine and theophylline (Theo-Dur) through CYP1A2 interaction; fluvoxamine and clozapine (Clozaril) through CYP1A2 inhibition; and fluvoxamine with alprazolam (Xanax) or clonazepam (Klonopin) through CYP3A4 inhibition. Fluoxetine and paroxetine also possess significant effects on the CYP2D6 isozyme, which may interfere with the efficacy of opiate analogs, such as codeine and hydrocodone, by blocking the conversion of these agents to their active form. Thus, coadministration of fluoxetine and

Table 27–2
CYP450 Inhibitory Potential of Commonly Prescribed Antidepressants

Relative Rank	CYP1A2	CYP2C	CYP2D6	CYP3A
Higher	Fluvoxamine (Luvox)	Fluoxetine Fluvoxamine	Bupropion Fluoxetine Paroxetine	Fluvoxamine Nefazodone Tricyclics
Moderate	Tertiary amine tricyclics	Sertraline	Secondary amine tricyclics	Fluoxetine
	Fluoxetine (Prozac)		Citalopram (Celexa) Escitalopram (Lexapro) Sertraline	Sertraline
Low or minimal	Bupropion (Wellbutrin) Mirtazapine (Remeron)	Paroxetine Venlafaxine (Effexor)	Fluoxetine Mirtazapine	Citalopram Escitalopram
	Nefazodone (Serzone) Paroxetine (Paxil) Sertraline (Zoloft) Venlafaxine		Nefazodone Venlafaxine	Mirtazapine Paroxetine Venlafaxine

CYP, cytochrome P450.

paroxetine with an opiate interferes with its analgesic effects. Sertraline, citalopram, and escitalopram are least likely to complicate treatment because of interactions.

The pharmacokinetics of vilazodone (5 to 80 mg) are dose-proportional. Steady-state plasma levels are achieved in about 3 days. Elimination of vilazodone is primarily by hepatic metabolism with a terminal half-life of approximately 25 hours.

Pharmacodynamics

Often, adequate clinical activity and saturation of the 5-HT transporters are achieved at starting dosages. As a rule, higher dosages do not increase antidepressant efficacy but may increase the risk of adverse effects.

Citalopram and escitalopram are the most selective inhibitors of serotonin reuptake, with very little inhibition of norepinephrine or dopamine reuptake and very low affinities for histamine H_1, γ-aminobutyric acid (GABA), or benzodiazepine receptors. The other SSRIs have a similar profile except that fluoxetine weakly inhibits norepinephrine reuptake and binds to 5-HT$_{2C}$ receptors, sertraline weakly inhibits norepinephrine and dopamine reuptake, and paroxetine has significant anticholinergic activity at higher dosages and binds to nitric oxide synthase. The most recently approved SSRI, vilazodone (Viibryd), has 5-HT$_{1A}$ receptor agonist properties. The clinical implications of the 5-HT$_{1A}$ receptor agonist effects are not yet evident.

A pharmacodynamic interaction appears to underlie the antidepressant effects of combined fluoxetine–olanzapine. When taken together, these drugs increase brain concentrations of norepinephrine. Concomitant use of SSRIs and drugs in the triptan class (sumatriptan [Imitrex], naratriptan [Amerge], rizatriptan [Maxalt], and zolmitriptan [Zomig]) may result in a serious pharmacodynamic interaction—the development of a serotonin syndrome (see Precautions and Adverse Reactions). However, many people use triptans while taking low doses of an SSRI for headache prophylaxis without adverse reaction. A similar reaction may occur when SSRIs are combined with tramadol (Ultram).

THERAPEUTIC INDICATIONS

Depression

In the United States, all SSRIs other than fluvoxamine have been approved by the FDA for treatment of depression. Several studies have found that antidepressants with serotonin–norepinephrine activity—drugs such as the MAOIs, TCAs, venlafaxine, and mirtazapine may produce higher rates of remission than SSRIs in head-to-head studies. The continued role of SSRIs as first-line treatments thus reflects their simplicity of use, safety, and broad spectrum of action.

Direct comparisons of individual SSRIs have not revealed any to be consistently superior to another. There nevertheless can be considerable diversity in response to the various SSRIs among individuals. For example, more than 50% of people who respond poorly to one SSRI will respond favorably to another. Thus, before shifting to non-SSRI antidepressants, it is most reasonable to try other agents in the SSRI class for persons who did not respond to the first SSRI.

Some clinicians have attempted to select a particular SSRI for a specific person on the basis of the drug's unique adverse effect profile. For example, thinking that fluoxetine is an activating and stimulating SSRI, they may assume it is a better choice for an abulic person than paroxetine, which is presumed to be a sedating SSRI. These differences, however, usually vary from person to person. Analyses of clinical trial data show that the SSRIs are more effective in patients with more severe symptoms of major depression than those with milder symptoms.

Suicide. The FDA has issued a black-box warning for antidepressants and suicidal thoughts and behavior in children and young adults. This warning is based on a decade-old analysis of clinical trial data. More recent, comprehensive reanalysis of data has shown that suicidal thoughts and behavior decreased over time for adult and geriatric patients treated with antidepressants as compared with placebo. No differences were found for youths. In adults, reduction in suicide ideation and attempts occurred through a reduction in depressive symptoms. In all age groups, severity of depression improved with medication and was significantly related to suicide ideation or behavior. It appears that SSRIs, as well as SNRIs, have a protective effect against suicide that is mediated by decreases in depressive symptoms with treatment. For youths, no significant effects of treatment on suicidal thoughts and behavior were found, although depression responded to treatment. No evidence of increased suicide risk was observed in youths receiving active medication. It is important to keep in mind that SSRIs, like all antidepressants, prevent potential suicides as a result of their primary action, the shortening and prevention of depressive episodes. In clinical practice, a few patients become especially anxious and agitated when started on an SSRI. The appearance of these symptoms could conceivably provoke or aggravate suicidal ideation. Thus, all depressed patients should be closely monitored during the period of maximum risk, the first few days and weeks they are taking SSRIs.

Use During Pregnancy and Breastfeeding. Rates of relapse of major depression during pregnancy among women who discontinue, attempt to discontinue, or modify their antidepressant regimens are extremely high. Rates range from 68% to 100% of patients. Thus, many women need to continue taking their medication during pregnancy and postpartum. The impact of maternal depression on infant development is unknown. There is no increased risk for major congenital malformations after exposure to SSRIs during pregnancy. Thus, the risk of relapse into depression when a newly pregnant mother is taken off SSRIs is severalfold higher than the risk to the fetus of exposure to SSRIs.

There is some evidence suggesting increased rates of special care nursery admissions after delivery for children of mothers taking SSRIs. There is also a potential for a discontinuation syndrome with paroxetine. However, there is an absence of clinically significant neonatal complications associated with SSRI use.

Studies that have followed children into their early school years have failed to find any perinatal complications, congenital fetal anomalies, decreases in global intelligence quotient (IQ), language delays, or specific behavioral problems attributable to the use of fluoxetine during pregnancy.

Postpartum depression (with or without psychotic features) affects a small percentage of mothers. Some clinicians start administering SSRIs if the postpartum blues extend beyond a few weeks or if a woman becomes depressed during pregnancy. The head starts afforded by starting SSRI administration during pregnancy if a woman is at risk for postpartum depression also protects the newborn, toward whom the woman may have harmful thoughts after parturition.

Babies whose mothers are taking an SSRI in the latter part of pregnancy may be at a slight risk of developing pulmonary hypertension. Data about the risk of this side effect are inconclusive but is estimated to involve 1 to 2 babies out of 1,000 births. Paroxetine should be avoided during pregnancy.

The FDA has classified paroxetine as the most problematic of the SSRI medications. In 2005, the FDA issued an alert that paroxetine increases the risk of birth defects, particularly heart defects, when women take it during the first 3 months of pregnancy. Paroxetine should usually not be taken during pregnancy, but for some women who have already been taking paroxetine, the benefits of continuing paroxetine may be greater than the potential risk to the baby. Women taking paroxetine who are pregnant, think they may be pregnant, or plan to become pregnant should talk to their physicians about the potential risks of taking paroxetine during pregnancy.

The FDA alert was based on the findings of studies that showed that women who took paroxetine during the first 3 months of pregnancy were about one and a half to two times as likely to have a baby with a heart defect as women who received other antidepressants and women in the general population. Most of the heart defects in these studies were not life-threatening, and happened mainly in the inside walls of the heart muscle where repairs can be done if needed (atrial and ventricular septal defects). Sometimes, these septal defects resolve without treatment. In one of the studies, the risk of heart defects in babies whose mothers had taken paroxetine early in pregnancy was 2%, compared to a 1% risk in the whole population. In the other study, the risk of heart defects in babies whose mothers had taken paroxetine in the first 3 months of pregnancy was 1.5% compared to 1% in babies whose mothers had taken other antidepressants in the first 3 months of pregnancy. This study also showed that women who took paroxetine in the first 3 months of pregnancy were about twice as likely to have a baby with any birth defect as women who took other antidepressants.

Very small amounts of SSRIs are found in breast milk and no harmful effects have been found in breastfed babies. Concentrations of sertraline and escitalopram are especially low in breast milk. However, in some cases, reported concentrations may be higher than average. No decision regarding the use of an SSRI is risk free. It is thus important to document that communication of potential risks to the patient has taken place.

Depression in Elderly and Medically Ill Persons. The SSRIs are safe and well tolerated when used to treat elderly and medically ill persons. As a class, they have little or no cardiotoxic, anticholinergic, antihistaminergic, or α-adrenergic adverse effects. Paroxetine does have some anticholinergic activity, which may lead to constipation and worsening of cognition. The SSRIs can produce subtle cognitive deficits, prolonged bleeding time, and hyponatremia, all of which may impact the health of this population. The SSRIs are effective in poststroke depression and dramatically reduce the symptom of crying.

Depression in Children. The use of SSRI antidepressants in children and adolescents has been controversial. Few studies have shown clear-cut benefits from the use of these drugs, and studies show that there may be an increase in suicidal or aggressive impulses. However, some children and adolescents do exhibit dramatic responses to these drugs in terms of depression and anxiety. Fluoxetine has most consistently demonstrated effectiveness in reducing symptoms of depressive disorder in both children and adolescents. This may be a function of the quality of the clinical trials involved. Sertraline has been shown to be effective in treating social anxiety disorder in this population, especially when combined with cognitive-behavioral therapy. Given the potential negative effect of untreated depression and anxiety in a young population and the uncertainty about many aspects of how children and adolescents might react to medication, any use of SSRIs should be undertaken only within the context of comprehensive management of the patient.

Anxiety Disorders

Obsessive-Compulsive Disorder. Fluvoxamine, paroxetine, sertraline, and fluoxetine are indicated for treatment of OCD in persons older than the age of 18 years. Fluvoxamine and sertraline have also been approved for treatment of children with OCD (ages 6 to 17 years). About 50% of persons with OCD begin to show symptoms in childhood or adolescence, and more than half of these respond favorably to medication. Beneficial responses can be dramatic. Long-term data support the model of OCD as a genetically determined, lifelong condition that is best treated continuously with drugs and cognitive-behavioral therapy from the onset of symptoms in childhood throughout the lifespan.

SSRI dosages for OCD may need to be higher than those required to treat depression. Although some response can be seen in the first few weeks of treatment, it may take several months for the maximum effects to become evident. Patients who fail to obtain adequate relief of their OCD symptoms with an SSRI often benefit from the addition of a small dose of risperidone (Risperdal). Apart from the extrapyramidal side effects of risperidone, patients should be monitored for increases in prolactin levels when this combination is used. Clinically, hyperprolactinemia may manifest as gynecomastia and galactorrhea (in both men and women) and loss of menses.

A number of disorders are now considered to be within the OCD spectrum. This includes a number of conditions and symptoms characterized by nonsuicidal self-mutilation, such as trichotillomania, eyebrow picking, nose picking, nail biting, compulsive picking of skin blemishes, and cutting. Patients with these behaviors benefit from treatment with SSRIs. Other spectrum disorders include compulsive gambling, compulsive shopping, hypochondriasis, and body dysmorphic disorder.

Panic Disorder. Paroxetine and sertraline are indicated for treatment of panic disorder, with or without agoraphobia. These agents work less rapidly than do the benzodiazepines alprazolam (Xanax) and clonazepam (Klonopin) but are far superior to the benzodiazepines for treatment of panic disorder with comorbid depression. Citalopram, fluvoxamine, and fluoxetine also may reduce spontaneous or induced panic attacks. Because fluoxetine can initially heighten anxiety symptoms, persons with panic disorder must begin taking small dosages (5 mg a day) and increase the dosage slowly. Low doses of benzodiazepines may be given to manage this side effect.

Social Anxiety Disorder. SSRIs are effective agents in the treatment of social phobia. They reduce both symptoms and disability. The response rate is comparable to that seen with the MAOI phenelzine (Nardil), the previous standard treatment. The SSRIs are safer to use than MAOIs or benzodiazepines.

Posttraumatic Stress Disorder. Pharmacotherapy for PTSD must target specific symptoms in three clusters: Re-experiencing, avoidance, and hyperarousal. For long-term treatment, SSRIs appear to have a broader spectrum of therapeutic effects on specific PTSD symptom clusters than do TCAs and MAOIs. Benzodiazepine augmentation is useful in the acute symptomatic state. The SSRIs are associated with marked improvement of both intrusive and avoidant symptoms.

Generalized Anxiety Disorder. The SSRIs may be useful for the treatment of specific phobias, generalized anxiety disorder, and separation anxiety disorder. A thorough, individualized evaluation is the first approach, with particular attention to identifying conditions amenable to drug therapy. In addition, cognitive-behavioral or other psychotherapies can be added for greater efficacy.

Bulimia Nervosa and Other Eating Disorders
Fluoxetine is indicated for treatment of bulimia, which is best done in the context of psychotherapy. Dosages of 60 mg a day are significantly more effective than 20 mg a day. In several well-controlled studies, fluoxetine in dosages of 60 mg a day was superior to placebo in reducing binge eating and induced vomiting. Some experts recommend an initial course of cognitive-behavioral therapy alone. If there is no response in 3 to 6 weeks, then fluoxetine administration is added. The appropriate duration of treatment with fluoxetine and psychotherapy has not been determined.

Fluvoxamine was not effective at a statistically significant level in one double-blind, placebo-controlled trial for inpatients with bulimia.

Anorexia Nervosa. Fluoxetine has been used in inpatient treatment of anorexia nervosa to attempt to control comorbid mood disturbances and obsessive-compulsive symptoms. However, at least two careful studies, one of 7 months and one of 24 months, failed to find that fluoxetine affected the overall outcome and the maintenance of weight. Effective treatments for anorexia include cognitive-behavioral, interpersonal, psychodynamic, and family therapies in addition to a trial with SSRIs.

Obesity. Fluoxetine, in combination with a behavioral program, has been shown to be only modestly beneficial for weight loss. A significant percentage of all persons who take SSRIs, including fluoxetine, lose weight initially but later may gain weight. However, all SSRIs may cause initial weight gain.

Premenstrual Dysphoric Disorder. PMDD is characterized by debilitating mood and behavioral changes in the week preceding menstruation that interfere with normal functioning. Sertraline, paroxetine, fluoxetine, and fluvoxamine have been reported to reduce the symptoms of PMDD. Controlled trials of fluoxetine and sertraline administered either throughout the cycle or only during the luteal phase (the 2-week period between ovulation and menstruation) showed both schedules to be equally effective.

An additional observation of unclear significance was that fluoxetine was associated with changing the duration of the menstrual period by more than 4 days, either lengthening or shortening it. The effects of SSRIs on menstrual cycle length are mostly unknown and may warrant careful monitoring in women of reproductive age.

Off-Label Uses

Premature Ejaculation.   The antiorgasmic effects of SSRIs make them useful as a treatment for men with premature ejaculation. The SSRIs permit intercourse for a significantly longer period and are reported to improve sexual satisfaction in couples in which the man has premature ejaculation. Fluoxetine and sertraline have been shown to be effective for this purpose.

Paraphilias.   The SSRIs may reduce obsessive-compulsive behavior in people with paraphilias. The SSRIs diminish the average time per day spent in unconventional sexual fantasies, urges, and activities. Evidence suggests a greater response for sexual obsessions than for paraphilic behavior.

Autism.   Obsessive-compulsive behavior, poor social relatedness, and aggression are prominent autistic features that may respond to serotonergic agents such as SSRIs and clomipramine. Sertraline and fluvoxamine have been shown in controlled and open-label trials to mitigate aggressiveness, self-injurious behavior, repetitive behaviors, some degree of language delay, and (rarely) lack of social relatedness in adults with autistic spectrum disorders. Fluoxetine has been reported to be effective for features of autism in children, adolescents, and adults.

Precautions and Adverse Reactions

SSRI side effects need to be considered in terms of their onset, duration, and severity. For example, nausea and jitteriness are early, generally mild, and time-limited side effects. Although SSRIs share common side-effect profiles, individual drugs in this class may cause a higher rate or carry a more severe risk of certain side effects depending on the patient.

Sexual Dysfunction

All SSRIs cause sexual dysfunction, and it is the most common adverse effect of SSRIs associated with long-term treatment. It has an estimated incidence of between 50% and 80%. The most common complaints are anorgasmia, inhibited orgasm, and decreased libido. Some studies suggest that sexual dysfunction is dose related, but this has not been clearly established. Unlike most of the other adverse effects of SSRIs, sexual inhibition rarely resolves in the first few weeks of use but usually continues as long as the drug is taken. In some cases, there may be improvement over time.

Strategies to counteract SSRI-induced sexual dysfunction are numerous, and none has been proven to be very effective. Some reports suggest decreasing the dosage or adding bupropion or amphetamine. Reports have described successful treatment of SSRI-induced sexual dysfunction with agents such as sildenafil (Viagra), which are used to treat erectile dysfunction. Ultimately, patients may need to be switched to antidepressants that do not interfere with sexual functioning, drugs such as mirtazapine or bupropion.

Gastrointestinal Adverse Effects

Gastrointestinal (GI) side effects are very common and are mediated largely through effects on the serotonin 5-HT$_3$ receptor. The most frequent GI complaints are nausea, diarrhea, anorexia, vomiting, flatulence, and dyspepsia. Sertraline and fluvoxamine produce the most intense GI symptoms. Delayed-release paroxetine, compared with the immediate-release preparation of paroxetine, has less intense GI side effects during the first week of treatment. However, paroxetine, because of its anticholinergic activity, frequently causes constipation. Nausea and loose stools are usually dose related and transient, usually resolving within a few weeks. Sometimes flatulence and diarrhea persist, especially during sertraline treatment. Initial anorexia may also occur and is most common with fluoxetine. SSRI-induced appetite and weight loss begin as soon as the drug is taken and peaks at 20 weeks, after which weight often returns to baseline. Up to one-third of persons taking SSRIs will gain weight, sometimes more than 20 lb. This effect is mediated through a metabolic mechanism, increase in appetite, or both. It happens gradually and is usually resistant to diet and exercise regimens. Paroxetine is associated with more frequent, more rapid, and more pronounced weight gain than the other SSRIs, especially among young women.

Cardiovascular Effects

All SSRIs can lengthen the QT interval in otherwise healthy people and cause drug-induced long QT syndrome, especially when taken in overdose. The risk of QTc prolongation increases when an antidepressant and an antipsychotic are used in combination, an increasingly common practice. Citalopram stands out as the SSRI with the most pronounced effect QT intervals. A QT study assessing the effects of 20- and 60-mg doses of citalopram on the QT interval in adults: Compared with placebo, found a maximum mean prolongation in the individually corrected QT intervals were 8.5 ms for 20-mg citalopram and 18.5 ms for 60 mg. For 40 mg, prolongation of the corrected QT interval was estimated to be 12.6 ms. Based on these findings, the FDA has issued the following recommendation regarding citalopram use:

- 20 mg/day is the maximum recommended dose for patients with hepatic impairment, who are older than 60 years of age, who are CYP2C19 poor metabolizers, or who are taking concomitant cimetidine.
- No longer prescribe at doses greater than 40 mg/day.
- Do not use in patients with congenital long QT syndrome.
- Correct hypokalemia and hypomagnesemia before administering citalopram.
- Monitor electrolytes monitored as clinically indicated.
- Consider more frequent EKGs in patients with CHF, bradyarrhythmias, or patients on concomitant medications that prolong the QT interval.

The fact that citalopram carries greater risk of causing fatal rhythm abnormalities seemed to be confirmed in a review of 469 SSRI poisoning admissions. Conversely, a study done at the Ann Arbor VAMC and the University of Michigan failed to confirm an increased risk for arrhythmias or death associated with daily doses of more than 40 mg. These findings do raise questions about the continued legitimacy of the FDA warning. Nevertheless, patients should be advised to contact their prescriber immediately if they experience signs and symptoms of an abnormal heart rate or rhythm while taking citalopram.

The effect of vilazodone (20, 40, 60, and 80 mg) on the QTc interval was evaluated and a small effect was observed. The upper bound of the 90% confidence interval for the largest placebo-adjusted, baseline-corrected QTc interval was below 10 ms, based on the individual correction method (QTcI). This is below the threshold for clinical concern. However, it is unknown whether 80 mg is adequate to represent a high clinical exposure condition.

Physicians should consider whether the benefits of androgen deprivation therapy outweigh the potential risks in SSRI-treated patients with prostate cancer, as reductions in androgen levels can cause QTc interval prolongation.

Dextromethorphan/quinidine (Nuedexta) is available as a treatment for pseudobulbar affect, which is defined by involuntary, sudden, and frequent episodes of laughing and/or crying that are generally out of proportion or inappropriate to the situation. Quinidine that can prolong the QT interval is a potent inhibitor of CYP2D6. It should not be used with other medications that prolong the QT interval and are metabolized by CYP2D6. This drug should be used with caution with any medications that can prolong the QT interval and inhibit CYP3A4, particularly in patients with cardiac disease.

Antepartum use of SSRIs is sometimes associated with QTc interval prolongation in exposed neonates. In a review of 52 newborns exposed to SSRIs in the immediate antepartum period and 52 matched control subjects, the mean QTc was significantly longer in the group of newborns exposed to antidepressants as compared with control subjects. Five (10%) newborns exposed to SSRIs had a markedly prolonged QTc interval (>460 ms) compared with none of the unexposed newborns. The longest QTc interval observed among exposed newborns was 543 ms. All of the drug-associated repolarization abnormalities normalized in subsequent electrocardiographic tracings.

Headaches

The incidence of headache in SSRI trials was 18% to 20%, only 1% point higher than the placebo rate. Fluoxetine is the most likely to cause headache. On the other hand, all SSRIs are effective prophylaxis against both migraine and tension-type headaches in many persons.

Central Nervous System Adverse Effects

Anxiety. Fluoxetine may cause anxiety, particularly in the first few weeks of treatment. However, these initial effects usually give way to an overall reduction in anxiety after a few weeks. Increased anxiety is caused considerably less frequently by paroxetine and escitalopram, which may be better choices if sedation is desired, as in mixed anxiety and depressive disorders.

Insomnia and Sedation. The major effect SSRIs exert in the area of insomnia and sedation is improved sleep resulting from treatment of depression and anxiety. However, as many as 25% of persons taking SSRIs note trouble sleeping, excessive somnolence, or overwhelming fatigue. Fluoxetine is the most likely to cause insomnia, for which reason it is often taken in the morning. Sertraline and fluvoxamine are about equally likely to cause insomnia as somnolence, and citalopram and especially paroxetine often cause somnolence. Escitalopram is more likely to interfere with sleep than its isomer, citalopram. Some persons benefit from taking their SSRI dose before going to bed, but others prefer to take it the morning. SSRI-induced insomnia can be treated with benzodiazepines, trazodone (Desyrel) (clinicians must explain the risk of priapism), or other sedating medicines. Significant SSRI-induced somnolence often requires switching to use of another SSRI or bupropion.

Other Sleep Effects. Many persons taking SSRIs report recalling extremely vivid dreams or nightmares. They describe sleep as "busy." Other sleep effects of the SSRIs include bruxism, restless legs, nocturnal myoclonus, and sweating.

Emotional Blunting. Emotional blunting is a largely overlooked but frequent side effect associated with chronic SSRI use. Patients report an inability to cry in response to emotional situations, a feeling of apathy or indifference, or a restriction in the intensity of emotional experiences. This side effect often leads to treatment discontinuation even when the drugs provide relief from depression or anxiety.

Yawning. Close clinical observation of patients taking SSRIs reveals an increase in yawning. This side effect is not a reflection of fatigue or poor nocturnal sleep but is the result of SSRI effects on the hypothalamus.

Seizures. Seizures have been reported in 0.1% to 0.2% of all patients treated with SSRIs, an incidence comparable to that reported with other antidepressants and not significantly different from that with placebo. Seizures are more frequent at the highest doses of SSRIs (e.g., fluoxetine 100 mg a day or higher).

Extrapyramidal Symptoms. The SSRIs may rarely cause akathisia, dystonia, tremor, cogwheel rigidity, torticollis, opisthotonos, gait disorders, and bradykinesia. Rare cases of tardive dyskinesia have been reported. Some people with well-controlled Parkinson's disease may experience acute worsening of their motor symptoms when they take SSRIs.

Anticholinergic Effects
Paroxetine has mild anticholinergic activity that causes dry mouth, constipation, and sedation in a dose-dependent fashion. Nevertheless, most persons taking paroxetine do not experience cholinergic adverse effects. Other SSRIs are associated with dry mouth, but this effect is not mediated by muscarinic activity.

Hematologic Adverse Effects
The SSRIs can cause functional impairment of platelet aggregation but not a reduction in platelet number. Easy bruising and excessive or prolonged bleeding manifest this pharmacologic effect. When patients exhibit these signs, a test for

bleeding time should be performed. Special monitoring is suggested when patients use SSRIs in conjunction with anticoagulants or aspirin. Concurrent use of SSRIs and NSAIDs is associated with a significantly increased risk of gastric bleeding. In cases where this combination is necessary, use of proton pump inhibitors should be considered.

Electrolyte and Glucose Disturbances
The SSRIs may acutely decrease glucose concentrations; therefore, diabetic patients should be carefully monitored. Long-term use may be associated with increased glucose levels, although it remains to be proven whether this is the result of a pharmacologic effect. It is possible that antidepressant users have other characteristics that raise their odds of developing diabetes, or are more likely to be diagnosed with diabetes or other medical conditions as a result of being in treatment for depression.

Cases of SSRI-associated hyponatremia and the syndrome of inappropriate antidiuretic hormone have been seen in patients, especially those who are older or treated with diuretics.

Endocrine and Allergic Reactions
The SSRIs can increase prolactin levels and cause mammoplasia and galactorrhea in both men and women. Breast changes are reversible upon discontinuation of the drug, but this may take several months to occur.

Various types of rashes appear in about 4% of all patients; in a small subset of these patients, the allergic reaction may generalize and involve the pulmonary system, resulting rarely in fibrotic damage and dyspnea. SSRI treatment may have to be discontinued in patients with drug-related rashes.

Serotonin Syndrome
Concurrent administration of an SSRI with an MAOI, L-tryptophan, or lithium can raise plasma serotonin concentrations to toxic levels, producing a constellation of symptoms called the *serotonin syndrome*. This serious and possibly fatal syndrome of serotonin overstimulation comprises, in order of appearance as the condition worsens, (1) diarrhea; (2) restlessness; (3) extreme agitation, hyperreflexia, and autonomic instability with possible rapid fluctuations in vital signs; (4) myoclonus, seizures, hyperthermia, uncontrollable shivering, and rigidity; and (5) delirium, coma, status epilepticus, cardiovascular collapse, and death.

Treatment of the serotonin syndrome consists of removing the offending agents and promptly instituting comprehensive supportive care with nitroglycerin, cyproheptadine, methysergide (Sansert), cooling blankets, chlorpromazine (Thorazine), dantrolene (Dantrium), benzodiazepines, anticonvulsants, mechanical ventilation, and paralyzing agents.

Sweating
Some patients experience sweating while being treated with SSRIs. The sweating is unrelated to ambient temperature. Nocturnal sweating may drench bed sheets and require a change of night clothes. Terazosin, 1 or 2 mg per day, is often dramatically effective in counteracting sweating.

Overdose

The adverse reactions associated with overdose of vilazodone at doses of 200 to 280 mg as observed in clinical trials included serotonin syndrome, lethargy, restlessness, hallucinations, and disorientation.

SSRI Withdrawal

The abrupt discontinuance of SSRI use, especially one with a shorter half-life such as paroxetine or fluvoxamine, has been associated with a withdrawal syndrome that may include dizziness, weakness, nausea, headache, rebound depression, anxiety, insomnia, poor concentration, upper respiratory symptoms, paresthesias, and migraine-like symptoms. It usually does not appear until after at least 6 weeks of treatment and usually resolves spontaneously in 3 weeks. Persons who experienced transient adverse effects in the first weeks of taking an SSRI are more likely to experience discontinuation symptoms.

Fluoxetine is the SSRI least likely to be associated with this syndrome because the half-life of its metabolite is more than 1 week, and it effectively tapers itself. Fluoxetine has therefore been used in some cases to treat the discontinuation syndrome caused by termination of other SSRIs. Nevertheless, a delayed and attenuated withdrawal syndrome occurs with fluoxetine as well.

DRUG INTERACTIONS

The SSRIs do not interfere with most other drugs. A serotonin syndrome (Table 27–3) can develop with concurrent administration of MAOIs, tryptophan, lithium (Eskalith), or other antidepressants that inhibit reuptake of serotonin. Fluoxetine, sertraline, and paroxetine can raise plasma concentrations of TCAs, which can cause clinical toxicity. A number of potential pharmacokinetic interactions have been described based on in vitro analyses of the CYP enzymes (see Table 1–2), but clinically relevant interactions are rare. SSRIs that inhibit CYP2D6 may interfere with the analgesic effects of hydrocodone and oxycodone. These drugs can also reduce the effectiveness of tamoxifen. Combined use of SSRIs and NSAIDs increases the risk of gastric bleeding.

The SSRIs, particularly fluvoxamine, should not be used with clozapine because it raises clozapine concentrations, increasing the risk of seizure. The SSRIs may increase the duration and severity of zolpidem (Ambien)-induced side effects, including hallucinations.

Fluoxetine

Fluoxetine can be administered with tricyclic drugs, but the clinician should use low dosages of the tricyclic drug. Because it is metabolized by the hepatic enzyme

Table 27–3
Serotonin Syndrome

Diarrhea	Myoclonus
Diaphoresis	Hyperactive reflexes
Tremor	Disorientation
Ataxia	Lability of mood

CYP2D6, fluoxetine may interfere with the metabolism of other drugs in the 7% of the population that has an inefficient isoform of this enzyme, the so-called poor metabolizers. Fluoxetine may slow down the metabolism of carbamazepine (Tegretol), antineoplastic agents, diazepam (Valium), and phenytoin (Dilantin). Drug interactions have been described for fluoxetine that may affect the plasma levels of benzodiazepines, antipsychotics, and lithium. Fluoxetine and other SSRIs may interact with warfarin (Coumadin) increasing the risk of bleeding and bruising.

Sertraline
Sertraline may displace warfarin from plasma proteins and may increase the prothrombin time. The drug interaction data on sertraline support a generally similar profile to that of fluoxetine, although sertraline does not interact as strongly with the CYP2D6 enzyme.

Paroxetine
Paroxetine has a higher risk for drug interactions than does either fluoxetine or sertraline because it is a more potent inhibitor of the CYP2D6 enzyme. Cimetidine (Tagamet) can increase the concentration of sertraline and paroxetine, and phenobarbital (Luminal) and phenytoin can decrease the concentration of paroxetine. Because of the potential for interference with the CYP2D6 enzyme, the coadministration of paroxetine with other antidepressants, phenothiazines, and antiarrhythmic drugs should be undertaken with caution. Paroxetine may increase the anticoagulant effect of warfarin. Coadministration of paroxetine and tramadol (Ultram) may precipitate a serotonin syndrome in elderly persons.

Fluvoxamine
Among the SSRIs, fluvoxamine appears to present the most risk for drug–drug interactions. Fluvoxamine is metabolized by the enzyme CYP3A4, which may be inhibited by ketoconazole (Nizoral). Fluvoxamine may increase the half-life of alprazolam (Xanax), triazolam (Halcion), and diazepam, and it should not be coadministered with these agents. Fluvoxamine may increase theophylline (Slo-Bid, Theo-Dur) levels threefold and warfarin levels twofold, with important clinical consequences; thus, the serum levels of the latter drugs should be closely monitored and the doses adjusted accordingly. Fluvoxamine raises concentrations and may increase the activity of clozapine, carbamazepine, methadone (Dolophine, Methadose), propranolol (Inderal), and diltiazem (Cardizem). Fluvoxamine has no significant interactions with lorazepam (Ativan) or digoxin (Lanoxin).

Citalopram
Citalopram is not a potent inhibitor of any CYP enzymes. Concurrent administration of cimetidine increases concentrations of citalopram by about 40%. Citalopram does not significantly affect the metabolism of, nor is its metabolism significantly affected by, digoxin, lithium, warfarin, carbamazepine, or imipramine (Tofranil). Citalopram increases the plasma concentrations of metoprolol twofold, but this usually has no effect on blood pressure or heart rate. Data on coadministration of citalopram and potent inhibitors of CYP3A4 or CYP2D6 are not available.

Escitalopram

Escitalopram is a moderate inhibitor of CYP2D6 and has been shown to significantly raise desipramine and metoprolol concentrations.

Vilazodone

Vilazodone dose should be reduced to 20 mg when coadministered with CYP3A4 strong inhibitors. Concomitant use with inducers of CYP3A4 can result in inadequate drug concentrations and may diminish effectiveness. The effect of CYP3A4 inducers on systemic exposure of vilazodone has not been evaluated.

LABORATORY INTERFERENCES

The SSRIs do not interfere with any laboratory tests.

DOSAGE AND CLINICAL GUIDELINES

Fluoxetine

Fluoxetine is available in 10- and 20-mg capsules, in a scored 10-mg tablet, as a 90-mg enteric-coated capsule for once-weekly administration, and as an oral concentrate (20 mg/5 mL). Fluoxetine is also marketed as Sarafem for PMDD. For depression, the initial dosage is usually 10 or 20 mg orally each day, usually given in the morning, because insomnia is a potential adverse effect of the drug. Fluoxetine should be taken with food to minimize the possible nausea. The long half-lives of the drug and its metabolite contribute to a 4-week period to reach steady-state concentrations. Twenty milligrams is often as effective as higher doses for treating depression. The maximum dosage recommended by the manufacturer is 80 mg a day. To minimize the early side effects of anxiety and restlessness, some clinicians initiate fluoxetine use at 5 to 10 mg a day, either with the scored 10-mg tablet or by using the liquid preparation. Alternatively, because of the long half-life of fluoxetine, its use can be initiated with an every-other-day administration schedule. The dosage of fluoxetine (and other SSRIs) that is effective in other indications may differ from the dosage generally used for depression.

Sertraline

Sertraline is available in scored 25-, 50-, and 100-mg tablets. For the initial treatment of depression, sertraline use should be initiated with a dosage of 50 mg once daily. To limit the GI effects, some clinicians begin at 25 mg a day and increase to 50 mg a day after 3 weeks. Patients who do not respond after 1 to 3 weeks may benefit from dosage increases of 50 mg every week, up to a maximum of 200 mg given once daily. Sertraline can be administered in the morning or the evening. Administration after eating may reduce the GI adverse effects. Sertraline oral concentrate (1 mL = 20 mg) has 12% alcohol content and must be diluted before use. When used to treat panic disorder, sertraline should be initiated at 25 mg to reduce the risk of provoking a panic attack.

Paroxetine

Immediate-release paroxetine is available in scored 20-mg tablets; in unscored 10-, 30-, and 40-mg tablets; and as an orange-flavored 10-mg/5-mL oral suspension. Paroxetine use for the treatment of depression is usually initiated at a dosage of 10 or

20 mg a day. An increase in the dosage should be considered when an adequate response is not seen in 1 to 3 weeks. At that point, the clinician can initiate upward dose titration in 10-mg increments at weekly intervals to a maximum of 50 mg a day. Persons who experience GI upset may benefit by taking the drug with food. Paroxetine can be taken initially as a single daily dose in the evening; higher dosages may be divided into two doses per day.

A delayed-release formulation of paroxetine, paroxetine CR, is available in 12.5-, 25-, and 37.5-mg tablets. The starting dosages of paroxetine CR are 25 mg per day for depression and 12.5 mg per day for panic disorder.

Paroxetine is the SSRI most likely to produce a discontinuation syndrome because plasma concentrations decrease rapidly in the absence of continuous dosing. To limit the development of symptoms of abrupt discontinuation, paroxetine use should be tapered gradually, with dosage reductions every 2 to 3 weeks.

Fluvoxamine

Fluvoxamine is the only SSRI not approved by the FDA as an antidepressant. It is indicated for social anxiety disorder and OCD. It is available in unscored 25-mg tablets and scored 50- and 100-mg tablets. The effective daily dosage range is 50 to 300 mg a day. A usual starting dosage is 50 mg once a day at bedtime for the first week, after which the dosage can be adjusted according to the adverse effects and clinical response. Dosages above 100 mg a day may be divided into twice-daily dosing. A temporary dosage reduction or slower upward titration may be necessary if nausea develops over the first 2 weeks of therapy. Although fluvoxamine can also be administered as a single evening dose to minimize its adverse effects, its short half-life may lead to interdose withdrawal. An extended-release formulation is available in 100- and 150-mg dose strengths. All fluvoxamine formulations should be swallowed with food without chewing the tablet. Abrupt discontinuation of fluvoxamine may cause a discontinuation syndrome owing to its short half-life.

Citalopram

Citalopram is available in 20- and 40-mg scored tablets and as a liquid (10 mg/ 5 mL). The usual starting dosage is 20 mg a day for the first week, after which it usually is increased to 40 mg a day. For elderly persons or persons with hepatic impairment, 20 mg a day is recommended, with an increase to 40 mg a day only if there is no response at 20 mg a day. Tablets should be taken once daily in either the morning or the evening with or without food.

Escitalopram

Escitalopram is available as 10- and 20-mg scored tablets, as well as an oral solution at a concentration of 5 mg/5 mL. The recommended dosage of escitalopram is 10 mg per day. In clinical trials, no additional benefit was noted when 20 mg per day was used.

Vilazodone

Vilazodone is available as 10-, 20- and 40-mg tablets. The recommended therapeutic dose of vilazodone is 40 mg once daily. Treatment should be titrated, starting with an initial dose of 10 mg once daily for 7 days, followed by 20 mg once daily for an additional 7 days, and then an increase to 40 mg once daily. Vilazodone should be taken with food. If vilazodone is taken without food, inadequate drug concentrations may result and the drug's effectiveness may be diminished. Vilazodone is not approved for use in children. The safety and efficacy of vilazodone in pediatric patients have not been studied. No dose adjustment is recommended on the basis of age. No dose adjustment is recommended in patients with mild or moderate hepatic impairment. Vilazodone has not been studied in patients with severe hepatic impairment. No dose adjustment is recommended in patients with mild, moderate, or severe renal impairment.

Pregnancy and Breastfeeding
With the exception of paroxetine, the SSRIs are safe to take during pregnancy when deemed necessary for treatment of the mother. There are no controlled human data regarding vilazodone use during pregnancy nor are there human data regarding drug concentrations in breast milk.

Transient QTc prolongation has been noted in newborns whose mother was being treated with an SSRI during pregnancy.

Loss of Efficacy
Some patients report a diminished response or total loss of response to SSRIs with recurrence of depressive symptoms while remaining on a full dose of medication. The exact mechanism of this so-called "poop-out" is unknown, but the phenomenon is very real. Potential remedies for the attenuation of response to SSRIs include increasing or decreasing the dosage, tapering drug use, and then rechallenging with the same medication, switching to another SSRI or non-SSRI antidepressant, and augmenting with bupropion or another augmentation agent.

VORTIOXETINE
Vortioxetine (Trintellix) is an atypical SSRI, FDA designated as a serotonin modulator and stimulator. It is only approved for the treatment of MDD in adults. Vortioxetine was investigated as a treatment for GAD but was found to be no better than placebo.

Pharmacodynamics
Vortioxetine is classified as a "serotonin modulator and stimulator." It has been shown to possess the following pharmacologic actions:

- Serotonin transporter blocker
- Norepinephrine transporter blocker
- 5-HT_{1A} receptor high-efficacy partial agonist/near-full agonist
- 5-HT_{1B} receptor partial agonist
- 5-HT_{1D} receptor antagonist
- 5-HT_{3A} receptor antagonist
- 5-HT_7 receptor antagonist
- β_1-Adrenergic receptor ligand

The clinical impact of these multiple receptor effects is not well understood.

Therapeutic Indications

Vortioxetine is approved for treatment of MDD in adults. There are no published data on the efficacy and safety of vortioxetine use in children and adolescents. It has been studied in elderly patients, with no evidence of unusual adverse events.

Pharmacokinetics

The pharmacologic activity of vortioxetine is entirely derived from the parent molecule. It has no active metabolites. It has a mean terminal half-life of about 66 hours. Vortioxetine reaches peak plasma concentration within 7 to 11 hours postadministration. Steady-state plasma concentrations are usually achieved within 2 weeks. It may be taken with or without food.

Vortioxetine is extensively metabolized, mainly through the CYP450 isozymes 2D6, 3A4/5, 2C19, 2C9, 2A6, 2C8, and 2B6. After oxidation, it undergoes glucuronic acid conjugation. It is converted to a pharmacologically inactive metabolite through CYP2D6 oxidation. Poor metabolizers of CYP2D6 have nearly twice the plasma concentration of vortioxetine than do extensive metabolizers. No significant impact on plasma protein binding or clearance has been demonstrated by hepatic or renal disease. Steady-state AUC and C_{max} of vortioxetine are increased when coadministered with bupropion, fluconazole, and ketoconazole. These are decreased when vortioxetine is used with rifampicin.

Precautions and Adverse Reactions

The most common side effects reported with vortioxetine are nausea, diarrhea, xerostomia, constipation, vomiting, flatulence, dizziness, and sexual dysfunction. Based on clinical trial data, the incidence of sexual dysfunction is reportedly higher in patients taking vortioxetine than in patients taking placebos but lower than in patients taking venlafaxine.

Pregnancy and Breastfeeding

Vortioxetine studies in animals have shown evidence of an increased occurrence of fetal damage, the significance of which is considered uncertain in humans. Use is not recommended unless clearly needed. Use during breastfeeding is not recommended and a decision should be made to discontinue breastfeeding or discontinue the drug, taking into account the importance of the drug to the mother. It is not known if it is excreted into human milk and effects on nursing infants are unknown.

Dosing

Patients typically initiate drug therapy at 10 mg daily, which may be subsequently increased to 20 mg daily. If 10 mg dosing is poorly tolerated, the dose can be lowered to 5 mg per day. Clinical trial data do not indicate a clinically significant difference response and remission rates at doses above 20 mg/day.

Available Formulations

In the United States, vortioxetine is available in 5-, 10-, 15-, and 20-mg tablets.

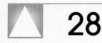

28

Second-Generation or Atypical Antipsychotics (Serotonin–Dopamine Antagonists, Modulators, and Similarly Acting Drugs)

INTRODUCTION

The second-generation antipsychotics (SGAs), the most widely prescribed agents for schizophrenia and other illnesses associated with psychotic symptoms, are actually a pharmacologically diverse group of compounds. Most of these drugs have received approval as monotherapy or adjunctive therapy in the treatment of bipolar disorder. Some have also been approved as adjuncts for antidepressants in the treatment of major depression without psychotic symptoms. One is exclusively used to treat psychosis associated with Parkinson's disease.

Initially, these agents were referred to as serotonin–dopamine antagonists (SDAs), based on the belief they could be differentiated from the dopamine receptor antagonists by their high affinity for serotonin 2A (5-HT$_{2A}$) as well as dopamine (D$_2$) receptors. This simplistic conceptualization is now questioned, and the term serotonin–dopamine antagonists (SDAs) has been replaced by the term second-generation antipsychotics (SGAs). The Food and Drug Administration (FDA) has more recently classified some of these drugs as modulators, to reflect their ability to control and alter neurotransmission. The fact is, the pharmacology of these drugs is complex, and individual drugs in this group have multiple neurotransmitter effects.

These drugs are also called atypical antipsychotics. The term *atypical* is also used because these drugs differ from the dopamine receptor antagonists (DRAs) in their side-effect profiles. Most notably, they have a lower risk of extrapyramidal side effects (EPS), and have spectra of action that are broader than those of the SGAs.

At least a dozen SGAs have been approved by the FDA. These include the following drugs: risperidone (Risperdal), risperidone IM long acting (Consta), olanzapine (Zyprexa), olanzapine for extended-release injectable suspension (Zyprexa, Relprevv), quetiapine (Seroquel), quetiapine XR (Seroquel XR), ziprasidone (Geodon), aripiprazole (Abilify), paliperidone (Invega), paliperidone palmitate (Invega, Invega Sustenna), asenapine (Saphris), lurasidone (Latuda), iloperidone (Fanapt), cariprazine (Vraylar), pimavanserin (Nuplazid), and clozapine (Clozaril). Pimavanserin is the only antipsychotic approved for the treatment of hallucinations and delusions associated with Parkinson's disease psychosis. It has no significant affinity for dopamine receptors and is not approved for treatment of other psychoses.

Although SGAs represent an improvement over the DRAs with respect to a lowered, but not absent, risk of EPS, most of the drugs in this group often produce substantial weight gain, which in turn increases the potential for development of diabetes mellitus.

MECHANISMS OF ACTION

The presumed antipsychotic effects of the SGAs are blockade of D_2 dopamine receptors. Where the SDAs differ from older antipsychotic drugs is their higher ratio interactions with serotonin receptor subtypes, most notably the 5-HT$_{2A}$ subtype, as well as with other neurotransmitter systems. It is hypothesized that these properties account for the distinct tolerability profiles associated with each of the SGAs. All SGAs have different chemical structures, receptor affinities, and side-effect profiles. No SGA is identical in its combination of receptor affinities, and the relative contribution of each receptor interaction to the clinical effects is unknown.

THERAPEUTIC INDICATIONS

Although initially approved for the treatment of schizophrenia and acute mania, some of these drugs have also been approved as adjunctive therapy in treatment-resistant depression and as adjunctive therapy in major depressive disorder. They are also useful in posttraumatic stress disorder and anxiety disorders, and although clinicians tend to use them in behavioral disturbances associated with dementia, all SGAs carry an FDA-boxed warning regarding adverse effects when used in elderly persons with dementia-related psychoses because elderly patients with dementia-related psychoses are at an increased risk (1.6 to 1.7 times) of death compared with placebo. All of these agents are considered first-line drugs for schizophrenia except clozapine, which may cause adverse hematologic effects that require weekly blood sampling.

Schizophrenia and Schizoaffective Disorder

The SDAs are effective for treating acute and chronic psychoses such as schizophrenia and schizoaffective disorder, in both adults and adolescents. SDAs are as good as or better than typical antipsychotics (DRAs) for the treatment of positive symptoms in schizophrenia and superior to DRAs for the treatment of negative symptoms. Compared with persons treated with DRAs, persons treated with SGAs have fewer relapses and require less frequent hospitalization, fewer emergency department visits, less phone contact with mental health professionals, and less treatment in day programs.

Because clozapine has potentially life-threatening adverse effects, it is appropriate only for patients with schizophrenia who are resistant to all other antipsychotics. Other indications for clozapine include treatment of persons with severe tardive dyskinesia—which can be reversed with high dosages in some cases—and those with a low threshold for EPS. Persons who tolerate clozapine have done well on long-term therapy. The effectiveness of clozapine may be increased by augmentation with risperidone, which raises clozapine concentrations and sometimes results in dramatic clinical improvement.

Mood Disorders

Many of the SGAs are FDA approved for treatment of acute mania. Some of these agents, including aripiprazole, olanzapine, quetiapine, lurasidone, and quetiapine XR, are also approved for the maintenance treatment in bipolar disorder as monotherapy or adjunctive therapy. Olanzapine in a fixed combination with fluoxetine

(Symbyax) has been approved for treatment-resistant depression and as a treatment for acute bipolar depression.

Other Indications

About 10% of schizophrenic patients exhibit outwardly aggressive or violent behavior and the SDAs are effective for treatment of such aggression. Other off-label indications include AIDS dementia, autistic spectrum disorders, Tourette's disorder, Huntington's disease, and Lesch–Nyhan syndrome. Risperidone and olanzapine have been used to control aggression and self-injury in children. These drugs have also been coadministered with sympathomimetics, such as methylphenidate (Ritalin) or dextroamphetamine (Dexedrine), to children with attention-deficit/hyperactivity disorder who are comorbid for either opposition-defiant disorder or conduct disorder. SGAs—especially olanzapine, quetiapine, and clozapine—are useful in persons who have severe tardive dyskinesia. The SDAs are also effective for treating psychotic depression and for psychosis secondary to head trauma, dementia, or treatment drugs.

Patients with treatment-resistant obsessive–compulsive disorder (OCD) have responded to the SGAs; however, a few persons treated with the SGAs have been noted to develop treatment-emergent symptoms of OCD. Some patients with borderline personality disorder may improve with the SGAs.

Some data suggest that treatment with conventional DRAs has protective effects against the progression of schizophrenia when used during the first episode of psychosis. Ongoing studies are looking at whether the use of SGAs in at-risk patients with early evidence of disease prevents deterioration, thus improving long-term outcome.

Adverse Effects

The SDAs share a similar spectrum of adverse reactions but differ considerably in terms of frequency or severity of their occurrence. Specific side effects that are more common with an individual SGA are emphasized in the discussion of each drug below.

Use in Pregnancy and Lactation

A large review of the reproductive safety of SGAs found that the drugs did not raise the risk of major malformations significantly beyond those observed in the general population or those using other psychotropic medications. SGAs are safe to use in breastfeeding, with the exception of clozapine.

RISPERIDONE (RISPERDAL)

Indications

Risperidone is indicated for the acute and maintenance treatment of schizophrenia in adults and for the treatment of schizophrenia in adolescents aged 13 to 17 years. Risperidone is also indicated for the short-term treatment of acute manic or mixed episodes associated with bipolar I disorder in adults and in children and adolescents aged 10 to 17 years. The combination of risperidone with lithium or valproate is indicated for the short-term treatment of acute manic or mixed episodes associated with bipolar I disorder.

Risperidone is also indicated for the treatment of irritability associated with autistic spectrum disorder in children and adolescents aged 5 to 16 years, including symptoms of aggression toward others, deliberate self-injuriousness, temper tantrums, and quickly changing moods.

Pharmacology

Risperidone undergoes extensive first-pass hepatic metabolism to 9-hydroxyrisperidone, a metabolite with equivalent antipsychotic activity. Peak plasma levels of the parent compound occur within 1 hour for the parent compound and 3 hours for the metabolite. Risperidone has a bioactivity of 70%. The combined half-life of risperidone and 9-hydroxyrisperidone averages 20 hours, so it is effective in once-daily dosing. Risperidone is an antagonist of the serotonin 5-HT$_{2A}$, dopamine D$_2$, α_1-, and α_2-adrenergic, and histamine H$_1$ receptors. It has a low affinity for α-adrenergic and muscarinic cholinergic receptors. Although it is as potent an antagonist of D$_2$ receptors as is haloperidol (Haldol), risperidone is much less likely than haloperidol to cause EPS in humans when the dose of Risperdal is below 6 mg per day.

Dosages

The recommended dose range and frequency of risperidone dosing have changed since the drug first came into clinical use. Risperidone is available in 0.25-, 0.5-, 1-, 2-, 3-, and 4-mg tablets and a 1-mg/mL oral solution. The initial dosage is usually 1 to 2 mg at night, which can then be increased to 4 mg per day. Positron emission tomography (PET) studies have shown that dosages of 1 to 4 mg per day provide the required D$_2$ blockade needed for a therapeutic effect. At first it was believed that because of its short elimination half-life, risperidone should be given twice a day, but studies have shown equal efficacy with once-a-day dosing. Dosages above 6 mg a day are associated with a higher incidence of adverse effects, particularly EPS. There is no correlation between plasma concentrations and therapeutic effect. Dosing guidelines for adolescents and children are different from those for adults, requiring lower starting dosages; higher dosages are associated with more adverse effects.

Side Effects

The EPS of risperidone are largely dosage dependent, and there has been a trend to using lower doses than initially recommended. Weight gain, anxiety, nausea and vomiting, rhinitis, erectile dysfunction, orgasmic dysfunction, and increased pigmentation are associated with risperidone use. The most common drug-related reasons for discontinuation of risperidone use are EPS, dizziness, hyperkinesias, somnolence, and nausea. Marked elevation of prolactin may occur. Weight gain occurs more commonly with risperidone use in children than in adults.

Risperidone is also available as an orally disintegrating tablet (Risperdal M-Tab), which is available in 0.5-, 1-, and 2-mg strengths, and in a depot formulation (Risperdal Consta), which is given as an intramuscular (IM) injection formulation every 2 weeks. The dose may be 25, 50, or 75 mg. Oral risperidone should be coadministered with Risperdal Consta for the first 3 weeks before being discontinued.

Drug Interactions

Inhibition of CYP2D6 by drugs such as paroxetine and fluoxetine can block the formation of risperidone's active metabolite. Risperidone is a weak inhibitor of CYP2D6 and has little effect on other drugs. Combined use of risperidone and selective serotonin reuptake inhibitors (SSRIs) may result in significant elevation of prolactin, with associated galactorrhea and breast enlargement.

PALIPERIDONE (INVEGA)

Indications

Paliperidone is indicated for the acute and maintenance treatment of schizophrenia. Paliperidone is also indicated for the acute treatment of schizoaffective disorder as monotherapy or as an adjunct to mood stabilizers, or antidepressants.

Pharmacology

Paliperidone is the major active metabolite of risperidone. Peak plasma concentrations (C_{max}) are achieved approximately 24 hours after dosing, and steady-state concentrations of paliperidone are attained within 4 or 5 days. The hepatic isoenzymes CYP2D6 and CYP3A4 play a limited role in the metabolism and elimination of paliperidone, so no dose adjustment is required in patients with mild or moderate hepatic impairment.

Dosage

Paliperidone is available in 3-, 6-, and 9-mg tablets. The recommended dosage is 6 mg once daily administered in the morning. It can be taken with or without food swallowed whole. It is also available as extended-release tablets, which are also available in 3-, 6-, and 9-mg tablets administered once daily. It is recommended that no more than 12 mg should be administered per day. A long-acting formulation of paliperidone (Invega Sustenna) is given by injection once a month. Invega Sustenna is available as a white to off-white sterile aqueous extended-release suspension for IM injection in dose strengths of 39-, 78-, 117-, 156-, and 234-mg paliperidone palmitate. The drug product hydrolyzes to the active moiety, paliperidone, resulting in dose strengths of 25, 50, 75, 100, and 150 mg of paliperidone, respectively.

Invega Sustenna is provided in a prefilled syringe with a plunger stopper and tip cap. The kit also contains two safety needles (a 1½-in, 22-gauge safety needle and a 1-in, 23-gauge safety needle). It has a half-life of 25 to 49 days. Monthly injections of 117 mg are recommended, although higher or lower dosages can be used depending on the clinical situation. The first two injections should be in the deltoid muscle because plasma concentrations are 28% higher with deltoid versus gluteal administration. Subsequent injections can alternate between gluteal and deltoid sites.

Side Effects

The dose of paliperidone should be reduced in patients with renal impairment. It may cause more sensitivity to temperature extremes such as very hot or cold conditions. Paliperidone may cause an increase in QT (QTc) interval and should be avoided in combination with other drugs that cause prolongation of QT interval. It may cause orthostatic hypotension, tachycardia, somnolence, akathisia, dystonia, EPS, and parkinsonism.

OLANZAPINE (ZYPREXA)

Indications

Olanzapine is indicated for the treatment of schizophrenia. Oral olanzapine is indicated for use as monotherapy for the acute treatment of manic or mixed episodes associated with bipolar I disorder and maintenance treatment of bipolar I disorder. Oral olanzapine is also indicated for the treatment of manic or mixed episodes associated with bipolar I disorder as an adjunct to lithium or valproate, and olanzapine can also be used in combination with fluoxetine (Symbyax) for the treatment of depressive episodes associated with bipolar I disorder.

Oral olanzapine and fluoxetine in combination (Symbyax) is indicated for the treatment of treatment-resistant depression. Olanzapine monotherapy is not indicated for the treatment of treatment-resistant depression.

Pharmacology

Approximately 85% of olanzapine is absorbed from the gastrointestinal (GI) tract, and about 40% of the dosage is inactivated by first-pass hepatic metabolism. Peak concentrations are reached in 5 hours, and the half-life averages 31 hours (range: 21 to 54 hours). It is given in once-daily dosing. In addition to 5-HT_{2A} and D_2 antagonism, olanzapine is an antagonist of the D_1, D_4, α_1, 5-HT_{1A}, muscarinic M_1 to M_5, and H_1 receptors.

Dosages

Olanzapine is available in 2.5-, 5-, 7.5-, 10-, 15-, and 20-mg oral and Zydis form (orally disintegrating) tablets. The initial dosage for treatment of psychosis is usually 5 or 10 mg and for treatment of acute mania is usually 10 or 15 mg given once daily. It is also available as 5-, 10-, 15-, and 20-mg orally disintegrating tablets that might be useful for patients who have difficulty swallowing pills or who "cheek" their medication.

A starting daily dose of 5 to 10 mg is recommended. After 1 week, the dosage can be raised to 10 mg a day. Given the long half-life, 1 week must be allowed to achieve each new steady-state blood level. Dosages in clinical use ranges vary, with 5 to 20 mg a day being most commonly used but 30 to 40 mg a day being needed in treatment-resistant patients. A word of caution, however, is that the higher dosages are associated with increased EPS and other adverse effects, and dosages above 20 mg a day were not studied in the pivotal trials that led to the approval of olanzapine. The parenteral form of olanzapine is indicated for the treatment of acute agitation associated with schizophrenia and bipolar disorder, and the IM dosage is 10 mg. Coadministration with benzodiazepines is not approved.

Other Formulations

Olanzapine is available as an extended-release injectable suspension (Relprevv), which is a long-acting atypical IM injection indicated for the treatment of schizophrenia. It is injected deeply in the gluteal region and should not be administered intravenously or subcutaneously, nor is it approved for deltoid administration. Before administering the injection, the administrator should aspirate the syringe for several seconds to ensure no blood is visible. It carries a boxed warning for postinjection delirium sedation syndrome (PDSS). Patients are at risk for severe sedation (including coma) and must be observed for 3 hours after each injection in a registered facility. In controlled studies, all patients with PDSS recovered, and there were no deaths reported. It is postulated that PDSS is secondary to increased levels of olanzapine secondary to accidental rupture of a blood vessel. Patients should be managed as clinically appropriate and, if necessary, monitored in a facility capable of resuscitation. The injection can be given every 2 or 4 weeks depending on the dosing guidelines.

Drug Interactions

Fluvoxamine (Luvox) and cimetidine (Tagamet) increase while carbamazepine and phenytoin decrease serum concentrations of olanzapine. Ethanol increases olanzapine absorption by more than 25%, leading to increased sedation. Olanzapine has little effect on the metabolism of other drugs.

Side Effects

Other than clozapine, olanzapine consistently causes a greater amount and more frequent weight gain than other atypicals. This effect is not dose related and continues over time. Clinical trial data suggest it peaks after 9 months, after which it may continue to increase more slowly. Somnolence, dry mouth, dizziness, constipation, dyspepsia, increased appetite, akathisia, and tremor are associated with olanzapine use. A small number of patients (2%) may need to discontinue use of the drug because of transaminase elevation. There is a dose-related risk of EPS. The manufacturer recommends "periodic" assessment of blood sugar and transaminases during treatment with olanzapine. There is an FDA-mandated warning about an increased risk of stroke among patients with dementia treated with SDAs, but this risk is small and is outweighed by improved behavioral control that treatment may produce.

QUETIAPINE (SEROQUEL)

Indications

Quetiapine is indicated for the treatment of schizophrenia, as well as the acute treatment of manic episodes associated with bipolar I disorder, both as monotherapy and as an adjunct to lithium or divalproex. It is also indicated as monotherapy for the acute treatment of depressive episodes associated with bipolar disorder and maintenance treatment of bipolar I disorder as an adjunct to lithium or divalproex.

Pharmacology

Quetiapine is structurally related to clozapine, but it differs markedly from that agent in biochemical effects. It is rapidly absorbed from the GI tract, with peak plasma concentrations reached in 1 to 2 hours. The steady-state half-life is about 7 hours, and optimal dosing is two or three times per day. Quetiapine, in addition to being an antagonist of D_2 and 5-HT$_2$, also blocks 5-HT$_6$, D_1 and H_1, and α_1 and α_2 receptors. It does not block muscarinic or benzodiazepine receptors. The receptor antagonism for quetiapine is generally lower than that for other antipsychotic drugs, and it is not associated with EPS.

Dosages

Quetiapine is available in 25-, 50-, 100-, 200-, 300-, and 400-mg tablets. Quetiapine dosing should begin at 25 mg twice daily, with doses then raised by 25 to 50 mg per dose every 2 to 3 days up to a target of 300 to 400 mg a day. Studies have shown efficacy in the range of 300 to 800 mg a day. In reality, more aggressive dosing is both tolerated and more effective. It has become evident that the target dose can be achieved more rapidly and that some patients benefit from dosages of as much as 1,200 to 1,600 mg a day. When used at higher doses, serial electrocardiograms (EKGs) should be performed. Despite its short elimination half-life, quetiapine can be given to many patients once a day. This is consistent with the observation that quetiapine receptor occupancy remains even when concentrations in the blood have markedly declined. Quetiapine in doses of 25 to 300 mg at night has been used for insomnia.

Other Formulations

Quetiapine XR has a comparable bioavailability to an equivalent dose of quetiapine administered two or three times daily. Quetiapine XR is given once daily preferably in the evening 3 to 4 hours before bedtime without food or a light meal to prevent an increase in C_{max}. The usual starting dose is 300 mg, and it may be increased to 400 to 800 mg.

It has all of the above indications and in addition is indicated for use as adjunctive therapy to antidepressants for the treatment of major depressive disorder (MDD).

Drug Interactions

The potential interactions between quetiapine and other drugs have been well studied. Phenytoin increases quetiapine clearance fivefold, no major pharmacokinetic interactions have been noted. Avoid use of quetiapine with drugs that increase the QT interval and in patients with risk factors for prolonged QT interval. The FDA has added a new warning about quetiapine cautioning prescribers about potential prolongation of the QT interval when above-recommended amounts of quetiapine are combined with specific drugs. The use of quetiapine should be avoided in combination with other drugs that are known to prolong QTc including Class 1A antiarrhythmics (e.g., quinidine, procainamide) or Class III antiarrhythmics (e.g., amiodarone, sotalol), antipsychotic medications (e.g., ziprasidone, chlorpromazine, thioridazine), antibiotics (e.g., gatifloxacin, moxifloxacin), or any other class of medications known to prolong the QTc interval (e.g., pentamidine, levomethadyl acetate, methadone). Quetiapine should also be avoided in circumstances that may increase the risk of occurrence of torsade de pointes and/or sudden death including (1) a history of cardiac arrhythmias such as bradycardia; (2) hypokalemia or hypomagnesemia; (3) concomitant use of other drugs that prolong the QTc interval; and (4) presence of congenital prolongation of the QT interval. Postmarketing cases also show increases in QT interval in patients who overdose on quetiapine.

Side Effects

Somnolence, postural hypotension, and dizziness are the most common adverse effects of quetiapine. These are usually transient and are best managed with initial gradual upward titration of the dosage. Quetiapine is the SDA least likely to cause EPS, regardless of dose. This makes it particularly useful in treating patients with Parkinson's disease who develop dopamine agonist–induced psychosis. Prolactin elevation is rare and both transient and mild when it occurs. Quetiapine is associated with modest transient weight gain in some persons, but some patients occasionally gain a considerable amount of weight. The relationship between quetiapine and the development of diabetes is not as clearly established as are the cases involving the use of olanzapine. Small increases in heart rate, constipation, and a transient increase in liver transaminases may also occur. Initial concerns about cataract formation, based on animal studies, have not been borne out since the drug has been in clinical use. Nevertheless, it might be prudent to test for lens abnormalities early in treatment and periodically thereafter.

ZIPRASIDONE (GEODON)

Indications

Ziprasidone is indicated for the treatment of schizophrenia. Ziprasidone is also indicated as monotherapy for the acute treatment of manic or mixed episodes associated with bipolar I disorder and as an adjunct to lithium or valproate for the maintenance treatment of bipolar I disorder.

Pharmacology

Peak plasma concentrations of ziprasidone are reached in 2 to 6 hours. Steady-state levels ranging from 5 to 10 hours are reached between the first and the third day of treatment. The mean terminal half-life at steady state ranges from 5 to 10 hours, which accounts for the recommendation that twice-daily dosing is necessary. Bioavailability doubles when ziprasidone is taken with food, and therefore should be taken with food.

Peak serum concentrations of IM ziprasidone occur after approximately 1 hour, with a half-life of 2 to 5 hours.

Ziprasidone, similar to the other SDAs, blocks 5-HT_{2A} and D_2 receptors. It is also an antagonist of 5-HT_{1D}, 5-HT_{2C}, D_3, D_4, α_1, and H_1 receptors. It has very low affinity for D_1, M_1, and α_2 receptors. Ziprasidone also has agonist activity at the serotonin 5-HT_{1A} receptors and is an SSRI and a norepinephrine reuptake inhibitor. This is consistent with clinical reports that ziprasidone has antidepressant-like effects in nonschizophrenic patients.

Dosages

Ziprasidone is available in 20-, 40-, 60-, and 80-mg capsules. Ziprasidone for IM use comes as a single-use 20-mg/mL vial. Oral ziprasidone dosing should be initiated at 40 mg a day divided into two daily doses. Studies have shown efficacy in the range of 80 to 160 mg a day, divided twice daily. In clinical practice, doses as high as 240 mg a day are being used. The recommended IM dosage is 10 to 20 mg every 2 hours for the 10-mg dose and every 4 hours for the 40-mg dose. The maximum total daily dose of IM ziprasidone is 40 mg.

Other than interactions with other drugs that prolong the QTc complex, ziprasidone appears to have low potential for clinically significant drug interactions.

Side Effects

Somnolence, headache, dizziness, nausea, and light-headedness are the most common adverse effects in patients taking ziprasidone. It has almost no significant effects outside the central nervous system, is associated with almost no weight gain, and does not cause sustained prolactin elevation. Concerns about prolongation of the QTc complex have deterred some clinicians from using ziprasidone as a first choice. The QTc interval has been shown to increase in patients treated with 40 and 120 mg per day, respectively. Ziprasidone is contraindicated in combination with other drugs known to prolong the QTc interval. These include, but are not limited to, dofetilide, sotalol, quinidine, other Class IA and III antiarrhythmics, mesoridazine, thioridazine, chlorpromazine, droperidol, pimozide, sparfloxacin, gatifloxacin, moxifloxacin, halofantrine, mefloquine, pentamidine, arsenic trioxide, levomethadyl acetate, dolasetron mesylate, probucol, and tacrolimus. Ziprasidone should be avoided in patients with congenital long QT syndrome and in patients with a history of cardiac arrhythmias.

ARIPIPRAZOLE (ABILIFY)

Aripiprazole is a potent $5-HT_{2A}$ antagonist and is indicated for the treatment of both schizophrenia and acute mania. It is also approved for augmentation of antidepressant agents in MDD. Aripiprazole is a D_2 antagonist, but can also act as a partial D_2 agonist. Partial D_2 agonists compete at D_2 receptors for endogenous dopamine, thereby producing a functional reduction of dopamine activity.

Indications

Aripiprazole is indicated for the treatment of schizophrenia. Short-term, 4- to 6-week studies comparing aripiprazole with haloperidol and risperidone in patients with schizophrenia and schizoaffective disorder have shown comparable efficacy. Dosages of 15, 20, and 30 mg a day were found to be effective. Long-term studies suggest that aripiprazole is effective as a maintenance treatment at a daily dose of 15 to 30 mg.

Aripiprazole is also indicated for the acute and maintenance treatment of manic and mixed episodes associated with bipolar I disorder. It is also used as an adjunctive therapy to either lithium or valproate for the acute treatment of manic and mixed episodes associated with bipolar I disorder.

Aripiprazole is indicated for use as an adjunctive therapy to antidepressants for the treatment of MDD. Aripiprazole is also indicated for the treatment of irritability associated with autistic disorder.

Pharmacology

Aripiprazole is well absorbed, reaching peak plasma concentrations after 3 to 5 hours. Absorption is not affected by food. The mean elimination half-life of aripiprazole is about 75 hours. It has a weakly active metabolite with a half-life of 96 hours. These relatively long half-lives make aripiprazole suitable for once-daily dosing. Clearance is reduced in elderly persons. Aripiprazole exhibits linear pharmacokinetics and is primarily metabolized by CYP3A4 and CYP2D6 enzymes. It is 99% protein bound. Aripiprazole is excreted in breast milk in lactating rats.

Mechanistically, aripiprazole acts as a modulator, rather than a blocker, and acts on both postsynaptic D_2 receptors and presynaptic autoreceptors. In theory, this mechanism addresses excessive limbic dopamine (hyperdopaminergic) activity, and decreased dopamine (hypordopaminergic) activity in frontal and prefrontal areas—abnormalities that are thought to be present in schizophrenia. The absence of complete D_2 blockade in the striatal areas would be expected to minimize EPS. Aripiprazole is an α_1-adrenergic receptor antagonist, which may cause some patients to experience orthostatic hypotension. Similar to the so-called atypical antipsychotic agents, aripiprazole is a $5-HT_{2A}$ antagonist.

Other Uses
A study of aggressive children and adolescents with oppositional-defiant disorder or conduct disorder found that there was a positive response in about 60% of the subjects. In this study, vomiting and somnolence led to a reduction in initial aripiprazole dosage.

Drug Interactions
Whereas carbamazepine and valproate reduce serum concentrations, ketoconazole, fluoxetine, paroxetine, and quinidine increase aripiprazole serum concentrations. Lithium and valproic acid, two drugs likely to be combined with aripiprazole when treating bipolar disorder, do not affect the steady-state concentrations of aripiprazole. Combined use with antihypertensives may cause hypotension. Drugs that inhibit CYP2D6 activity reduce aripiprazole elimination.

Dosage and Clinical Guidelines
Aripiprazole is available as 5-, 10-, 15-, 20-, and 30-mg tablets. The effective dosage range is 10 to 30 mg per day. Although the starting dosage is 10 to 15 mg per day, problems with nausea, insomnia, and akathisia have led to use of lower than recommended starting dosages of aripiprazole. Many clinicians find that an initial dose of 5 mg increases tolerability. The FDA has approved aripiprazole as the first drug to have a digital ingestion tracking system. MyCite, the name of that formulation has an ingestible sensor embedded in the pill that records that the medication was taken. It is available in 2-, 5-, 10-, 15-, 20- and 30-mg tablets.

Side Effects
The most commonly reported side effects of aripiprazole are headache, somnolence, agitation, dyspepsia, anxiety, and nausea. Although it is not a frequent cause of EPS, aripiprazole does cause akathisia-like activation. Described as restlessness or agitation, it can be highly distressing and often leads to discontinuation of medication. Insomnia is another common complaint. Data so far do not indicate that weight gain or diabetes mellitus has an increased incidence with aripiprazole (Abilify). Prolactin elevation does not typically occur. Aripiprazole does not cause significant QTc interval changes. There have been reports of seizures.

ASENAPINE (SAPHRIS)
Pharmacology
Asenapine has an affinity for several receptors, including serotonin ($5-HT_{2A}$ and $5-HT_{2C}$), noradrenergic (α_2 and α_1), dopaminergic (D_3 and D_4 receptors is higher

than its affinity for D_2 receptors), and histamine (H_1). It has negligible affinity for muscarinic-1 cholinergic receptors and hence less incidence of dry mouth, blurred vision, constipation, and urinary retention. The bioavailability is 35% via sublingual (preferred) route and achieves peak plasma concentration in 1 hour. It is metabolized through glucuronidation and oxidative metabolism by CYP1A2, so coadministration with fluvoxamine and other CYP1A2 inhibitors should be done cautiously.

Indications
Asenapine is approved for the acute treatment of adults with schizophrenia and acute treatment of manic or mixed episodes associated with bipolar I disorder with or without psychotic features in adults.

Dosage
Asenapine is available as 5- and 10-mg sublingual tablets, and should be placed under the tongue. This is because the bioavailability of asenapine is less than 2% when swallowed, but is 35% when absorbed sublingually. It dissolves in saliva within seconds and is absorbed through the oral mucosa. Sublingual administration avoids first-pass hepatic metabolism. Patients should be advised to avoid drinking or eating for 10 minutes after taking asenapine because this may lower the blood levels. The recommended starting and target dose for schizophrenia is 5 mg twice a day. In bipolar disorder, the patient may be started on 10 mg twice a day, and if necessary, the dosage may be lowered to 5 mg twice a day depending on the tolerability issues. In acute schizophrenia treatment, there is no evidence of added benefit with a 10-mg BID dose, but there is a clear increase in certain adverse reactions. In both bipolar I disorder and schizophrenia, the maximum dose should not exceed 10 mg BID. The safety of doses above 10 mg BID has not been evaluated in clinical studies.

Side Effects
The most common side effects observed in schizophrenic and bipolar disorders are somnolence, dizziness, EPS other than akathisia, and increased weight. In clinical trials, the mean weight gain after 52 weeks is 0.9 kg and there were no clinically relevant differences in lipid profile and blood glucose after 52 weeks. In clinical trials, asenapine was found to increase the QTc interval in a range of 2 to 5 ms compared to placebo. No patients treated with asenapine experienced QTc increases ≥60 ms from baseline measurements, nor did any experience a QTc of ≥500 ms. Nevertheless, asenapine should be avoided in combination with other drugs known to prolong QTc interval, in patients with congenital prolongation of QT interval or a history of cardiac arrhythmias, and in circumstances that may increase the occurrence of torsades de pointes. Asenapine can elevate prolactin levels, and the elevation can persist during chronic administration. Galactorrhea, amenorrhea, gynecomastia, and impotence may occur.

CARIPRAZINE (VRAYLAR)
Pharmacology
Cariprazine is a dopamine D_2 and D_3 receptor partial agonist, with higher affinity for D_3 receptors, as opposed to the D_2 antagonism.

Indications

Cariprazine is indicated in adults for the acute treatment of manic or mixed episodes associated with bipolar I disorder and the treatment of schizophrenia.

Dosages

Cariprazine is available as 1.5-, 3-, 4-, and 6-mg capsules. The dosage range is 1.5 to 6 mg a day in schizophrenia. The starting dose is 1.5 mg a day. The dose may be increased to 3 mg on day 2. Further dose adjustments can be made in 1.5- to 3-mg increments. The dosage range for bipolar disorder is 3 to 6 mg a day. The starting dose is 1.5 mg a day and should be increased to 3 mg on day 2. Further dose adjustments can be made in 1.5- to 3-mg increments. When a strong CYP3A4 inhibitor is added when a patient is already on a stable dose of cariprazine, reduce the current cariprazine dose by 50%. For those patients taking cariprazine 4.5 mg/day, the dose should be reduced to 1.5 or 3 mg daily. For patients taking 1.5 mg daily, the dosing regimen should be adjusted to every other day. When a CYP3A4 inhibitor is discontinued, cariprazine dosage may need to be increased. When initiating cariprazine while already on a strong CYP3A4 inhibitor, use cariprazine 1.5 mg on days 1 and 3, with no dose on day 2. After day 4 the dose should be administered at 1.5 mg/day, then increased to a maximum of 3 mg/day. When a CYP3A4 inhibitor is discontinued, cariprazine dosage may need to be increased. Concomitant with CYP3A4 inducers administration has not been evaluated. Use of cariprazine is not recommended in patients with severe liver disease.

Side Effects

The most common side effects of cariprazine are extrapyramidal, especially akathisia. Also seen are insomnia, weight gain, sedation, nausea, dizziness, vomiting, and anxiety. Compared to other SGAs, cariprazine is less likely to impact metabolic variables or prolactin levels. It does not increase the QT interval. Some constipation may occur.

BREXPIPRAZOLE (REXULTI)

Pharmacology

Brexpiprazole is a D_2 dopamine partial agonist called serotonin–dopamine activity modulator (SDAM).

Indications

It is indicated for use as an adjunctive therapy to antidepressants for the treatment of major depressive disorder and for the treatment of schizophrenia.

Dosages

Brexpiprazole is available as 0.25-, 0.5-, 1-, 2-, 3-, and 4-mg tablets. The recommended starting dosage for brexpiprazole as adjunctive treatment for MDD is 0.5 or 1 mg once daily, taken orally. The recommended target brexpiprazole dosage to treat schizophrenia is 2 to 4 mg once daily.

Side Effects

Common side effects of brexpiprazole reported in clinical trials include weight gain, agitation, distress, restlessness, constipation, fatigue, runny or stuffy nose, increased appetite, headache, drowsiness, tremor, dizziness, and anxiety.

Interactions

Brexpiprazole interacts with strong/moderate CYP2D6 or CYP3A4 inhibitors or strong CYP3A4 inducers.

Use in Pregnancy and Breastfeeding

Because it is a relatively new drug, it should be avoided in pregnant or nursing women. The effects of brexpiprazole on a fetus are still unknown, and it is unknown if brexpiprazole passes into breast milk or if it can affect a nursing infant.

PIMAVANSERIN (NUPLAZID)

Pharmacology

The mechanism of action of pimavanserin in the treatment of hallucinations and delusions associated with Parkinson's disease psychosis is not well understood. It is postulated that the effect of pimavanserin could be mediated through a combination of inverse agonist and antagonist activity at serotonin 5-HT_{2A} receptors and to a lesser extent at serotonin 5-HT_{2C} receptors.

Indications

Pimavanserin is approved for the treatment of hallucinations and delusions associated with Parkinson's disease psychosis. It is not indicated for treatment of schizophrenia or bipolar disorder.

Dosages

The drug should be administered as 34 mg (taken as two 17-mg tablets) once daily. It is only available as 17-mg tablets. There is no need for titration.

Side Effects

Common side effects include nausea, constipation, swelling of the extremities, walking abnormally (gait disturbance), hallucinations, and confusion.

Interactions

Coadministration of many drugs needs to be avoided or requires dosage adjustments. Strong CYP3A4 inhibitors, such as itraconazole, ketoconazole, clarithromycin, and indinavir, potentiate its effects. When using these drugs, its dose should be reduced by 50%. Strong CYP3A4 inducers, such as rifampin, carbamazepine, phenytoin, and St. John's wort, antagonize Pimavanserin. When patients are taking these compounds, monitor for reduced efficacy. Avoid concomitant use with other drugs known to prolong QT interval including Class 1A (e.g., quinidine, procainamide, disopyramide) or Class 3 antiarrhythmics (e.g., amiodarone, sotalol), certain antipsychotics (e.g., ziprasidone, chlorpromazine, thioridazine), and certain antibiotics (e.g., gatifloxacin, moxifloxacin).

CLOZAPINE (CLOZARIL)

Pharmacology

Clozapine is rapidly absorbed, with peak plasma levels reached in about 2 hours. Steady state is achieved in less than 1 week if twice-daily dosing is used. The elimination half-life is about 12 hours. Clozapine has two major metabolites, one of which, N-dimethyl clozapine, may have some pharmacologic activities. Clozapine is an antagonist of 5-HT_{2A}, D_1, D_3, D_4, and α (especially α_1) receptors. It has relatively low potency as a D_2 receptor antagonist. Data from PET scanning show whereas that 10 mg of haloperidol produces 80% occupancy of striatal D_2 receptors, clinically effective dosages of clozapine occupy only 40% to 50% of striatal D_2 receptors. This difference in D_2 receptor occupancy is probably why clozapine does not cause EPS. It has also been postulated that clozapine and other SDAs bind more loosely to the D_2 receptor, and as a result of this "fast dissociation," more normal dopamine neurotransmission is possible.

Indications

In addition to being the most effective drug treatment for patients who have failed standard therapies, clozapine has been shown to benefit patients with severe tardive dyskinesia. Clozapine suppresses these dyskinesias, but the abnormal movements return when clozapine is discontinued. This is true even though clozapine, on rare occasions, may cause tardive dyskinesia. Other clinical situations in which clozapine may be used include the treatment of psychotic patients who are intolerant of EPS caused by other agents, treatment-resistant mania, severe psychotic depression, idiopathic Parkinson's disease, Huntington's disease, and suicidal patients with schizophrenia or schizoaffective disorder. Other treatment-resistant disorders that have demonstrated response to clozapine include pervasive developmental disorder, autism of childhood, and OCD (either alone or in combination with an SSRI). Used by itself, clozapine may very rarely induce obsessive–compulsive symptoms.

Dosages

Clozapine is available in 25- and 100-mg tablets. The initial dosage is usually 25 mg one or two times daily, although a conservative initial dosage is 12.5 mg twice daily. The dosage can then be raised gradually (25 mg a day every 2 or 3 days) to 300 mg a day in divided doses, usually two or three times daily. Dosages up to 900 mg a day can be used. Testing for blood concentrations of clozapine may be helpful in patients who fail to respond. Studies have found that plasma concentrations greater than 350 mg/mL are associated with a better likelihood of response.

Drug Interactions

Clozapine should not be used with any other drug that is associated with the development of agranulocytosis or bone marrow suppression. Such drugs include carbamazepine, phenytoin, propylthiouracil, sulfonamides, and captopril (Capoten). Lithium combined with clozapine may increase the risk of seizures, confusion, and movement disorders. Lithium should not be used in combination with clozapine by persons who have experienced an episode of neuroleptic malignant syndrome.

Clomipramine (Anafranil) can increase the risk of seizure by lowering the seizure threshold and by increasing clozapine plasma concentrations. Risperidone, fluoxetine, paroxetine, and fluvoxamine increase serum concentrations of clozapine. Addition of paroxetine may precipitate clozapine-associated neutropenia.

Side Effects

The most common drug-related adverse effects are sedation, dizziness, syncope, tachycardia, hypotension, EKG changes, nausea, and vomiting. Other common adverse effects include fatigue, weight gain, various GI symptoms (most commonly constipation), anticholinergic effects, and subjective muscle weakness. Sialorrhea, or hypersalivation, is a side effect that begins early in treatment and is most evident at night. Patients report that their pillows are drenched with saliva. This side effect is most likely the result of impairment of swallowing. Although there are reports that clonidine or amitriptyline may help reduce hypersalivation, the most practical solution is to put a towel over the pillow.

The risk of seizures is about 4% in patients taking dosages above 600 mg a day. Leukopenia, granulocytopenia, agranulocytosis, and fever occur in about 1% of patients. During the first year of treatment, there is a 0.73% risk of clozapine-induced agranulocytosis. The risk during the second year is 0.07%. For neutropenia, the risk is 2.32% and 0.69% during the first and second years of treatment, respectively. The only contraindications to the use of clozapine are a white blood cell (WBC) count below 3,500 cells/mm^3; a previous bone marrow disorder; a history of agranulocytosis during clozapine treatment; or the use of another drug that is known to suppress the bone marrow, such as carbamazepine (Tegretol).

During the first 6 months of treatment, weekly WBC counts are indicated to monitor the patient for the development of agranulocytosis. If the WBC count remains normal, the frequency of testing can be decreased to every 2 weeks. Although monitoring is expensive, early indication of agranulocytosis can prevent a fatal outcome. Clozapine should be discontinued if the WBC count is below 3,000 cells/mm^3 or the granulocyte count is below 1,500/mm^3. In addition, a hematologic consultation should be obtained, and obtaining bone marrow sample should be considered. Persons with agranulocytosis should not be reexposed to the drug. To avoid situations in which a physician or a patient fails to comply with the required blood tests, clozapine cannot be dispensed without proof of monitoring.

Patients exhibiting symptoms of chest pain, shortness of breath, fever, or tachypnea should be immediately evaluated for myocarditis or cardiomyopathy, an infrequent but serious adverse effect ending in death. Serial creatine phosphokinase with myocardial band fractions (CPK-MB), troponin levels, and EKG are recommended with immediate discontinuation of clozapine.

ILOPERIDONE (FANAPT)

Indications

Iloperidone (Fanapt) is indicated for the acute treatment of schizophrenia in adults. The safety and efficacy of iloperidone in children and adolescents has not been established.

Pharmacology

Iloperidone is not a derivative of another antipsychotic agent. It has complex multiple antagonist effects on several neurotransmitter systems. Iloperidone has a strong affinity for dopamine D_3 receptors, followed by decreasing affinities of α_{2C}-noradrenergic, 5-HT$_{1A}$, D_{2A}, and 5-HT$_6$ receptors. Iloperidone has a low affinity for histaminergic receptors. As with other antipsychotics, the clinical significance of this receptor binding affinity is unknown.

Iloperidone has a peak concentration of 2 to 4 hours and a half-life that is dependent on hepatic isoenzyme metabolism. It is metabolized primarily through CYP2D6 and CYP3A4, and the dosage should be reduced by half when administered concomitantly with strong inhibitors of these two isoenzymes. The half-life is 18 to 26 hours in CYP2D6 extensive metabolizers and is 31 to 37 hours in CYP2D6 poor metabolizers. Of note, approximately 7% to 10% of whites and 3% to 8% of African Americans lack the capacity to metabolize CYP2D6 substrates; hence, dosing should be done with this caveat in mind. Iloperidone should be used with caution in persons with severe hepatic impairment.

Side Effects

Iloperidone prolongs the QT interval and may be associated with arrhythmia and sudden death. Iloperidone prolongs the QTc interval by 9 ms at dosages of 12 mg twice daily. Concurrent use with other agents that prolong the QTc interval may result in additive effects on the QTc interval. The concurrent use of iloperidone with agents that prolong the QTc interval may result in potentially life-threatening cardiac arrhythmias, including torsades de pointes. Concurrent administration of other drugs that are known to prolong the QTc interval should be avoided. Cardiovascular disease, hypokalemia, hypomagnesemia, bradycardia, congenital prolongation of the QT interval, and concurrent use of inhibitors of CYPP-450-3A4 or CYPP-450-2D6, which metabolize iloperidone, may increase the risk of QT prolongation.

The most common adverse effects reported are dizziness, dry mouth, fatigue, sedation, tachycardia, and orthostatic hypotension (depending on dosing and titration). Despite being a strong D_2 antagonist, the rate of EPS and akathisia are similar to those of placebo. The mean weight gain in short- and long-term trials is 2.1 kg. Due to its relatively limited use, there is no accurate understanding of iloperidone's effects on weight and lipids. Some patients exhibit elevated prolactin levels. Three cases of priapism have been reported in the premarketing phase.

Dosing

Iloperidone must be titrated slowly to avoid orthostatic hypotension. It is available in a titration pack, and the effective dose (12 mg) should be reached in approximately 4 days based on a twice-a-day dosing schedule. It is usually started on day 1 at 1 mg twice a day and increased daily on a twice-a-day schedule to reach 12 mg by day 4. The maximum recommended dose is 12 mg twice a day (24 mg a day) and can be administered without regard to food.

LURASIDONE (LATUDA)

Indications

Lurasidone HCL is an oral, once daily, atypical antipsychotic indicated for the treatment of patients with schizophrenia. To date there has not been extensive clinical experience with lurasidone.

Side Effects

The most commonly observed adverse reactions associated with the use of lurasidone are similar to those seen with other new-generation antipsychotics. These include, but are not limited to somnolence, akathisia, nausea, parkinsonism, and agitation. Based on clinical trial data, lurasidone appears to cause less weight gain and metabolic changes than the two other most recently approved SDAs, asenapine, and iloperidone. Whether this is in fact the case will await more extensive clinical experience with the drug.

Drug Interactions

When coadministration of lurasidone with a moderate CYP3A4 inhibitor such as diltiazem is considered, the dose should not exceed 40 mg per day. Lurasidone should not be used in combination with a strong CYP3A4 inhibitor (e.g., ketoconazole). Lurasidone also should not be used in combination with a strong CYP3A4 inducer (e.g., rifampin).

Dosages

Lurasidone is available as 20-, 40-, 80-, and 120-mg tablets. Initial dose titration is not required. The recommended starting dose is 40 mg once daily, and the medication should be taken with food. It has been shown to be effective in a dose range of 40 to 120 mg per day. While there is no proven added benefit with the 120 mg per day dose, there may be a dose-related increase in adverse reactions. Still, some patients may benefit from the maximum recommended dose of 160 mg per day. Dose adjustment is recommended in patients with renal impairment. The dose in moderate to severe renal impairment should not exceed 80 mg per day. The dose in severe hepatic impairment patients should not exceed 40 mg per day.

CLINICAL GUIDELINES FOR SGAs

All SGAs, with the exception of pimavanserin and clozapine, are indicated for the management of an initial psychotic episode. Pimavanserin is used only for psychosis in Parkinson's disease, generally a late-onset clinical manifestation. Clozapine is reserved for persons who are refractory to all other antipsychotic drugs. If a person does not respond to the first SGA, other SGAs should be tried. The choice of drug should be based on the patient's clinical status and history of response to medication. Recent studies have challenged the notion that SGAs require 4 to 6 weeks to reach full effectiveness, and it may take up to 8 weeks for the full clinical effects of an SGA to become apparent. The newer meta-analysis suggests that the apparent benefits may be seen as early as 2 to 3 weeks, and early response or failure is an indicator of subsequent response or failure. Nevertheless, it is acceptable practice to augment an SGA with a high-potency DRA or benzodiazepine in the first few weeks of use. Lorazepam (Ativan) 1 to 2 mg orally or IM can be used as needed for acute agitation. Once effective, dosages can be lowered as tolerated. Clinical improvement may take 6 months of treatment with SDAs in some particularly treatment-refractory persons.

Use of all SGAs must be initiated at low dosages and gradually tapered upward to therapeutic dosages. The gradual increase in dosage is necessitated by the potential development of adverse effects. If a person stops taking an SGA for more than 36 hours, drug use should be resumed at the initial titration schedule. After the decision to terminate olanzapine or clozapine use, dosages should be tapered whenever possible to avoid cholinergic rebound symptoms such as diaphoresis, flushing, diarrhea, and hyperactivity.

After a clinician has determined that a trial of an SGA is warranted for a particular person, the risks and benefits of SGA treatment must be explained to the person and the family. In the case of clozapine, an informed consent procedure should be documented in the person's chart. The patient's history should include information about blood disorders, epilepsy, cardiovascular disease, hepatic and renal diseases, and drug abuse. The presence of a hepatic or renal disease necessitates using low starting dosages of the drug. The physical examination should include supine and standing blood pressure measurements to screen for orthostatic hypotension. The laboratory examination should include an EKG; several complete blood counts with WBC counts, which can then be averaged; and liver and renal function tests. Periodic monitoring of blood glucose, lipids, and body weight is recommended.

Although the transition from a DRA to an SGA may be made abruptly, it is wiser to taper off the DRA slowly while titrating up the SGA. Clozapine and olanzapine both have anticholinergic effects, and the transition from one to the other can usually be accomplished with little risk of cholinergic rebound. The transition from risperidone to olanzapine is best accomplished by tapering the risperidone off over 3 weeks while simultaneously beginning olanzapine at 10 mg a day. Risperidone, quetiapine, and ziprasidone lack anticholinergic effects, and the abrupt transition from a DRA, olanzapine, or clozapine to one of these agents may cause cholinergic rebound, which consists of excessive salivation, nausea, vomiting, and diarrhea. The risk of cholinergic rebound can be mitigated by initially augmenting risperidone, quetiapine, or ziprasidone with an anticholinergic drug, which is then tapered off slowly. Any initiation and termination of SGA use should be accomplished gradually.

It is wise to overlap administration of the new drug with the old drug. Of interest, some people have a more robust clinical response while taking the two agents during the transition and then regressing on monotherapy with the newer drug. Little is known about the effectiveness and safety of a strategy of combining one SGA with another SGA or with a DRA.

Persons receiving regular injections of depot formulations of a DRA who are to switch to SDA use are given the first dose of the SDA on the day the next injection is due.

Persons who developed agranulocytosis while taking clozapine can safely switch to olanzapine use, although initiation of olanzapine use in the midst of clozapine-induced agranulocytosis can prolong the time of recovery from the usual 3 to 4 days

Table 28–1
Comparison of Usual Dosing^a for Some Available Second-Generation Antipsychotics in Schizophrenia

Antipsychotic	Typical Starting Dosage	Maintenance Therapy Dose Range	Titration	Maximum Recommended Dosage
Aripiprazole (Abilify)	10–15-mg tablets once a day	10–30 mg/day	Dosage increases should not be made before 2 weeks.	30 mg/day
Asenapine (Saphris)	5 mg twice a day	10 mg twice a day	Titration not necessary.	20 mg/day
Clozapine (Clozaril)	12.5-mg tablets once or twice a day	150–300 mg/day in divided doses or 200 mg as a single dose in the evening	The dosage should be increased to 25–50 mg on the 2nd day. Further increases may be made in daily increments of 25–50 mg to a target dosage of 300–450 mg/day. Subsequent dosage increases should be made no more than once or twice weekly in increments of no more than 100 mg.	900 mg/day
Iloperidone (Fanapt)	1 mg twice a day	12–24 mg a day in divided dose	Start at 1 mg twice a day then move to 2, 4, 6, 8 and 12 mg twice a day. Do this over the course of 7 days.	24 mg/day
Lurasidone (Latuda)	40 mg/day	40–80 mg/day	Titration not necessary.	120 mg/day
Olanzapine (Zyprexa)	5–10 mg/day tablets or orally disintegrating tablets	10–20 mg/day	Dosage increments of 5 mg once a day are recommended when required at intervals of not less than 1 week.	20 mg/day
Paliperidone (Invega)	3–9-mg extended-release tablets once a day	3–6 mg/day	Plasma concentration rises to a peak approximately 24 hours after dosing.	12 mg/day
Quetiapine (Seroquel)	25-mg tablets twice a day	Lowest dose needed to maintain remission	Increase in increments of 25–50 mg 2 or 3 times a day on the 2nd and the 3rd day, as tolerated, to a target dosage of 500 mg daily by the 4th day (given in 2 or 3 doses/day). Further dosage adjustments, if required, should be of 25–50 mg twice a day and occur at intervals of not fewer than 2 days.	800 mg/day
Risperidone (Risperdal)	1-mg tablet and oral solution once a day	2–6 mg once a day	Starting dose: 25 mg every 2 weeks.	50 mg for 2 weeks

(continued)

Table 28–1—continued
Comparison of Usual Dosing[a] for Some Available Second-Generation Antipsychotics in Schizophrenia

Antipsychotic	Typical Starting Dosage	Maintenance Therapy Dose Range	Titration	Maximum Recommended Dosage
Risperidone IM long acting (Consta)	25–50-mg IM injection every 2 weeks	Start with oral risperidone for 3 weeks	Increase to 2 mg once a day on the 2nd day and 4 mg once a day on the 3rd day. In some patients, a slower titration may be appropriate. When dosage adjustments are necessary, further dosage increments of 1–2 mg/day at intervals of not less than 1 week are recommended.	1–6 mg/day
Ziprasidone (Geodon)	20-mg capsules twice a day with food	20–80 mg twice a day	Dosage adjustments based on individual clinical status may be made at intervals of not fewer than 2 days.	80 mg twice a day
Ziprasidone (IM)	For acute agitation: 10–20 mg, as required, up to a maximum of 40 mg/day	Not applicable	For acute agitation: Doses of 10 mg may be administered every 2 hours, and doses of 20 mg may be administered every 4 hours up to a maximum of 40 mg/day.	For acute agitation: 40 mg/day, for not more than 3 consecutive days
Cariprazine (Vraylar)	1.5 mg/day	3–6 mg once a day	Initial dose can be increased in 1.5 mg increments, depending on tolerability.	6 mg/day
Brexpiprazole (Rexulti)	1 mg/day through day 4	2–4 mg/day	Can titrate to 2 mg/day on day 5, and 4 mg/day on day 8.	4 mg/day
Pimavanserin (Nuplazid)	17 or 34 mg once a day	34 mg once a day	No titration.	34 mg/day

Note: Information taken from US Prescribing Information for individual agents.
[a]Dosage adjustments may be required in special populations.
IM, Intramuscular.

up to 11 to 12 days. It is prudent to wait for resolution of agranulocytosis before initiating olanzapine use. Emergence or recurrence of agranulocytosis has not been reported with olanzapine, even in persons who developed it while taking clozapine.

Olanzapine and clozapine appear to account for most cases of weight gain and drug-induced diabetes mellitus. The other agents pose a smaller risk of these side effects; nevertheless, the FDA has requested that all SGAs carry a warning label that patients taking the drugs be monitored closely and has recommended the following factors be considered for all patients prescribed SGAs.

1. Personal and family history of obesity, diabetes, dyslipidemia, hypertension, and cardiovascular disease
2. Weight and height (so that body mass index can be calculated)
3. Waist circumference (at the level of the umbilicus)
4. Blood pressure
5. Fasting plasma glucose level
6. Fasting lipid profile

Patients with pre-existing diabetes should have regular monitoring, including HgA1c and in some cases insulin levels. Among these drugs, clozapine sits apart. It is not considered a first-line agent because of side effects and need for weekly blood tests. Although highly effective in treating both mania and depression, clozapine does not have an FDA indication for these conditions.

SGA use by pregnant women has not been studied, but consideration should be given to the potential of risperidone to raise prolactin concentrations, sometimes up to three to four times the upper limit of the normal range. Because the drugs can be excreted in breast milk, they should not be taken by nursing mothers. The dosages for selected SDAs are given in Table 28–1.

29

Sympathomimetic Drugs: Modafinil, Armodafinil, and Atomoxetine

INTRODUCTION

Sympathomimetic drugs, or as they also called stimulant drugs, enhance motivation, attention, concentration, wakefulness, and stimulate the cardiovascular system. They also suppress appetite and interfere with sleep. These drugs achieve these effects by activating the sympathetic central nervous system (CNS) through effects on endogenous catecholamines. Several chemical classes are included in this group.

Currently these drugs are most commonly used to treat symptoms of poor concentration and hyperactivity in children and adults with attention-deficit/hyperactivity disorder (ADHD). Paradoxically, many patients with ADHD find that these drugs can have a calming effect. Sympathomimetics are also approved for use in increasing alertness in narcolepsy.

Amphetamines were the first stimulants to be synthesized. They were created in the late 19th century and were used by Bavarian soldiers in the mid-1880s to maintain wakefulness, alertness, energy, and confidence in combat. They have been used in a similar fashion in most wars since then. They were not widely used clinically until the 1930s when they were marketed as Benzedrine inhalers for relief of nasal congestion. When their psychostimulant effects were noted, these drugs were used to treat sleepiness associated with narcolepsy. They have been classified as controlled drugs because of their rapid onset, immediate behavioral effects, and propensity to develop tolerance, which leads to the risk of abuse and dependence in vulnerable individuals. Their manufacture, distribution, and use are regulated by state and federal agencies.

Sympathomimetics have also been found effective in treating certain cognitive disorders that result in secondary depression or profound apathy (e.g., acquired immunodeficiency syndrome [AIDS], multiple sclerosis, poststroke depression and dementia, closed head injury) as well as in the augmentation of antidepressant medications in specific treatment-resistant depressions. Curiously, all amphetamines have long been used to facilitate weight loss, but only one formulation, Evekeo, has been approved by the FDA as an adjunct in a regimen of weight reduction.

Even though it is not a psychostimulant, atomoxetine (Strattera) is included in this chapter because it is approved to treat ADHD. Similarly, Modafinil (Provigil) and Armodafinil (Nuvigil) are discussed in this chapter because both are wakefulness-promoting agents with behavioral actions similar to psychostimulants. Pharmacologically, they are not classified as psychostimulants, but are used off-label to treat ADHD. Modafinil is a racemic compound. Modafinil and its R-enantiomer, armodafinil, exert clinical effects by enhancing catecholamine neurotransmission. Modafinil has been found to activate lateral hypothalamus orexin (hypocretin) neurons. However, because its pharmacologic profile is unique from stimulants, it is not classified as such. In addition to the wake-promoting effects, modafinil increases motor activity, euphoria, and alterations in perception, emotions, and cognition typical of CNS stimulants. Both drugs have similar clinical effects and side effects.

PHARMACOLOGIC ACTIONS

All of these drugs are well absorbed from the gastrointestinal tract. Amphetamine (Adderall) and dextroamphetamine (Dexedrine, Dextrostat) reach peak plasma concentrations in 2 to 3 hours and have a half-life of about 6 hours, thereby necessitating once- or twice-daily dosing. Methylphenidate is available in immediate-release (Ritalin), sustained-release (Ritalin SR), and extended-release (Concerta, Quillivant XR) formulations. Immediate-release methylphenidate reaches peak plasma concentrations in 1 to 2 hours and has a short half-life of 2 to 3 hours, thereby necessitating multiple-daily dosing. The sustained-release formulation reaches peak plasma concentrations in 4 to 5 hours and doubles the effective half-life of methylphenidate. The extended-release formulation reaches peak plasma concentrations in 6 to 8 hours and is designed to be effective for 12 hours in once-daily dosing. Dexmethylphenidate (Focalin) reaches peak plasma concentration in about 3 hours and is prescribed twice daily.

Lisdexamfetamine dimesylate, also known as L-lysine-D-amphetamine (Vyvanse), is an amphetamine prodrug. In this formulation, dextroamphetamine is coupled with the amino acid L-lysine. Lisdexamfetamine becomes active upon cleavage of the lysine portion of the molecule by enzymes in the red blood cells. This results in the gradual release of dextroamphetamine into the bloodstream. Apart from having an extended duration of action, this type of formulation reduces its abuse potential. It is the only prodrug of its kind. Lisdexamfetamine is indicated for the treatment of ADHD in children 6 to 12 years and in adults as an integral part of a total treatment program that may include other measures (i.e., psychological, educational, social). The safety and efficacy of lisdexamfetamine dimesylate in patients 3 to 5 years old has not been established. In contrast to Adderall, which contains approximately 75% dextroamphetamine and 25% levoamphetamine, lisdexamfetamine is a single, dextro-enantiomer amphetamine molecule. In most cases this makes the drug better tolerated, but there are some patients who experience greater benefit from the mixed isomer preparation. Another amphetamine formulation is for all-day symptom control in Mydayis. It is indicated for patients 13 years of age or older. Mydayis consists of long-acting, triple-bead, mixed amphetamine salts—equal amounts (by weight) of four salts: dextroamphetamine sulfate and amphetamine sulfate, dextroamphetamine saccharate and amphetamine aspartate monohydrate. This results in a 3:1 mixture of dextro- to levoamphetamine base equivalent. In clinical studies, Mydayis was found to significantly improve ADHD symptoms in subjects when compared to a placebo, starting at 2 to 4 hours post dose and lasting up to 16 hours.

Methylphenidate, dextroamphetamine, and amphetamine are indirectly acting sympathomimetics, with the primary effect causing the release of catecholamines from presynaptic neurons. Their clinical effectiveness is associated with increased release of both dopamine and norepinephrine. Dextroamphetamine and methylphenidate are also weak inhibitors of catecholamine reuptake and inhibitors of monoamine oxidase.

For modafinil, the specific mechanism of action is unknown. Narcolepsy–cataplexy results from deficiency of hypocretin, a hypothalamic neuropeptide. Hypocretin-producing neurons are activated after modafinil administration. Modafinil does not appear to work through a dopaminergic mechanism. It does have α_1-adrenergic agonist properties, which may account for its alerting effects, because the wakefulness induced by modafinil can be attenuated by prazosin, an α_1-adrenergic antagonist. Some evidence suggests that modafinil has some norepinephrine reuptake blocking effects. Armodafinil (Nuvigil) is the R-enantiomer of modafinil. Both drugs have similar clinical effects and side effects.

THERAPEUTIC INDICATIONS

Attention-Deficit/Hyperactivity Disorder

Sympathomimetics are the first-line drugs for treatment of ADHD in children and are effective about 75% of the time. Methylphenidate and dextroamphetamine are equally effective and work within 15 to 30 minutes. Pemoline (Cylert) requires 3 to 4 weeks to reach its full efficacy; however, it is rarely used because of toxicity. Sympathomimetic drugs decrease hyperactivity, increase attentiveness, and reduce impulsivity. They may also reduce comorbid oppositional behaviors associated with ADHD. Many persons take these drugs throughout their schooling and beyond. In responsive persons, use of a sympathomimetic may be a critical determinant of scholastic success.

Sympathomimetics improve the core ADHD symptoms of hyperactivity, impulsivity, and inattentiveness and permit improved social interactions with teachers, family, other adults, and peers. The success of long-term treatment of ADHD with sympathomimetics, which are efficacious for most of the various constellations of ADHD symptoms present from childhood to adulthood, supports a model in which ADHD results from a genetically determined neurochemical imbalance that requires lifelong pharmacologic management.

Methylphenidate is the most commonly used initial agent, at a dosage of 5 to 10 mg every 3 to 4 hours. Dosages may be increased to a maximum of 20 mg four times daily or 1 mg/kg a day. Use of the 20-mg sustained-release formulation to achieve 6 hours of benefit and eliminate the need for dosing at school is supported by many experts, although other authorities believe it is less effective than the immediate-release formulation. Dextroamphetamine is about twice as potent as methylphenidate on a per milligram basis and provides 6 to 8 hours of benefit. Some 70% of nonresponders to one sympathomimetic may benefit from another. All of the sympathomimetic drugs should be tried before switching to drugs of a different class. The previous dictum that sympathomimetics worsen tics and therefore should be avoided by persons with comorbid ADHD and tic disorders has been questioned. Small dosages of sympathomimetics do not appear to cause an increase in the frequency and severity of tics. Alternatives to sympathomimetics for ADHD include bupropion (Wellbutrin), venlafaxine (Effexor), guanfacine (Tenex), clonidine (Catapres), and tricyclic drugs. Multiple trials have demonstrated the clinical effectiveness of modafinil on the core symptoms of inattention, hyperactivity, and impulsivity, both at school and at home.

Short-term use of the sympathomimetics induces a euphoric feeling; however, tolerance develops for both the euphoric feeling and the sympathomimetic activity.

Narcolepsy and Hypersomnolence

Narcolepsy consists of sudden sleep attacks (*narcolepsy*), sudden loss of postural tone (*cataplexy*), loss of voluntary motor control going into (hypnagogic) or coming out of (hypnopompic) sleep (*sleep paralysis*), and hypnagogic or hypnopompic *hallucinations*. Sympathomimetics reduce narcoleptic sleep attacks and improve wakefulness in other types of hypersomnolent states. Modafinil is approved as an antisomnolence agent for treatment of narcolepsy, for people who cannot adjust to night shift work, and for those who do not sleep well because of obstructive sleep apnea.

Other sympathomimetics are also used to maintain wakefulness and accuracy of motor performance in persons subject to sleep deprivation, such as pilots and military personnel. Persons with narcolepsy, unlike persons with ADHD, may develop tolerance for the therapeutic effects of the sympathomimetics.

In direct comparison with amphetamine-like drugs, modafinil is equally effective at maintaining wakefulness, with a lower risk of excessive activation.

Depressive Disorders

Sympathomimetics may be used for treatment-resistant depressive disorders, usually as augmentation of standard antidepressant drug therapy. Possible indications for use of sympathomimetics as monotherapy include depression in elderly persons, who are at increased risk for adverse effects from standard antidepressant drugs; depression in medically ill persons, especially persons with AIDS; obtundation caused by chronic use of opioids; and clinical situations in which a rapid response is important but for which electroconvulsive therapy is contraindicated. Depressed patients with abulia and anergia may also benefit.

Dextroamphetamine may be useful in differentiating pseudodementia of depression from dementia. A depressed person generally responds to a 5-mg dose with increased alertness and improved cognition. Sympathomimetics are thought to provide only short-term benefit (2 to 4 weeks) for depression because most persons rapidly develop tolerance for the antidepressant effects of the drugs. However, some clinicians report that long-term treatment with sympathomimetics can benefit some persons.

Encephalopathy Caused by Brain Injury

Sympathomimetics increase alertness, cognition, motivation, and motor performance in persons with neurologic deficits caused by strokes, trauma, tumors, or chronic infections. Treatment with sympathomimetics may permit earlier and more robust participation in rehabilitative programs. Poststroke lethargy and apathy may respond to long-term use of sympathomimetics.

Obesity

Sympathomimetics are used in the treatment of obesity because of their anorexia-inducing effects. Because tolerance develops for the anorectic effects and because of the drugs' high abuse potential, their use for this indication is limited. Of the sympathomimetic drugs, phentermine (Adipex-P, Fastin) is the most widely used for appetite suppression. Phentermine was the second half of "fen-phen," an off-label combination of fenfluramine and phentermine, widely used to promote weight loss until fenfluramine and dexfenfluramine were withdrawn from commercial availability because of an association with cardiac valvular insufficiency, primary pulmonary hypertension, and irreversible loss of cerebral serotoninergic nerve fibers. The toxicity of fenfluramine is attributed to the fact that it stimulates release of massive amounts of serotonin from nerve endings, a mechanism of action not shared by phentermine. Use of phentermine alone has not been reported to cause the same adverse effects as those caused by fenfluramine or dexfenfluramine.

Careful limitation of caloric intake and judicious exercise are at the core of any successful weight loss program. Sympathomimetic drugs facilitate loss of, at most, an additional fraction of a pound per week. Sympathomimetic drugs are effective appetite suppressants only for the first few weeks of use; then the anorexigenic effects tend to decrease.

Fatigue

Between 70% and 90% of individuals with multiple sclerosis experience fatigue. Modafinil, armodafinil, amphetamines, methylphenidate, and the dopamine receptor agonist amantadine (Symmetrel) are sometimes effective in combating this symptom. Other causes of fatigue such as chronic fatigue syndrome respond to stimulants in many cases.

PRECAUTIONS AND ADVERSE REACTIONS

The most common adverse effects associated with amphetamine-like drugs are stomach pain, anxiety, irritability, insomnia, tachycardia, cardiac arrhythmias, and dysphoria. Sympathomimetics cause a decreased appetite, although tolerance usually develops for this effect. The treatment of common adverse effects in children with ADHD is usually straightforward (Table 29–1). The drugs can also cause increases in heart rate and blood pressure (BP) and may cause palpitations. Less common adverse effects include the possible induction of movement disorders, such as tics, Tourette's disorder–like symptoms, and dyskinesias, all of which are often self-limited over 7 to 10 days. If a person taking a sympathomimetic develops one of these movement disorders, a correlation between the dose of the medication and the severity of the disorder must be firmly established before adjustments are made in the medication dosage. In severe cases, augmentation with risperidone (Risperdal), clonidine (Catapres), or guanfacine (Tenex) is necessary. Methylphenidate may worsen tics in one-third of persons; these persons fall into two groups: Those whose methylphenidate-induced tics resolve immediately upon metabolism of the dosage and a smaller group in whom methylphenidate appears to trigger tics that persist for several months but eventually resolve spontaneously.

Table 29-1
Management of Common Stimulant-Induced Adverse Effects in Attention-Deficit/Hyperactivity Disorder

Adverse Effect	Management
Anorexia, nausea, weight loss	• Administer stimulant with meals. • Use caloric-enhanced supplements. Discourage forcing meals.
Insomnia, nightmares	• Administer stimulants earlier in day. • Change to short-acting preparations. • Discontinue afternoon or evening dosing. • Consider adjunctive treatment (e.g., antihistamines, clonidine, antidepressants).
Dizziness	• Monitor BP. • Encourage fluid intake. • Change to long-acting form.
Rebound phenomena	• Overlap stimulant dosing. • Change to long-acting preparation or combine long- and short-acting preparations. • Consider adjunctive or alternative treatment (e.g., clonidine, antidepressants).
Irritability	• Assess timing of phenomena (during peak or withdrawal phase). • Evaluate comorbid symptoms. • Reduce dose. • Consider adjunctive or alternative treatment (e.g., lithium, antidepressants, anticonvulsants).
Dysphoria, moodiness, agitation	• Consider comorbid diagnosis (e.g., mood disorder). • Reduce dosage or change to long-acting preparation. • Consider adjunctive or alternative treatment (e.g., lithium, anticonvulsants, antidepressants).

BP, blood pressure.
From Wilens TE, Blederman J. The stimulants. In: Shaffer D, ed. *The Psychiatric Clinics of North America: Pediatric Psychopharmacology.* Philadelphia, PA: Saunders; 1992, with permission.

Longitudinal studies do not indicate that sympathomimetics cause growth suppression. Sympathomimetics may exacerbate glaucoma, hypertension, cardiovascular disorders, hyperthyroidism, anxiety disorders, psychotic disorders, and seizure disorders.

High dosages of sympathomimetics can cause dry mouth, pupillary dilation, bruxism, formication, excessive ebullience, restlessness, emotional lability, and occasionally seizures. Long-term use of high dosages can cause a delusional disorder that resembles paranoid schizophrenia. Seizures can be treated with benzodiazepines, cardiac effects with β-adrenergic receptor antagonists, fever with cooling blankets, and delirium with dopamine receptor antagonists (DRAs). Overdosages of sympathomimetics result in hypertension, tachycardia, hyperthermia, toxic psychosis, delirium, hyperpyrexia, convulsions, coma, chest pain, arrhythmia, heart block, hyper- or hypotension, shock, and nausea. Toxic effects of amphetamines can be seen at 30 mg, but idiosyncratic toxicity can occur at doses as low as 2 mg. Conversely, survival has been reported up to 500 mg.

The most limiting adverse effect of sympathomimetics is their association with psychological and physical dependence. At the doses used for treatment of ADHD, development of psychological dependence virtually never occurs. A larger concern is the presence of adolescent or adult cohabitants who might confiscate the supply of sympathomimetics for abuse or sale.

USE IN PREGNANCY AND LACTATION

When weighing the potential risks and benefits of different treatment strategies for ADHD in young women of reproductive age and in pregnant women, it is important to consider that there might be a small increase in the risk of cardiac malformations associated with intrauterine exposure to methylphenidate. No association has observed between amphetamines and any congenital or cardiac malformations. Both dextroamphetamine and methylphenidate pass into the breast milk. It is not known whether modafinil or armodafinil do.

DRUG INTERACTIONS

The coadministration of sympathomimetics and tricyclic or tetracyclic antidepressants, warfarin (Coumadin), primidone (Mysoline), phenobarbital (Luminal), phenytoin (Dilantin), or phenylbutazone (Butazolidin) decreases the metabolism of these compounds, resulting in increased plasma levels. Sympathomimetics decrease the therapeutic efficacy of many antihypertensive drugs, especially guanethidine (Esimil, Ismelin). The sympathomimetics should be used with extreme caution with monoamine oxidase inhibitors (MAOIs).

LABORATORY INTERFERENCES

Dextroamphetamine may elevate plasma corticosteroid levels and interfere with some assay methods for urinary corticosteroids.

DOSAGE AND ADMINISTRATION

Many psychiatrists believe that amphetamine use has been overly regulated by governmental authorities. Amphetamines are listed as schedule II drugs by the Drug Enforcement Agency. Some states keep a registry of patients who receive amphetamines. Such mandates worry both patients and physicians about breaches in confidentiality, and physicians are concerned that their prescribing practices may be misinterpreted by official agencies. Consequently, some physicians may withhold prescription of sympathomimetics, even from persons who may benefit from the medications.

The dosage ranges and the available preparations for sympathomimetics are presented in Table 29–2. Vyvanse dosing is a special case, because many patients are switched to this formulation after being treated with other stimulants. A conversion table is shown in Table 29–3. It is available in 20-, 30-, 40-, 50-, 60-, and 70-mg capsules. Dosage should be individualized according to the therapeutic needs and response of the patient. Lisdexamfetamine (Vyvanse) should be administered at the lowest effective dosage. In patients who are either starting treatment for the first time or switching from another medication, 30 mg once daily in the morning is the recommended dose. Dosages may go up or down in 10- or 20-mg increments in intervals of approximately 1 week. Afternoon doses should be avoided because of the potential for insomnia. The drug may be taken with or without food.

Dextroamphetamine, methylphenidate, amphetamine, benzphetamine, and methamphetamine are schedule II drugs and in some states require triplicate prescriptions. Phendimetrazine (Adipost, Bontril) and phenmetrazine (Prelude) are schedule III drugs, and modafinil, armodafinil, phentermine, diethylpropion (Tenuate), and mazindol (Mazanor, Sanorex) are schedule IV drugs.

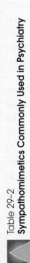

Table 29-2
Sympathomimetics Commonly Used in Psychiatry

Generic Name	Trade Name	Preparations	Initial Daily Dose	Usual Daily Dose for ADHD[a]	Usual Daily Dose for Disorders Associated With Excessive Daytime Somnolence	Maximum Daily Dose
Amphetamine–dextroamphetamine	Adderall	5-, 10-, 20-, and 30-mg tablets	5–10 mg	20–30 mg	5–60 mg	Children: 40 mg Adults: 60 mg
Armodafinil	Nuvigil	50-, 150-, and 250-mg tablets	50–150 mg	150–250 mg	250 mg	Children: 80 mg Adults: 100 mg
Atomoxetine	Strattera	10-, 18-, 25-, 40-, and 60-mg tablets	20 mg	40–80 mg	Not used	20 mg
Dexmethylphenidate	Focalin	2.5-, 5-, and 10-mg capsules	5 mg	5–20 mg	Not used	Children: 40 mg Adults: 60 mg
Dextroamphetamine	Dexedrine, Dextrostat	5-, 10-, and 15-mg ER capsules; 5- and 10-mg tablets	5–10 mg	20–30 mg	5–60 mg	70 mg
Lisdexamfetamine	Vyvanse	20-, 30-, 40-, 50-, 60- and 70-mg capsules	20–30 mg			Adults: 50 mg/day Pediatrics: 25 mg/day
Equal amounts (by weight) of: dextroamphetamine sulfate and amphetamine sulfate, dextroamphetamine saccharate and amphetamine aspartate monohydrate. This results in a 3:1 mixture of dextro- to levoamphetamine base equivalent.	Mydayis	Each pill contains equal portions of the following: amphetamine aspartate, amphetamine sulfate, dextroamphetamine saccharate, and dextroamphetamine capsules: • 12.5 mg • 25 mg • 37.5 mg • 50 mg	12.5 mg once daily in the morning upon awakening.	12.5–50 mg/day	Not used	
Methamphetamine	Desoxyn	5-mg tablets; 5-, 10-, and 15-mg XR tablets	5–10 mg	20–25 mg	Not generally used	45 mg
Methylphenidate	Ritalin, Methidate, Methylin, Attenade	5-, 10-, and 20-mg tablets; 10- and 20-mg SR tablets	5–10 mg	5–60 mg	20–30 mg	Children: 80 mg Adults: 90 mg
	Concerta	18- and 36-mg ER tablets	18 mg	18–54 mg	Not yet established	54 mg
Methylphenidate hydrochloride	Quillivant XR		20 mg			60 mg
Modafinil	Provigil	100- and 200-mg tablets	100 mg		400 mg	400 mg

[a]For children 6 years of age and older.
[b]Obstructive sleep apnea, narcolepsy, and shift work disorder.
ER, extended release; SR, sustained release.

239

Table 29–3
Lisdexamfetamine (Vyvanse) Dosage Equivalency Conversions

Vyvanse and Adderall XR		
Vyvanse (mg)	**Adderall XR (mg)**	
20	5	
30	10	
40	15	
50	20	
60	25	
70	30	
Vyvanse, Adderall IR, and Dexedrine		
Vyvanse (mg)	**Adderall IR (mg)**	**Dexedrine (mg)**
70	30	22.5
50	20	15
30	10	7.5

XR, extended release; IR, immediate release.

Pretreatment evaluation should include an evaluation of the person's cardiac function, with particular attention to the presence of hypertension or tachyarrhythmias. The clinician should also examine the person for the presence of movement disorders, such as tics and dyskinesia, because these conditions can be exacerbated by the administration of sympathomimetics. If tics are present, many experts will not prescribe sympathomimetics but will instead choose clonidine or antidepressants. However, recent data indicate that sympathomimetics may cause only a mild increase in motor tics and may actually suppress vocal tics. Liver function and renal function should be assessed, and dosages of sympathomimetics should be reduced for persons with impaired metabolism.

Persons with ADHD can take immediate-release methylphenidate at 8 AM, 12 noon, and 4 PM. Dextroamphetamine, Adderall, sustained-release methylphenidate, or 18 mg of extended-release methylphenidate may be taken once at 8 AM. The starting dose of methylphenidate ranges from 2.5 mg of regular to 20 mg of the sustained-release formulation. If this is inadequate, it may be increased to a maximum dose of 80 mg in children and 90 mg daily in adults. The dosage of dextroamphetamine is 2.5 to 40 mg a day up to 0.5 mg/kg a day.

Quillivant XR (methylphenidate hydrochloride) is a once-daily, extended-release liquid formulation of methylphenidate HCL. Quillivant XR is supplied as a liquid solution designed for oral administration. Quillivant XR is taken once a day. The recommended dose for patients 6 years and above is 20 mg orally once daily in the morning with or without food. The dose may be titrated weekly in increments of 10 to 20 mg. Daily doses above 60 mg have not been studied and are not recommended. Before administering the dose, vigorously shake the bottle of Quillivant XR for at least 10 seconds, to ensure that the proper dose is administered. The clinical effects of the drug are evident from 45 minutes to 12 hours after dosing.

The starting dosage of modafinil is 200 mg in the morning in medically healthy individuals and 100 mg in the morning in persons with hepatic impairment. Some persons take a second 100- or 200-mg dose in the afternoon. The maximum recommended daily dosage is 400 mg, although dosages of 600 to 1,200 mg a day have been used safely. Adverse effects become prominent at dosages above 400 mg a day. Compared with amphetamine like drugs, modafinil promotes wakefulness but produces less attentiveness and less irritability. Modafinil and armodafinil are generally well tolerated. Adverse events include headache, nausea, and nervousness.

Some persons with excessive daytime sleepiness extend the activity of the morning modafinil dose with an afternoon dose of methylphenidate. Armodafinil is virtually identical to modafinil, but is dosed differently, the dosing range being 50 to 250 mg daily. The pharmacokinetics of modafinil may be altered in older males and in patients with chronic hepatic impairment. In vitro, modafinil has been shown to inhibit the cytochrome P450 (CYP) isoenzyme CYP2C19 (moderately potent, reversible inhibition), modestly induce CYP1A2, CYP3A4/5, and CYP2B6, and suppress CYP2C9.

ATOMOXETINE (STRATTERA)

Atomoxetine is the first nonstimulant drug to be approved by the FDA as a treatment of ADHD in children, adolescents, and adults. It is included in this chapter because it shares this indication with the stimulants described above.

Pharmacologic Actions

Atomoxetine is believed to produce a therapeutic effect through selective inhibition of the presynaptic norepinephrine transporter. It is well absorbed after oral administration and is minimally affected by food. High-fat meals may decrease the rate but not the extent of absorption. Maximum plasma concentrations are reached after approximately 1 to 2 hours. At therapeutic concentrations, 98% of atomoxetine in plasma is bound to protein, mainly albumin. Atomoxetine has a half-life of approximately 5 hours and is metabolized principally by the CYP2D6 pathway. Poor metabolizers of this compound reach a fivefold higher area under the curve and fivefold higher peak plasma concentration than normal or extensive metabolizers. This is important to consider in patients receiving medications that inhibit the CYP2D6 enzyme. For example, the antidepressant-like pharmacology of atomoxetine has led to its use as an add-on to selective serotonin reuptake inhibitors (SSRIs) or other antidepressants. Drugs such as fluoxetine (Prozac), paroxetine (Paxil), and bupropion (Wellbutrin) are CYP2D6 inhibitors and may raise atomoxetine levels.

Therapeutic Indications

Atomoxetine is used for the treatment of ADHD. It should be considered for use in patients who find stimulants too activating or who experience other intolerable side effects. Because atomoxetine has no abuse potential, it is a reasonable choice in the treatment of patients with both ADHD and substance abuse, patients who complain of ADHD symptoms but are suspected of seeking stimulant drugs, and patients who are in recovery.

Atomoxetine may enhance cognition when used to treat patients with schizophrenia. It may also be used as an alternative or add-on to antidepressants in patients who fail to respond to standard therapies.

Precautions and Adverse Reactions

Common side effects of atomoxetine include abdominal discomfort, decreased appetite with resulting weight loss, sexual dysfunction, dizziness, vertigo, irritability, and mood swings. Minor increases in BP and heart rate have also been observed. There have been cases of severe liver injury in a small number of patients taking atomoxetine. The drug should be discontinued in patients with jaundice (yellowing of the skin or whites of the eyes, itching) or laboratory evidence of liver injury. Atomoxetine should not be taken at the same time, or within 2 weeks of taking, as an MAOI or by patients with narrow-angle glaucoma.

The effects of overdose greater than twice the maximum recommended daily dose in humans are unknown. No specific information is available on the treatment of overdose with atomoxetine.

Dosage and Clinical Guidelines

Atomoxetine is available as 10-, 18-, 25-, 40-, and 60-mg capsules. In children and adolescents who weigh up to 70 kg in body weight, atomoxetine should be initiated at a total daily dose of approximately 0.5 mg/kg and increased after a minimum of 3 days to a target total daily dose of approximately 1.2 mg/kg administered either as a single daily dose in the morning or as evenly divided doses in the morning and late afternoon or early evening. The total daily dose in smaller children and adolescents should not exceed 1.4 mg/kg or 100 mg, whichever is less. Dosing of children and adolescents, who weigh more than 70 kg, and adults should start at a total daily dose of 40 mg and then be increased after a minimum of 3 days to a target total daily dose of approximately 80 mg. The doses can be administered either as a single daily dose in the morning or as evenly divided doses in the morning and late afternoon or early evening. After 2 to 4 additional weeks, the dose may be increased to a maximum of 100 mg in patients who have not achieved an optimal response. The maximum recommended total daily dose in children and adolescents over 70 kg and adults is 100 mg.

30

Thyroid Hormones

INTRODUCTION

Thyroid hormones—levothyroxine (Synthroid, Levothroid, Levoxine) and liothyronine (Cytomel)—are used in psychiatry either alone or as augmentation to treat persons with depression or rapid-cycling bipolar I disorder. They can convert an antidepressant-nonresponsive person into an antidepressant-responsive person. Thyroid hormones are also used as replacement therapy for persons treated with lithium (Eskalith) who have developed a hypothyroid state. Successful use of thyroid hormone as an intervention for treatment-resistant patients was first reported in the early 1970s. Study results since then have been mixed; however, most show that patients taking triiodothyronine (T_3) are twice as likely to respond to antidepressant treatment versus placebo. These studies have found that augmentation with T_3 is effective with tricyclic antidepressants and selective serotonin reuptake inhibitors (SSRIs). Nevertheless, many endocrinologists object to the use of thyroid hormones as antidepressant augmentation agents, citing such risks as osteoporosis and cardiac arrhythmias.

PHARMACOLOGIC ACTIONS

Thyroid hormones are administered orally, and their absorption from the gastrointestinal tract is variable. Absorption is increased if the drug is administered on an empty stomach. In the brain, thyroxine (T_4) crosses the blood–brain barrier and diffuses into neurons, where it is converted into T_3, which is the physiologically active form. The half-life of T_4 is 6 to 7 days, and that of T_3 is 1 to 2 days.

The mechanism of action for thyroid hormone effects on antidepressant efficacy is unknown. Thyroid hormone binds to intracellular receptors that regulate the transcription of a wide range of genes, including several receptors for neurotransmitters.

THERAPEUTIC INDICATIONS

The major indication for thyroid hormones in psychiatry is as an adjuvant to antidepressants. There is no clear correlation between the laboratory measures of thyroid function and the response to thyroid hormone supplementation of antidepressants. If a patient has not responded to a 6-week course of antidepressants at appropriate dosages, adjuvant therapy with either lithium or a thyroid hormone is an alternative. Most clinicians use adjuvant lithium before trying a thyroid hormone. Several controlled trials have indicated that liothyronine use converts about 50% of antidepressant nonresponders to responders.

The dosage of liothyronine is 25 or 50 μg a day added to the patient's antidepressant regimen. Liothyronine has been used primarily as an adjuvant for tricyclic drugs; however, evidence suggests that liothyronine augments the effects of all of the antidepressant drugs.

Thyroid hormones have not been shown to cause particular problems in pediatric or geriatric patients; however, the hormones should be used with caution in elderly persons, who may have occult heart disease.

PRECAUTIONS AND ADVERSE REACTIONS

At the dosages usually used for augmentation—25 to 50 μg a day—adverse effects occur infrequently. The most common adverse effects associated with thyroid hormones are transient headache, weight loss, palpitations, nervousness, diarrhea, abdominal cramps, sweating, tachycardia, increased blood pressure, tremors, and insomnia. Osteoporosis may also occur with long-term treatment, but this has not been found in studies involving liothyronine augmentation. Overdoses of thyroid hormones can lead to cardiac failure and death.

Thyroid hormones should not be taken by persons with cardiac disease, angina, or hypertension. The hormones are contraindicated in thyrotoxicosis and uncorrected adrenal insufficiency and in persons with acute myocardial infarctions.

USE IN PREGNANCY AND LACTATION

Thyroid hormones can be administered safely to pregnant women, provided that laboratory thyroid indexes are monitored. Thyroid hormones are minimally excreted in breast milk and have not been shown to cause problems in nursing babies.

DRUG INTERACTIONS

Thyroid hormones can potentiate the effects of warfarin (Coumadin) and other anticoagulants by increasing the catabolism of clotting factors. They may increase the insulin requirement for diabetic persons and the digitalis requirement for persons with cardiac disease. Thyroid hormones should not be coadministered with sympathomimetics, ketamine (Ketalar), or maprotiline (Ludiomil) because of the risk of cardiac decompensation. Administration of SSRIs, tricyclic and tetracyclic drugs, lithium, or carbamazepine (Tegretol) can mildly lower serum T_4 and raise serum thyrotropin concentrations in euthyroid persons or persons taking thyroid replacements. This interaction warrants close serum monitoring and may require an increase in the dosage or initiation of thyroid hormone supplementation.

LABORATORY INTERFERENCES

Levothyroxine has not been reported to interfere with any laboratory test other than thyroid function indexes. Liothyronine, however, suppresses the release of endogenous T_4, thereby lowering the result of any thyroid function test that depends on the measure of T_4.

THYROID FUNCTION TESTS

Several thyroid function tests are available, including tests for T_4 by competitive protein binding (T_4 [D]) and by radioimmunoassay (T_4 RIA) involving a specific antigen–antibody reaction. Over 90% of T_4 is bound to serum protein and is responsible for thyroid-stimulating hormone (TSH) secretion and cellular metabolism. Other thyroid measures include the free T_4 index (FT_4I), T_3 uptake, and total serum T_3 measured by radioimmunoassay (T_3 RIA). Those tests are used to rule out hypothyroidism, which can be associated with symptoms of depression. In some studies, up to 10% of patients complaining of depression and associated fatigue had incipient hypothyroid disease. Lithium can cause hypothyroidism and, more rarely, hyperthyroidism. Neonatal hypothyroidism results in intellectual disability and is preventable if the diagnosis is made at birth.

Thyrotropin-Releasing Hormone Stimulation Test

The thyrotropin-releasing hormone (TRH) stimulation test is indicated for patients who have marginally abnormal thyroid test results with suspected subclinical hypothyroidism, which may account for clinical depression. It is also used in patients with possible lithium-induced hypothyroidism. The procedure entails an intravenous injection of 500 mg of protirelin (TRH), which produces a sharp increase in serum TSH levels measured at 15, 30, 60, and 90 minutes. An increase in serum TSH of 5 to 25 mIU/mL above the baseline is normal. An increase of less than 7 mIU/mL is considered a blunted response, which may correlate with a diagnosis of depression. Eight percent of all patients with depression have some thyroid illness.

DOSAGE AND CLINICAL GUIDELINES

Liothyronine is available in 5-, 25-, and 50-μg tablets. Levothyroxine is available in 12.5-, 25-, 50-, 75-, 88-, 100-, 112-, 125-, 150-, 175-, 200-, and 300-μg tablets; it is also available in a 200- and 500-μg parenteral form. The dosage of liothyronine is 25 or 50 μg a day added to the person's antidepressant regimen. Liothyronine has been used as an adjuvant for all of the available antidepressant drugs. An adequate trial of liothyronine supplementation should last 2 to 3 weeks. If liothyronine supplementation is successful, it should be continued for 2 months and then tapered off at the rate of 12.5 μg a day every 3 to 7 days.

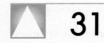

31
Tricyclics and Tetracyclics

INTRODUCTION

The observation in 1957 that imipramine (Tofranil) had antidepressant effects led to the development of a new class of antidepressant compounds, the tricyclics (TCAs). In turn, the finding that imipramine blocked reuptake of norepinephrine led to research into the role of catecholamines in depression. After the introduction of imipramine, several other antidepressant compounds were developed that shared a basic tricyclic structure and had relatively similar effects. Later, other heterocyclic compounds were also marketed that were somewhat similar in structure and that had relatively comparable secondary properties. At one time, amitriptyline (Elavil, Endep) and imipramine were the two most commonly prescribed antidepressants in the United States, but because of their anticholinergic and antihistaminic side effects, their use declined, and nortriptyline (Aventyl, Pamelor) and desipramine (Norpramin, Pertofrane) became more popular. Nortriptyline has the least effect on orthostatic hypotension, and desipramine is the least anticholinergic. Although introduced as antidepressants, the therapeutic indications for these agents have grown to include panic disorder, generalized anxiety disorder, posttraumatic stress disorder (PTSD), obsessive-compulsive disorder (OCD), and pain syndromes. The introduction of newer antidepressant agents with more selective actions on neurotransmitters or with unique mechanisms of action has sharply reduced the prescribing of TCAs and tetracyclics. The improved safety profiles of the newer drugs, especially when taken in overdose, also contributed to the decline in use of the older drugs. Nevertheless, the TCAs and tetracyclics remain unsurpassed in terms of their antidepressant efficacy. Table 31–1 lists TCA and tetracyclic drugs and their available preparations.

PHARMACOLOGIC ACTIONS

The absorption of most TCAs is complete after oral administration, and there is significant metabolism from the first-pass effect. Peak plasma concentrations occur within 2 to 8 hours, and the half-lives of the TCAs vary from 10 to 70 hours; nortriptyline, maprotiline (Ludiomil), and particularly protriptyline (Vivactil) can have longer half-lives. The long half-lives allow all the compounds to be given once daily; 5 to 7 days is needed to reach steady-state plasma concentrations. Imipramine pamoate (Tofranil) is a depot form of the drug for intramuscular (IM) administration; indications for the use of this preparation are limited.

The TCAs undergo hepatic metabolism by the CYP450 enzyme system. Clinically relevant drug interactions may result from competition for enzyme CYP2D6 among TCAs and quinidine, cimetidine (Tagamet), fluoxetine (Prozac), sertraline (Zoloft), paroxetine (Paxil), phenothiazines, carbamazepine (Tegretol), and the type IC antiarrhythmics propafenone (Rythmol) and flecainide (Tambocor). Concomitant administration of TCAs and these inhibitors may slow down the metabolism and raise the plasma concentrations of TCAs. Additionally, genetic variations in the

Table 31–1
Tricyclic and Tetracyclic Drug Preparations

Drug	Tablets (mg)	Capsules (mg)	Parenteral (mg/mL)	Solution
Imipramine (Tofranil)	10, 25, and 50	75, 100, 125, and 150	12.5	—
Desipramine (Norpramin, Pertofrane)	10, 25, 50, 75, 100, and 150	—	—	—
Trimipramine (Surmontil)	—	25, 50, and 100	—	—
Amitriptyline (Elavil)	10, 25, 50, 75, 100, and 150	—	10	—
Nortriptyline (Aventyl, Pamelor)	—	10, 25, 50, and 75	—	10 mg/5 mL
Protriptyline (Vivactil)	5 and 10	—	—	—
Amoxapine (Asendin)	25, 50, 100, and 150	—	—	—
Doxepin (Sinequan)	—	10, 25, 50, 75, 100, and 150	—	10 mg/mL
Maprotiline (Ludiomil)	25, 50, and 75	—	—	—
Clomipramine (Anafranil)	—	25, 50, and 75	—	—

activity of CYP2D6 may account for up to a 40-fold difference in plasma TCA concentrations in different persons. The dosage of the TCA may need to be adjusted to correct changes in the rate of hepatic TCA metabolism.

The TCAs block the transporter site for norepinephrine and serotonin, thus increasing synaptic concentrations of these neurotransmitters. Each drug differs in its affinity for each of these transporters, with clomipramine (Anafranil) being the most serotonin selective and desipramine the most norepinephrine selective of the TCAs. Secondary effects of the TCAs include antagonism at the muscarinic acetyl-choline, histamine H_1, and α_1- and α_2-adrenergic receptors. The potency of these effects on other receptors largely determines the side-effect profile of each drug. Amoxapine, nortriptyline, desipramine, and maprotiline have the least anticholinergic activity; doxepin has the most antihistaminergic activity. Although they are more likely to cause constipation, sedation, dry mouth, or light-headedness than the selective serotonin reuptake inhibitors (SSRIs), the TCAs are less prone to cause sexual dysfunction, significant long-term weight gain, and sleep disturbances than the SSRIs. The half-life and plasma clearance for most TCAs are very similar.

THERAPEUTIC INDICATIONS

Each of the following indications is also an indication for the SSRIs, which have widely replaced the TCAs in clinical practice. However, the TCAs represent a reasonable alternative for persons who cannot tolerate the adverse effects of the SSRIs.

Major Depressive Disorder

The treatment of a major depressive episode and the prophylactic treatment of major depressive disorder are the principal indications for using TCAs. Although the TCAs are effective in the treatment of depression in persons with bipolar I disorder, they are more likely to induce mania, hypomania, or cycling than the newer antidepressants, most notably the SSRIs and bupropion. It is thus not advised that TCAs be routinely used to treat depression associated with bipolar I or bipolar II disorder.

Melancholic features, prior major depressive episodes, and a family history of depressive disorders increase the likelihood of a therapeutic response. All of the available TCAs are equally effective in the treatment of depressive disorders. In the case of an individual person, however, one tricyclic or tetracyclic may be effective, and another one may be ineffective. The treatment of a major depressive episode with psychotic features almost always requires the coadministration of an antipsychotic drug and an antidepressant.

Although it is used worldwide as an antidepressant, clomipramine is only approved in the United States for the treatment of OCD.

Panic Disorder with Agoraphobia
Imipramine is the TCA most studied for panic disorder with agoraphobia, but other TCAs are also effective when taken at the usual antidepressant dosages. Because of the potential initial anxiogenic effects of the TCAs, starting dosages should be small, and the dosage should be titrated upward slowly. Small doses of benzodiazepines may be used initially to deal with this side effect.

Generalized Anxiety Disorder
The use of doxepin for the treatment of anxiety disorders is approved by the Food and Drug Administration. Some research data show that imipramine may also be useful. Although rarely used anymore, a chlordiazepoxide–amitriptyline combination (Limbitrol) is available for mixed anxiety and depressive disorders.

Obsessive-Compulsive Disorder
OCD appears to respond specifically to clomipramine, as well as the SSRIs. Some improvement is usually seen in 2 to 4 weeks, but a further reduction in symptoms may continue for the first 4 to 5 months of treatment. None of the other TCAs appear to be nearly as effective as clomipramine for treatment of this disorder. Clomipramine may also be a drug of choice for depressed persons with marked obsessive features.

Pain
The TCAs are widely used to treat chronic neuropathic pain and in prophylaxis of migraine headache. Amitriptyline is the TCA most often used in this role. During treatment of pain, doses are generally lower than those used in depression; for example, 75 mg of amitriptyline may be effective. These effects also appear more rapidly.

Other Disorders
Childhood enuresis is often treated with imipramine. Peptic ulcer disease can be treated with doxepin, which has marked antihistaminergic effects. Other indications for the TCAs are narcolepsy, nightmare disorder, and PTSD. The drugs are sometimes used for treatment of children and adolescents with attention-deficit/hyperactivity disorder, sleepwalking disorder, separation anxiety disorder, and sleep terror disorder. Clomipramine has also been used to treat premature ejaculation, movement disorders, and compulsive behavior in children with autistic disorders; however, because the TCAs have caused sudden death in several children and adolescents, they should not be used in children.

PRECAUTIONS AND ADVERSE REACTIONS

The TCAs are associated with a wide range of problematic side effects and can be lethal when taken in overdose.

Psychiatric Effects

The TCAs can induce a switch to mania or hypomania in susceptible individuals. The TCAs may also exacerbate psychotic disorders in susceptible persons. At high plasma concentrations (levels above 300 ng/mL), the anticholinergic effects of the TCAs can cause confusion or delirium. Patients with dementia are particularly vulnerable to this development.

Anticholinergic Effects

Anticholinergic effects often limit the tolerable dosage to relatively low ranges. Some persons may develop a tolerance for the anticholinergic effects with continued treatment. Anticholinergic effects include dry mouth, constipation, blurred vision, delirium, and urinary retention. Sugarless gum, candy, or fluoride lozenges can alleviate dry mouth. Bethanechol (Urecholine), 25 to 50 mg three or four times a day, may reduce urinary hesitancy and may be helpful in erectile dysfunction when the drug is taken 30 minutes before sexual intercourse. Narrow-angle glaucoma can also be aggravated by anticholinergic drugs, and the precipitation of glaucoma requires emergency treatment with a miotic agent. The TCAs should be avoided in persons with narrow-angle glaucoma, and an SSRI should be substituted. Severe anticholinergic effects can lead to a central nervous system (CNS) anticholinergic syndrome with confusion and delirium, especially if the TCAs are administered with dopamine receptor antagonists (DRAs) or anticholinergic drugs. IM or intravenous physostigmine (Antilirium, Eserine) is used to diagnose and treat anticholinergic delirium.

Cardiac Effects

When administered in their usual therapeutic dosages the TCAs may cause tachycardia, flattened T waves, prolonged QT intervals, and depressed ST segments in the electrocardiographic (EKG) recording. Imipramine has a quinidine-like effect at therapeutic plasma concentrations and may reduce the number of premature ventricular contractions. Because the drugs prolong conduction time, their use in persons with pre-existing conduction defects is contraindicated. In persons with a history of any type of heart disease, the TCAs should be used only after SSRIs or other newer antidepressants have been found ineffective, and if used, they should be introduced at low dosages, with gradual increases in dosage and monitoring of cardiac functions. All of the TCAs can cause tachycardia, which may persist for months and is one of the most common reasons for drug discontinuation, especially in younger persons. At high plasma concentrations, as seen in overdoses, the drugs become arrhythmogenic.

Other Autonomic Effects

Orthostatic hypotension is the most common cardiovascular autonomic adverse effect and the most common reason TCAs are discontinued. It can result in falls and injuries in affected persons. Nortriptyline may be the drug least likely to cause this problem. Orthostatic hypotension is treated with avoidance of caffeine, intake of at least 2 L of fluid per day, and addition of salt to the diet unless the person is being treated for hypertension. In persons taking antihypertensive agents, reduction of the dosage may reduce the risk of orthostatic hypotension. Other possible autonomic effects are profuse sweating, palpitations, and increased blood pressure (BP). Although some persons respond to fludrocortisone (Florinef), 0.02 to 0.05 mg twice a day, substitution of an SSRI is preferable to addition of a potentially toxic mineralocorticoid such as fludrocortisone. The TCAs' use should be discontinued several days before elective surgery because of the occurrence of hypertensive episodes during surgery in persons receiving TCAs.

Sedation

Sedation is a common effect of the TCAs and may be welcomed if sleeplessness has been a problem. The sedative effect of the TCAs is a result of anticholinergic and antihistaminergic activities. Amitriptyline, trimipramine, and doxepin are the most sedating agents; imipramine, amoxapine, nortriptyline, and maprotiline are less sedating; and desipramine and protriptyline are the least sedating agents.

Neurologic Effects

A fine, rapid tremor may occur. Myoclonic twitches and tremors of the tongue and the upper extremities are common. Rare effects include speech blockage, paresthesia, peroneal palsies, and ataxia.

Amoxapine is unique in causing parkinsonian symptoms, akathisia, and even dyskinesia because of the dopaminergic blocking activity of one of its metabolites. Amoxapine may also cause neuroleptic malignant syndrome in rare cases. Maprotiline may cause seizures when the dosage is increased too quickly or is kept at high levels for too long. Clomipramine and amoxapine may lower the seizure threshold more than other drugs in the class. As a class, however, the TCAs have a relatively low risk for inducing seizures, except in persons who are at risk for seizures (e.g., persons with epilepsy and those with brain lesions). Although the TCAs can still be used by such persons, the initial dosages should be lower than usual, and subsequent dosage increases should be gradual.

Allergic and Hematologic Effects

Exanthematous rashes are seen in 4% to 5% of all persons treated with maprotiline. Jaundice is rare. Agranulocytosis, leukocytosis, leukopenia, and eosinophilia are rare complications of TCA treatment. However, a person who has a sore throat or a fever during the first few months of TCA treatment should have a complete blood count (CBC) done immediately.

Hepatic Effects

Mild and self-limited increases in serum transaminase concentrations may occur and should be monitored. The TCAs can also produce a fulminant acute hepatitis in 0.1% to 1% of persons. This can be life threatening, and the antidepressant should be discontinued.

Other Adverse Effects

Modest weight gain is common. Amoxapine exerts a DRA effect and may cause hyperprolactinemia, impotence, galactorrhea, anorgasmia, and ejaculatory disturbances. Other TCAs have also been associated with gynecomastia and amenorrhea. The syndrome of inappropriate secretion of antidiuretic hormone has also been reported with TCAs. Other effects include nausea, vomiting, and hepatitis.

Use in Pregnancy and Lactation. A definitive link between the tricyclic compounds and tetracyclic compounds and teratogenic effects has not been established, but isolated reports of morphogenesis have been reported. TCAs cross the placenta, and neonatal drug withdrawal can occur. This syndrome includes tachypnea, cyanosis, irritability, and poor sucking reflex. If possible, tricyclic and tetracyclic medications should be discontinued 1 week before delivery. Recently, norepinephrine and serotonin transporters have been identified in the placenta and appear to play an important role in the clearance of these amines in the fetus. The understanding of the effects of reuptake inhibitors on these transporters during pregnancy is limited, but one study compared intelligence and language development in 80 children exposed to TCAs during pregnancy with 84 children exposed to other nonteratogenic agents and found no deleterious effects of the TCAs. The TCAs are excreted in breast milk at concentrations similar to plasma. The actual quantity delivered, however, is small, so drug levels in the infant are usually undetectable or very low. Because the risk of relapse is a serious concern in patients with recurrent depression and these risks may be increased during pregnancy or the postpartum period, the risks and benefits of continuing or withdrawing treatment need to be discussed with the patient and weighed carefully.

Precautions

The TCAs may cause a withdrawal syndrome in newborns, consisting of tachypnea, cyanosis, irritability, and poor sucking reflex. The drugs do pass into breast milk but at concentrations that are usually undetectable in the infant's plasma. The drugs should be used with caution in persons with hepatic and renal diseases. The TCAs should not be administered during a course of electroconvulsive therapy, primarily because of the risk of serious adverse cardiac effects.

DRUG INTERACTIONS

Monoamine Oxidase Inhibitors

The TCAs should not be taken within 14 days of administration of a monoamine oxidase inhibitor.

Antihypertensives

The TCAs block the therapeutic effects of antihypertensive medication. The antihypertensive effects of the β-adrenergic receptor antagonists (e.g., propranolol [Inderal] and clonidine [Catapres]) may be blocked by the TCAs. The coadministration of a TCA and α-methyldopa (Aldomet) may cause behavioral agitation.

Antiarrhythmic Drugs

The antiarrhythmic properties of TCAs can be additive to those of quinidine, an effect that is further exacerbated by the inhibition of TCA metabolism by quinidine.

Dopamine Receptor Antagonists

Concurrent administration of TCAs and DRAs increases the plasma concentrations of both drugs. Desipramine plasma concentrations may increase twofold during concurrent administration with perphenazine (Trilafon). The DRAs also add to the anticholinergic and sedative effects of the TCAs. Concomitant use of serotonindopamine antagonists also increases those effects.

Central Nervous System Depressants

Opioids, alcohol, anxiolytics, hypnotics, and over-the-counter cold medications have additive effects by causing CNS depression when coadministered with TCAs. Persons should be advised to avoid driving or using dangerous equipment if sedated by TCAs.

Sympathomimetics

Tricyclic drug use with sympathomimetic drugs may cause serious cardiovascular effects.

Oral Contraceptives

Birth control pills may decrease TCA plasma concentrations through the induction of hepatic enzymes.

Other Drug Interactions

Nicotine may reduce TCA concentrations. Plasma concentrations may also be lowered by ascorbic acid, ammonium chloride, barbiturates, cigarette smoking, carbamazepine, chloral hydrate, lithium (Eskalith), and primidone (Mysoline). TCA plasma concentrations may be increased by concurrent use of acetazolamide (Diamox), sodium bicarbonate, acetylsalicylic acid, cimetidine, thiazide diuretics, fluoxetine, paroxetine, and fluvoxamine (Luvox). Plasma concentrations of the TCAs may rise three- to fourfold when administered concurrently with fluoxetine, fluvoxamine, and paroxetine.

LABORATORY INTERFERENCES

The tricyclic compounds are present at low concentrations and are not likely to interfere with other laboratory assays. It is possible that they may interfere with the determination of conventional neuroleptic blood concentrations because of their structural similarity and the low concentrations of some neuroleptics.

DOSAGE AND CLINICAL GUIDELINES

Persons who intend to take TCAs should undergo routine physical and laboratory examinations, including a CBC, a white blood cell count with differential, and serum electrolytes with liver function tests. An EKG should be obtained for all persons, especially women older than 40 years of age and men older than 30 years of age. The TCAs are contraindicated in persons with a QT_c greater than 450 ms. The initial dose should be small and should be raised gradually. Because of the availability of highly effective alternatives to TCAs, a newer agent should be used if there is any medical condition that may interact adversely with the TCAs.

Elderly persons and children are more sensitive to TCA adverse effects than are young adults. In children, the EKG should be regularly monitored during use of a TCA.

Table 31–2
General Information for the Tricyclic and Tetracyclic Antidepressants

Generic Name	Trade Name	Usual Adult Dosage Range (mg/day)	Therapeutic Plasma Concentrations (μg/mL)
Imipramine	Tofranil	150–300	150–300^a
Desipramine	Norpramin, Pertofrane	150–300	150–300^a
Trimipramine	Surmontil	150–300	?
Amitriptyline	Elavil, Endep	150–300	100–250^b
Nortriptyline	Pamelor, Aventyl	50–150	50–150^a (maximum)
Protriptyline	Vivactil	15–60	75–250
Amoxapine	Asendin	150–400	?
Doxepin	Adapin, Sinequan	150–300	100–250^a
Maprotiline	Ludiomil	150–230	150–300^a
Clomipramine	Anafranil	130–250	?

^{a}Exact range may vary among laboratories.
^{b}Includes parent compound and desmethyl metabolite.
?, Therapeutic plasma levels unknown.

The available preparations of TCAs are presented in Table 31–1. The dosages and therapeutic blood levels for the TCAs vary among the drugs (Table 31–2). With the exception of protriptyline, all of the TCAs should be started at 25 mg a day and increased as tolerated. Divided doses at first reduce the severity of the adverse effects, although most of the dosage should be given at night to help induce sleep if a sedating drug such as amitriptyline is used. Eventually, the entire daily dose can be given at bedtime. A common clinical mistake is to stop increasing the dosage when the person is tolerating the drug but taking less than the maximum therapeutic dose and does not show clinical improvement. The clinician should routinely assess the person's pulse and orthostatic changes in BP while the dosage is being increased.

Nortriptyline use should be started at 25 mg a day. Most patients need only 75 mg a day to achieve a blood level of 100 mg/nL. However, the dosage may be raised to 150 mg a day if needed. Amoxapine use should be started at 150 mg a day and raised to 400 mg a day. Protriptyline use should be started at 15 mg a day and raised to 60 mg a day. Maprotiline has been associated with an increased incidence of seizures if the dosage is raised too quickly or is maintained at too high a level. Maprotiline use should be started at 25 mg a day and increased over 4 weeks to 225 mg a day. It should be kept at that level for only 6 weeks and then be reduced to 175 to 200 mg a day.

Persons with chronic pain may be particularly sensitive to adverse effects when TCA use is started. Therefore, treatment should begin with low dosages that are raised in small increments. However, persons with chronic pain may experience relief on long-term low-dosage therapy, such as amitriptyline or nortriptyline at 10 to 75 mg a day.

The TCAs should be avoided in children, except as a last resort. Dosing guidelines in children for imipramine include initiation at 1.5 mg/kg a day. The dosage can be titrated to no more than 5 mg/kg a day. In enuresis, the dosage is usually 50 to 100 mg a day taken at bedtime. Clomipramine use can be initiated at 50 mg a day and increased to no more than 3 or 200 mg a day.

When TCA treatment is discontinued, the dosage should first be decreased to three-fourths the maximal dosage for a month. At that time, if no symptoms are present, drug use can be tapered by 25 mg (5 mg for protriptyline) every 4 to 7 days. Slow tapering avoids a cholinergic rebound syndrome consisting of nausea, upset stomach, sweating, headache, neck pain, and vomiting. This syndrome can be treated by reinstituting a small dosage of the drug and tapering more slowly than before. Several case reports note the appearance of rebound mania or hypomania after the abrupt discontinuation of TCA use.

Plasma Concentrations and Therapeutic Drug Monitoring

Clinical determinations of plasma concentrations should be conducted after 5 to 7 days on the same dosage of medication and 8 to 12 hours after the last dose. Because of variations in absorption and metabolism, there may be a 30- to 50-fold difference in the plasma concentrations in persons given the same dosage of a TCA. Nortriptyline is unique in its association with a therapeutic window—that is, plasma concentrations below 50 ng/mL or above 150 ng/mL may reduce its efficacy.

Plasma concentrations may be useful in confirming compliance, assessing reasons for drug failures, and documenting effective plasma concentrations for future treatment. Clinicians should always treat the person and not the plasma concentration. Some persons have adequate clinical responses with seemingly subtherapeutic plasma concentrations, and other persons only respond at supratherapeutic plasma concentrations without experiencing adverse effects. The latter situation, however, should alert the clinician to monitor the person's condition with, for example, serial EKG recordings.

Overdose Attempts

Overdose attempts with TCAs are serious and can often be fatal. Prescriptions for these drugs should be nonrefillable and for no longer than a week at a time for patients at risk for suicide. Amoxapine may be more likely than the other TCAs to result in death when taken in overdose. The newer antidepressants are safer in overdose.

Symptoms of overdose include agitation, delirium, convulsions, hyperactive deep tendon reflexes, bowel and bladder paralysis, dysregulation of BP and temperature, and mydriasis. The patient then progresses to coma and perhaps respiratory depression. Cardiac arrhythmias may not respond to treatment. Because of the long half-lives of TCAs, the patients are at risk of cardiac arrhythmias for 3 to 4 days after the overdose, so they should be monitored in an intensive care medical setting.

32 ▲

Valproate

INTRODUCTION

Originally used as an anticonvulsant, valproate (Depakene, Depakote), or valproic acid, is also approved for the treatment of manic episodes associated with bipolar I disorder and is one of the most widely prescribed mood stabilizers in psychiatry. It has a rapid onset of action and is well tolerated, and numerous studies have found that it reduces the frequency and intensity of recurrent manic episodes over extended periods of time. Even though lithium is still considered as the first-line treatment for bipolar disorder, many patients cannot tolerate lithium or develop renal complications, and valproate is often a good alternative treatment.

CHEMISTRY

Valproate is a simple-chain branch carboxylic acid. It is called valproic acid because it is rapidly converted to the acid form in the stomach. Multiple formulations of valproic acid are marketed. These include valproic acid (Depakene); divalproex sodium (Depakote), an enteric-coated delayed-release 1:1 mixture of valproic acid and sodium valproate available in tablet and sprinkle formulation (can be opened and spread on food); and sodium valproate injection (Depacon). An extended-release preparation is also available. Each of these is therapeutically equivalent because at physiologic pH, valproic acid dissociates into valproate ion.

PHARMACOLOGIC ACTIONS

Regardless of how it is formulated, valproate is rapidly and completely absorbed 1 to 2 hours after oral administration, with peak concentrations occurring 4 to 5 hours after oral administration. The plasma half-life of valproate is 10 to 16 hours. Valproate is highly protein bound. Protein binding becomes saturated at higher dosages, and concentrations of therapeutically effective free valproate increase at serum concentrations above 50 to 100 μg/mL. The unbound portion of valproate is considered to be pharmacologically active and can cross the blood–brain barrier. The extended-release preparation produces lower peak concentrations and higher minimum concentrations and can be given once a day. Valproate is metabolized primarily by hepatic glucuronidation and mitochondrial β oxidation.

The biochemical basis of valproate's therapeutic effects remains poorly understood. Postulated mechanisms include enhancement of γ-aminobutyric acid (GABA) activity, modulation of voltage-sensitive sodium channels, and action on extrahypothalamic neuropeptides.

THERAPEUTIC INDICATIONS

Valproate is currently approved as monotherapy or adjunctive therapy of complex partial seizures, monotherapy and adjunctive therapy of simple and complex absence seizures, and adjunctive therapy for patients with multiple seizures that include absence seizures. Divalproex has additional indications for prophylaxis of migraine.

Bipolar I Disorder

Acute Mania. About two-thirds of persons with acute mania respond to valproate. The majority of patients with mania usually respond within 1 to 4 days after achieving valproate serum concentrations above 50 μg/mL. Antimanic response is generally associated with levels greater than 50 μg/mL, in a range of 50 to 150 μg/mL. Using gradual dosing strategies, this serum concentration may be achieved within 1 week of initiation of dosing, but rapid oral loading strategies achieve therapeutic serum concentrations in 1 day and can control manic symptoms within 5 days. The short-term antimanic effects of valproate can be augmented with addition of lithium, carbamazepine (Tegretol), serotonin–dopamine antagonists (SDAs), or dopamine receptor antagonists (DRAs). Numerous studies have suggested that the irritable manic subtype respond significantly better to divalproex than lithium or placebo. Because of its more favorable profile of cognitive, dermatologic, thyroid, and renal adverse effects, valproate is preferred to lithium for treatment of acute mania in children and elderly persons.

Acute Bipolar Depression. Valproate possesses some activity as a short-term treatment of depressive episodes in bipolar I disorder, but this effect is far less pronounced than for treatment of manic episodes. Among depressive symptoms, valproate is more effective for treatment of agitation than dysphoria. In clinical practice, valproate is most often used as add-on therapy to an antidepressant to prevent the development of mania or rapid cycling.

Prophylaxis. Studies suggest that valproate is effective in the prophylactic treatment of bipolar I disorder, resulting in fewer, less severe, and shorter manic episodes. In direct comparison, valproate is at least as effective as lithium and is better tolerated than lithium. It may be particularly effective in persons with rapid-cycling and ultrarapid-cycling bipolar disorders, dysphoric or mixed mania, and mania caused by a general medical condition as well as in persons who have comorbid substance abuse or panic attacks and in persons who have not had complete favorable responses to lithium treatment.

Schizophrenia and Schizoaffective Disorder

Valproate may accelerate response to antipsychotic therapy in patients with schizophrenia or schizoaffective disorder. Valproate alone is generally less effective in schizoaffective disorder than in bipolar I disorder. Valproate alone is ineffective for treatment of psychotic symptoms and is typically used in combination with other drugs in patients with these symptoms.

Other Mental Disorders

Valproate has been studied for possible efficacy in a broad range of psychiatric disorders. These include alcohol withdrawal and relapse prevention, panic disorder, posttraumatic stress disorder, impulse control disorder, borderline personality disorder, and behavioral agitation and dementia. Evidence supporting use in these cases is weak, and any observed therapeutic effects may be related to treatment of comorbid bipolar disorder.

PRECAUTIONS AND ADVERSE REACTIONS

Although valproate treatment is generally well tolerated and safe, it carries quite a few black-box warnings and other warnings (Table 32–1). The two most serious adverse effects of valproate treatment affect the pancreas and liver. Risk factors for potentially fatal hepatotoxicity include young age (younger than 3 years); concurrent use of phenobarbital; and the presence of neurologic disorders, especially inborn errors of metabolism. The rate of fatal hepatotoxicity in persons who have been treated with only valproate is 0.85 per 100,000 persons; no persons older than the age of 10 years have been reported to have died from hepatotoxicity. Therefore, the risk of this adverse reaction in adult psychiatric patients is low. Nevertheless, if symptoms of lethargy, malaise, anorexia, nausea and vomiting, edema, and abdominal pain occur in a person treated with valproate, the clinician must consider the possibility of severe hepatotoxicity. A modest increase in liver function test results does not correlate with the development of serious hepatotoxicity. Rare cases of pancreatitis have been reported; they occur most often in the first 6 months of treatment, and the condition occasionally results in death. Pancreatic function can be assessed and followed with serum amylase concentrations. Other potentially serious consequences of treatment include hyperammonemia-induced encephalopathy and thrombocytopenia. Thrombocytopenia and platelet

Table 32-1
Black-Box Warnings and Other Warnings for Valproate

More Serious Side Effect	Management Considerations
Hepatotoxicity	Rare, idiosyncratic event Estimated risk: 1:118,000 (adults) Greatest risk profile (polypharmacy, younger than 2 years of age, mental retardation): 1:800
Pancreatitis	Rare, similar pattern to hepatotoxicity Incidence in clinical trial data is 2 in 2,416 (0.0008%) Postmarketing surveillance shows no increased incidence Relapse with rechallenge Asymptomatic amylase not predictive
Hyperammonemia	Rare; more common in combination with carbamazepine (Tegretol) Associated with coarse tremor and may respond to L-carnitine administration
Associated with urea cycle disorders	Discontinue valproate and protein intake Assess underlying urea cycle disorder Divalproex is contraindicated in patients with urea cycle disorders
Teratogenicity	Neural tube defect: 1–4% with valproate Preconceptual education and folate–vitamin B complex supplementation for all young women of childbearing potential
Somnolence in elderly persons	Slower titration than conventional doses Regular monitoring of fluid and nutritional intake
Thrombocytopenia	Decrease dose if clinically symptomatic (i.e., bruising, bleeding gums) Thrombocytopenia more likely with valproate levels ≥110 μg/mL (women) and ≥135 μg/mL (men)

dysfunction occur most commonly at high dosages and result in the prolongation of bleeding times.

USE IN PREGNANCY AND LACTATION

There are multiple concerns regarding the use of valproate during pregnancy. Women who require valproate therapy should therefore inform their physicians if they intend to become pregnant. First trimester use of valproate has been associated with a 3% to 5% risk of neural tube defects, as well as an increased risk of other malformations affecting the heart and other organ systems. Multiple reports have also indicated that in utero exposure to valproate may also negatively affect cognitive development in children of mothers who take valproate during pregnancy. They have lower IQ scores at age 6 compared to those exposed to other antiepileptic drugs. Fetal valproate exposure has dose-dependent associations with reduced cognitive abilities across a range of domains at 6 years of age. Valproate exposure may also increase the risk of autistic spectrum disorder.

Valproate is also associated with teratogenicity, most notably neural tube defects (e.g., spina bifida). The risk is about 1% to 4% of all women who take valproate during the first trimester of the pregnancy. The risk of valproate-induced neural tube defects can be reduced with daily folic acid supplements (1 to 4 mg a day). All women with childbearing potential who take the drug should be given folic acid supplements. Infants breastfed by mothers taking valproate develop serum valproate concentrations 1% to 10% of maternal serum concentrations, but no data suggest that this poses a risk to the infant. Valproate is not contraindicated in nursing mothers. Clinicians should not administer the drug to persons with hepatic diseases. Valproate may be especially problematic for adolescent and young women. Cases of polycystic ovarian disease have been reported in women using valproate. Even when the full syndromal criteria for this syndrome are not met, many of these women develop menstrual irregularities, hair loss, and hirsutism. These effects are thought to result from a metabolic syndrome that is driven by insulin resistance and hyperinsulinemia.

The common adverse effects associated with valproate (Table 32–2) are those affecting the gastrointestinal (GI) system, such as nausea, vomiting, dyspepsia, and diarrhea. The GI effects are generally most common in the first month of treatment, particularly if the dosage is increased rapidly. Unbuffered valproic acid (Depakene) is more likely to cause GI symptoms than the enteric-coated "sprinkle" or the delayed-release divalproex sodium formulations. Other common adverse effects involve the nervous system, such as sedation, ataxia, dysarthria, and tremor. Valproate-induced tremor may respond well to treatment with β-adrenergic receptor antagonists or gabapentin. Treatment of the other neurologic adverse effects usually requires lowering the valproate dosage.

Weight gain is a common adverse effect, especially in long-term treatment, and can best be treated by strict limitation of caloric intake. Hair loss may occur in 5% to 10% of all persons treated, and rare cases of complete loss of body hair have been reported. Some clinicians have recommended treatment of valproate-associated hair loss with vitamin supplements that contain zinc and selenium. Five percent to 40% of persons

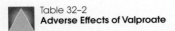

Table 32–2
Adverse Effects of Valproate

Common
  GI irritation
  Nausea
  Sedation
  Tremor
  Weight gain
  Hair loss
Uncommon
  Vomiting
  Diarrhea
  Ataxia
  Dysarthria
  Persistent elevation of hepatic transaminases
Rare
  Fatal hepatotoxicity (primarily in pediatric patients)
  Reversible thrombocytopenia
  Platelet dysfunction
  Coagulation disturbances
  Edema
  Hemorrhagic pancreatitis
  Agranulocytosis
  Encephalopathy and coma
  Respiratory muscle weakness and respiratory failure

GI, gastrointestinal.

experience a persistent but clinically insignificant elevation in liver transaminases up to three times the upper limit of normal, which is usually asymptomatic and resolves after discontinuation of the drug. High dosages of valproate (above 1,000 mg a day) may rarely produce mild to moderate hyponatremia, most likely because of some degree of the syndrome of secretion of inappropriate antidiuretic hormone, which is reversible upon lowering of the dosage. Overdoses of valproate can lead to coma and death.

DRUG INTERACTIONS

Valproate is commonly prescribed as part of a regimen involving other psychotropic agents. The only consistent drug interaction with lithium, if both drugs are maintained in their respective therapeutic ranges, is the exacerbation of drug-induced tremors, which can usually be treated with β-receptor antagonists. The combination of valproate and DRAs may result in increased sedation, as can be seen when valproate is added to any central nervous system (CNS) depressant (e.g., alcohol), and an increased severity of extrapyramidal symptoms, which usually responds to treatment with antiparkinsonian drugs. Valproate can usually be safely combined with carbamazepine or SDAs. Perhaps the most worrisome interaction of valproate and a psychotropic drug involves lamotrigine. Since the approval of lamotrigine for the treatment of bipolar disorder, the likelihood that patients will be treated with both agents has increased. Valproate more than doubles lamotrigine concentrations, increasing the risk of a serious rash (Stevens–Johnson syndrome, and toxic epidermal necrolysis).

Table 32–3
Interactions of Valproate with Other Drugs

Drug	Interactions Reported with Valproate
Lithium	Increased tremor
Antipsychotics	Increased sedation; increased extrapyramidal effects; delirium and stupor (single report)
Clozapine	Increased sedation; confusional syndrome (single report)
Carbamazepine	Acute psychosis (single report); ataxia, nausea, lethargy (single report); may decrease valproate serum concentrations
Antidepressants	Amitriptyline and fluoxetine may increase valproate serum concentrations
Diazepam	Serum concentration increased by valproate
Clonazepam	Absence status (rare; reported only in patients with pre-existing epilepsy)
Phenytoin	Serum concentration decreased by valproate
Phenobarbital	Serum concentration increased by valproate; increased sedation
Other CNS depressants	Increased sedation
Anticoagulants	Possible potentiation of effect

CNS, central nervous system.

The plasma concentrations of carbamazepine, diazepam (Valium), amitriptyline (Elavil), nortriptyline (Pamelor), and phenobarbital (Luminal) may also be increased when these drugs are coadministered with valproate, and the plasma concentrations of phenytoin (Dilantin) and desipramine (Norpramin) may be decreased when they are combined with valproate. The plasma concentrations of valproate may be decreased when the drug is coadministered with carbamazepine and may be increased when coadministered with guanfacine (Tenex), amitriptyline, or fluoxetine (Prozac). Valproate can be displaced from plasma proteins by carbamazepine, diazepam, and aspirin. Persons who are treated with anticoagulants (e.g., aspirin and warfarin [Coumadin]) should also be monitored when valproate use is initiated to assess the development of any undesired augmentation of the anticoagulation effects. Interactions of valproate with other drugs are listed in Table 32–3.

LABORATORY INTERFERENCES

Valproate may cause laboratory increase of serum-free fatty acids. Valproate metabolites may produce a false-positive test result for urinary ketones as well as falsely abnormal thyroid function test results.

DOSAGE AND CLINICAL GUIDELINES

When starting valproate therapy, a baseline hepatic panel, complete blood cell and platelet counts, and pregnancy testing should be ordered. Additional testing should include amylase and coagulation studies if baseline pancreatic disease or coagulopathy is suspected. In addition to baseline laboratory tests, hepatic transaminase concentrations should be obtained 1 month after initiation of therapy and every 6 to 24 months thereafter. However, because even frequent monitoring may not predict serious organ toxicity, it is more prudent to reinforce the need for prompt evaluation of any illnesses when reviewing the instructions with patients. Asymptomatic elevation of transaminase concentrations up to three times the upper limit of normal

Table 32-4
Recommended Laboratory Tests During Valproate Therapy

Before treatment
  Standard chemistry screen with special attention to liver function tests
  CBC, including WBC and platelet count
During treatment
  Liver function tests at 1 month; then every 6-24 months if no abnormalities are found
  Complete blood work with platelet count at 1 month; then every 6-24 months if findings
    are normal
Liver function test results become abnormal
  Mild transaminase elevation (less than three times normal): monitoring every 1-2 weeks; if stable
    and patient is responding to valproate, results are monitored monthly to every 3 months
  Pronounced transaminase elevation (more than three times normal): dosage reduction or
    discontinuation of valproate; increase dose or rechallenge if transaminases normalize and if
    the patient is a valproate responder

CBC, complete blood count; WBC, white blood cell.

are common and do not require any change in dosage. Table 32–4 lists the recommended laboratory tests for valproate treatment.

Valproate is available in a number of formulations (Table 32–5). For treatment of acute mania, an oral loading strategy of initiation with 20 to 30 mg/kg a day can be used to accelerate control of symptoms. This is usually well tolerated but can cause excessive sedation and tremor in elderly persons. Agitated behavior can be rapidly stabilized with intravenous infusion of valproate. If acute mania is absent, it is best to initiate drug treatment gradually to minimize the common adverse effects of nausea, vomiting, and sedation. The dose on the first day should be 250 mg administered with a meal. The dosage can be raised up to 250 mg orally three times daily over the course of 3 to 6 days. The plasma concentrations can be assessed in the morning before the first daily dose is administered. Therapeutic plasma concentrations for the control of seizures range between 50 and 150 μg/mL, but concentrations up to 200 μg/mL are usually well tolerated. It is reasonable to use the same range for the treatment of mental disorders; most of the controlled studies have used 50 to 125 μg/mL. Most persons attain therapeutic plasma concentrations on a dosage between 1,200 and 1,500 mg a day in divided doses. After a person's symptoms are well controlled, the full daily dose can be taken all at once before sleep.

Table 32-5
Valproate Preparations Available in the United States

Generic Name	Trade Name, Form (Doses)	Time to Peak
Valproate sodium injection	Depacon injection (100 mg valproic acid/mL)	1 hour
Valproic acid	Depakene, syrup (250 mg/5 mL)	1-2 hours
	Depakene, capsules (250 mg)	1-2 hours
Divalproex sodium	Depakote, delayed-released tablets (125, 250, 500 mg)	3-8 hours
Divalproex sodium-coated particles in capsules	Depakote, sprinkle capsules (125 mg)	Compared with divalproex tablets, divalproex sprinkle has earlier onset and slower absorption, with slightly lower peak plasma concentration

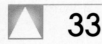 **33**

Nutritional Supplements and Medical Foods

INTRODUCTION

Some of the herbal and dietary supplements that are being marketed today are purported to have psychoactive properties. A number have even shown promise in the treatment of certain psychiatric symptoms. While certain compounds may be beneficial, in many cases the quantity and quality of data have been insufficient to make definitive conclusions. Nevertheless, some patients prefer to use these substances in place of, or in conjunction with, standard pharmaceutical treatments. If electing to use herbal drugs or nutritional supplements, bear in mind that their use may come at the expense of proven interventions and that adverse effects are possible. Though more research is needed, information published to date is still of clinical interest in diagnosing and treating patients who may be taking dietary supplements.

Additionally, herbal and nonherbal supplements may augment or antagonize the actions of prescription and nonprescription drugs. Thus, it is important for clinicians to remain informed on the latest research involving these substances. Because of the paucity of clinical trials, the clinician must be extraordinarily alert to the possibility of adverse effects as a result of drug–drug interactions, especially if psychotropic agents are prescribed, because many phytomedicinals have ingredients that produce physiologic changes in the body.

NUTRITIONAL SUPPLEMENTS

In the United States, the term nutritional supplement is used interchangeably with the term dietary supplement. The Dietary Supplement Health and Education Act (DSHEA) of 1994 defined nutritional supplements as items taken by mouth that contain a "dietary ingredient" meant to supplement the diet. These ingredients may include vitamins, minerals, herbs, botanicals, amino acids, and substances such as enzymes, tissues, glandulars, and metabolites. By law such products must be labeled as supplements and may not be marketed as conventional food.

DSHEA places dietary supplements in a special category and therefore the regulations governing them are more lax than those for prescription and over-the-counter drugs. Unlike pharmaceutical drugs, nutritional supplements are not required to seek the approval of the Food and Drug Administration (FDA), and the FDA does not evaluate their effectiveness. Because dietary supplements are not regulated by the FDA, the contents and quality on store shelves vary dramatically. Contamination, mislabeling, and misidentification of herbs and supplements are important problems. See Table 33–1 for a list of dietary supplements used in psychiatry.

MEDICAL FOODS

In recent years the FDA has introduced a new category of nutritional supplement called "medical foods." According to the FDA, the term medical food, as defined in the

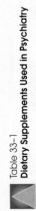

Table 33-1
Dietary Supplements Used in Psychiatry

Name	Ingredients/ What Is It?	Uses	Adverse Effects	Interactions	Dosage	Comments
Docosahexaenoic acid (DHA)	Omega-3 polyunsaturated fatty acid	ADD, dyslexia, cognitive impairment, dementia	Anticoagulant properties, mild GI distress	Warfarin	Varies with indication	Stop using prior to surgery
Choline	Choline	Fetal brain development, manic conditions, cognitive disorders, tardive dyskinesia, cancers	Restrict in patients with primary genetic trimethylaminuria, sweating, hypotension, depression	Methotrexate, works with B₆, B₁₂, and folic acid in metabolism of homocysteine	300–1,200 mg BID doses >3 g associated with fishy body odor	Needed for structure and function of all cells
L-α-Glyceryl-phosphorylcholine (α-GPC)	Derived from soy lecithin	To increase growth hormone secretion, cognitive disorders	None known	None known	500 mg–1 g daily	Remains poorly understood
Phosphatidylcholine	Phospholipid that is part of cell membranes	Manic conditions, Alzheimer's disease, and cognitive disorders, tardive dyskinesia	Diarrhea, steatorrhea in those with malabsorption, avoid with antiphospholipid antibody syndrome	None known	3–9 g/day in divided doses	Soybeans, sunflower, and rapeseed are major sources
Phosphatidylserine	Phospholipid isolated from soya and egg yolks	Cognitive impairment including Alzheimer's disease, may reverse memory problems	Avoid with antiphospholipid antibody syndrome, GI side effects	None known	For soya-derived variety, 100 mg TID	Type derived from bovine brain carries hypothetical risk of bovine spongiform encephalopathy

(continued)

Table 33-1—*continued*
Dietary Supplements Used in Psychiatry

Name	Ingredients/ What Is It?	Uses	Adverse Effects	Interactions	Dosage	Comments
Zinc	Metallic element	Immune impairment, wound healing, cognitive disorders, prevention of neural tube defects	GI distress, high doses can cause copper deficiency, immunosuppression	Bisphosphonates, quinolones, tetracycline, penicillamine, copper, cysteine-containing foods, caffeine, iron	Typical dose 15 mg/day, adverse effects >30 mg	Claims that zinc can prevent and treat the common cold are supported in some studies but not in others; more research needed
Acetyl-L-carnitine	Acetyl ester of L-carnitine	Neuroprotection, Alzheimer's disease, Down's syndrome, strokes, antiaging, depression in geriatric patients	Mild GI distress, seizures, increased agitation in some with Alzheimer's disease	Nucleoside analogs, valproic acid, and pivalic acid-containing antibiotics	500 mg–2 g daily in divided doses	Found in small amounts in milk and meat
Huperzine A	Plant alkaloid derived from Chinese club moss	Alzheimer's disease, age-related memory loss, inflammatory disorders	Seizures, arrhythmias, asthma, irritable bowel disease	Acetylcholinesterase inhibitors and cholinergic drugs	60–200 µg/day	*Huperzia serrata* has been used in Chinese folk medicine for the treatment of fevers and inflammation
NADH (nicotinamide adenine dinucleotide)	Dinucleotide located in mitochondria and cytosol of cells	Parkinson's disease, Alzheimer's disease, chronic fatigue, CV disease	GI distress	None known	5 mg/day or 5 mg BID	Precursor of NADH is nicotinic acid
S-Adenosyl-L-methionine (SAMe)	Metabolite of essential amino acid L-methionine	Mood elevation, osteoarthritis	Hypomania, hyperactive muscle movement, caution in patients with cancer	None known	200–1,600 mg daily in divided doses	Several trials demonstrate some efficacy in the treatment of depression

Name	Description	Uses	Cautions/Adverse effects	Drug interactions	Dosage	Notes
5-Hydroxytryptophan (5-HTP)	Immediate precursor of serotonin	Depression, obesity, insomnia, fibromyalgia, headaches	Possible risk of serotonin syndrome in those with carcinoid tumors or taking MAOIs	SSRIs, MAOIs, methyldopa, St. John's wort, phenoxybenzamine, 5-HT antagonists, 5-HT receptor agonists	100 mg–2 g daily, safer with carbidopa	5-HTP along with carbidopa is used in Europe for the treatment of depression
Folinic acid (Leucovorin)		Depression Prevention of side effects of methotrexate				
Phenylalanine	Essential amino acid	Depression, analgesia, vitiligo	Contraindicated in patients with PKU, may exacerbate tardive dyskinesia or hypertension	MAOIs and neuroleptic drugs	Comes in 2 forms: 500 mg–1.5 g daily for DL-phenylalanine, 375 mg–2.25 g for DL-phenylalanine	Found in vegetables, juices, yogurt, and miso
Myoinositol	Major nutritionally active form of inositol	Depression, panic attacks, OCD	Caution in patients with bipolar disorder, GI distress	Possible additive effects with SSRIs and 5-HT receptor agonists (sumatriptan)	12 g in divided doses for depression and panic attacks	Studies have *not* shown effectiveness in treating Alzheimer's disease, autism, or schizophrenia
Vinpocetine	Semisynthetic derivative of vincamine (plant derivative)	Cerebral ischemic stroke, dementias	GI distress, dizziness, insomnia, dry mouth, tachycardia, hypotension, flushing	Warfarin	5–10 mg daily with food, no more than 20 mg/day	Used in Europe, Mexico, and Japan as pharmaceutical agent for treatment of cerebrovascular and cognitive disorders

(continued)

Table 33-1—continued
Dietary Supplements Used in Psychiatry

Name	Ingredients/ What Is It?	Uses	Adverse Effects	Interactions	Dosage	Comments
Vitamin E family	Essential fat-soluble vitamin, family made of tocopherols and tocotrienols	Immune-enhancing, antioxidant, some cancers, protection in CV disease, neurologic disorders, diabetes, premenstrual syndrome	May increase bleeding in those with propensity to bleed, possible increased risk of hemorrhagic stroke, thrombophlebitis	Warfarin, antiplatelet drugs, neomycin, may be additive with statins.	Depends on form: tocotrienols, 200–300 mg daily with food; tocopherols, 200 mg/day	Stop members of vitamin E family 1 month prior to surgical procedures
Glycine	Amino acid	Schizophrenia, alleviating spasticity, and seizures	Avoid in those who are anuric or have hepatic failure	Additive with antispasmodics	1 g/day in divided doses for supplement; 40–90 g/day for schizophrenia	
Melatonin	Hormone of pineal gland	Insomnia, sleep disturbances, jet lag, cancer	May inhibit ovulation in 1 g doses, seizures, grogginess, depression, headache, amnesia	Aspirin, NSAIDs, β-blockers, INH, sedating drugs, corticosteroids, valerian, kava kava, 5-HTP, alcohol	0.3–3 hs for short periods of time	Melatonin sets the timing of circadian rhythms and regulates seasonal responses
Fish oil	Lipids found in fish	Bipolar disorder, lowering triglycerides, hypertension, decrease blood clotting	Caution in hemophiliacs, mild GI upset, "fishy"-smelling excretions	Coumadin, aspirin, NSAIDs, garlic, ginkgo	Varies depending on form and indication—usually about 3–5 g daily	Stop prior to any surgical procedure

ADD, attention-deficit disorder; CV, cardiovascular; OCD, obsessive-compulsive disorder; GI, gastrointestinal; MAOIs, monoamine oxidase inhibitors; SSRIs, selective serotonin reuptake inhibitors; NSAIDs, nonsteroidal anti-inflammatory drugs; INH, Isoniazid; 5-HTP, 5-hydroxytryptophan; PKU, phenylketonuria. Table by Mercedes Blackstone, MD.

Orphan Drug Act, is "a food which is formulated to be consumed or administered enterally under the supervision of a physician and which is intended for the specific dietary management of a disease or condition for which distinctive nutritional requirements, based on recognized scientific principles, are established by medical evaluation."

A clear distinction can be made between the regulatory classifications of medical foods and dietary supplements. Medical foods must be shown, by medical evaluation, to meet the distinctive nutritional needs of a specific population of patients with a specific disease being targeted. Dietary supplements, on the other hand, are intended for normal, healthy adults and may not require proof of efficacy of the finished product. Medical foods are distinguished from the broader category of foods for special dietary use and from foods that make health claims by the requirement that medical foods are to be used under medical supervision.

Medical foods do not have to undergo premarket approval by FDA. But medical food firms must comply with other requirements, such as good manufacturing practices and registration of food facilities. Medical foods do have some additional regulations that dietary supplements do not because medical foods are intended to treat illnesses. For example, a compliance program requires annual inspections of all medical food manufacturers.

In summary, to be considered a medical food a product must, at a minimum, meet the following criteria: (1) The product must be a food for oral or tube feeding; (2) the product must be labeled for the dietary management of a specific medical disorder, disease, or condition for which there is distinctive nutritional requirements; and (3) the product must be intended to be used under medical supervision. The most common medical foods with psychoactive claims are listed in Table 33–2.

PHYTOMEDICINALS

The term phytomedicinals (from the Greek *phyto,* meaning plant) refers to herb and plant preparations that are used or have been used for centuries for the treatment of a variety of medical conditions. Phytomedicinals are categorized as dietary supplements and not drug products, and are therefore exempt from the regulations that govern prescriptions and over-the-counter medications. Manufacturers of phytomedicinals are not required to provide the FDA with safety information before marketing a product or give the FDA postmarketing safety reports. Thousands of herbal drugs are being marketed today; the most common with psychoactive properties are listed in Table 33–3. Ingredients, to the extent they have been identified, are listed, as indications, adverse events, dosages, and comments, particularly on interactions with commonly prescribed drugs used in psychiatry. For example, St. John's wort (*wort* is an old English word meaning root or herb), which is used to treat depression, decreases the effectiveness of certain psychotropic drugs such as amitriptyline, alprazolam, paroxetine, and sertraline, among others. Kava kava, which is used to treat anxiety states, has been associated with liver toxicity.

Adverse Effects

Adverse effects are possible, and toxic interactions with other drugs may occur with all phytomedicinals, dietary supplements, and medicinal foods. Adulteration is possible, especially with phytomedicinals. There are few or no consistent standard

Table 33–2
Some Common Medical Foods

Medical Food	Indication	Mechanism of Action
Caprylic-triglyceride (Axona)	Alzheimer's disease	Increases plasma concentration of ketones as an alternative energy source in the brain; metabolized in the liver.
L-methylfolate (Deplin)	Depression	Regulates synthesis of serotonin, norepinephrine, and dopamine; adjunctive to SSRIs; 15 mg/day.
S-adenosyl-L-methionine (SAMe)	Depression	Naturally occurring molecule involved in synthesis of hormones and neurotransmitters including serotonin and norepinephrine.
L-Tryptophan	Sleep disturbance Depression	Essential amino acid; precursor of serotonin; reduces sleep latency; usual dose 4–5 g/day.
Omega-3 fatty acid	Depression Cognition	Eicosapentaenoic (EPA) and docosahexaenoic (DHA) acids; direct effect on lipid metabolism; used for augmentation of antidepressant drugs.
Theramine (Sentra)	Sleep disturbances Cognitive enhancer	Cholinergic modulator; increases acetylcholine and glutamate.
N-Acetylcysteine	Depression Obsessive-compulsive disorder	Amino acid that attenuates glutamatergic neurotransmission; used to augment SSRIs.
L-Tyrosine	Depression	Amino acid precursor to biogenic amines epinephrine and norepinephrine.
Glycine	Depression	Amino acid that activates N-methyl-D-aspartate (NMDA) receptors; may facilitate excitatory transmission in the brain.
Citicoline	Alzheimer's disease Ischemic brain injury	Choline donor involved in synthesis of brain phospholipids and acetylcholine; 300–1,000 mg/day; may improve memory.
Acetyl-L-carnitine (Alcar)	Alzheimer's disease Memory loss	Antioxidant that may prevent oxidative damage in the brain.

SSRIs, selective serotonin reuptake inhibitors.

preparations available for most herbs. Medical foods are not tested by the FDA; however, strict voluntary compliance is required. Safety profiles and knowledge of adverse effects of most of these substances have not been studied rigorously, however. Because of the paucity of clinical trials, all of these agents should be avoided during pregnancy; some herbs may act as abortifacients, for example. Because most of these substances or their metabolites are secreted in breast milk, they are contraindicated during lactation.

Clinicians should always attempt to obtain a history of herbal use or the use of medical foods or nutritional supplements during the psychiatric evaluation.

It is important to be nonjudgmental in dealing with patients who use these substances. Many do so for various reasons: (1) As part of their cultural tradition, (2) because they mistrust physicians or are dissatisfied with conventional medicine, or (3) because they experience relief of symptoms with the particular substance. Because patients will be more cooperative with traditional psychiatric treatments if they are allowed to continue using their preparations, psychiatrists should try to keep an open mind and not attribute all effects to suggestion. If psychotropic agents are prescribed, the clinician must be extraordinarily alert to the possibility of adverse effects as a result of drug–drug interactions because many of these compounds have ingredients that produce actual physiologic changes in the body.

Table 33-3

Phytomedicinals with Psychoactive Effects

Name	Ingredients	Use	Adverse Effects[a]	Interactions	Dosage[a]	Comments
Arctic weed, golden root	MAOI and β-endorphin	Anxiolytic, mood enhancer, antidepressant	No side effect yet documented in trials		100 mg BID-200 mg TID	Use caution with drugs that mimic MAOIs
Areca, areca nut, betel nut, L. Areca catechu	Arecoline, guvacoline	For alteration of consciousness to reduce pain and elevate mood	Parasympathomimetic overload: increased salivation, tremors, bradycardia, GI spasms, ulcers of the mouth	Avoid with parasympathomimetic drugs; atropine-like compounds reduce effect	Undetermined; 8–10 g is toxic dose for humans	Used by chewing the nut; used in the past as a chewing balm for gum disease and as a vermifuge; long-term use may result in malignant tumors of the oral cavity
Ashwagandha	Also called Indian Winter Cherry or Indian Ginseng, native to India. Flavonoids	Antioxidant, may decrease anxiety levels. Improved libido in men and women May lower levels of the stress hormone, cortisol	Drowsiness and sleepiness	None	Dosage is 1 tablet twice daily before meals with a gradual increase to 4 tablets per day	None
Belladonna, L. Atropa belladonna, deadly nightshade	Atropine, scopolamine, flavonoids[b]	Anxiolytic	Tachycardia, arrhythmias, xerostomia, mydriasis, difficulties with micturition and constipation	Synergistic with anticholinergic drugs; avoid with TCAs, amantadine, and quinidine	0.05–0.10 mg a day; maximum single dose is 0.20 mg BID	Has a strong smell, tastes sharp and bitter, and is poisonous
Biota, Platycladus orientalis	Plant derivative	Used as a sedative. Other uses are to treat heart palpitations, panic, night sweats, and constipation. May be useful in ADHD	No known adverse effects	None	No clear established doses exist	None

(continued)

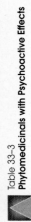

Table 33-3—*continued*
Phytomedicinals with Psychoactive Effects

Name	Ingredients	Use	Adverse Effects[a]	Interactions	Dosage[a]	Comments
Bitter orange flower, *Citrus aurantium*	Flavonoids, limonene	Sedative, anxiolytic, hypnotic	Photosensitization	Undetermined	Tincture, 2-3 g/day; drug, 4-6 g/day; extract, 1-2 g/day	Contradictory evidence; some refer to it as a gastric stimulant
Black cohosh, *L. Cimicifuga racemosa*	Triterpenes, Isoferulic acid	For PMS, menopausal symptoms, dysmenorrhea	Weight gain, GI disturbances	Possible adverse interaction with male or female hormones	1-2 g/day; over 5 g can cause vomiting, headache, dizziness, cardiovascular collapse	Estrogen-like effects questionable because root may act as an estrogen receptor blocker
Black haw, cramp bark, *L. Viburnum prunifolium*	Scopoletin, flavonoids, caffeic acids, triterpenes	Sedative, antispasmodic action on uterus; for dysmenorrhea	Undetermined	Anticoagulant-enhanced effects	1-3 g/day	Insufficient data
California poppy, *L. Eschscholtzia californica*	Isoquinoline alkaloids, cyanogenic glycosides	Sedative, hypnotic, anxiolytic; for depression	Lethargy	Combination of California poppy, valerian, St. John's wort, and passion flowers can result in agitation.	2 g/day	Clinical or experimental documentation of effects is unavailable
Casein	Casein peptides	Used antistress agent. May improve sleep	Usually consumed though milk products. May interact with antihypertensive medicine and lower the blood pressure. May cause drowsiness and should be avoided when taking alcohol or benzodiazepines	None	1-2 tablets once or twice daily	

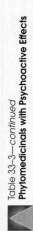

Catnip, L. *Nepeta cataria*	Valeric acid	Sedative, antispasmodic; for migraine	Headache, malaise, nausea, hallucinogenic effects	Undetermined	Undetermined	Delirium produced in children
Chamomile, L. *Matricaria chamomilla*	Flavonoids	Sedative, anxiolytic	Allergic reaction	Undetermined	2–4 g/day	May be GABAergic
Coastal water hyssop		Anxiolytic, sedative, epilepsy, asthma	Mild GI discomfort	May stimulate	300–450 mg QID	Insufficient data
Cordyceps sinensis	A genus of fungi that includes about 400 described species, found primarily in the high altitudes of the Tibetan plateau in China. Antioxidant	Has been used for weakness, fatigue, to improve sexual drive in the elderly	GI discomfort, dry mouth, and nausea	None	Dosage in ranges of 3–6 g daily	None
Corydalis, L. *Corydalis cava*	Isoquinoline alkaloids	Sedative, antidepressant; for mild depression	Hallucination, lethargy	Undetermined	Undetermined	Clonic spasms and muscular tremor with overdose
Cyclamen, L. *Cyclamen europaeum*	Triterpene	Anxiolytic; for menstrual complaints	Small doses (e.g., 300 mg) can lead to nausea, vomiting, and diarrhea	Undetermined	Undetermined	High doses can lead to respiratory collapse
Echinacea, L. *Echinacea purpurea*	Flavonoids, polysaccharides, caffeic acid derivatives, alkamides	Stimulates immune system; for lethargy, malaise, respiratory infections and lower UTIs	Allergic reaction, fever, nausea, vomiting	Undetermined	1–3 g/day	Use in HIV and AIDS patients is controversial; may not be effective in coryza

(continued)

Table 33-3—continued
Phytomedicinals with Psychoactive Effects

Name	Ingredients	Use	Adverse Effects[a]	Interactions	Dosage[a]	Comments
Ephedra, ma-huang *L. Ephedra sinica*	Ephedrine, pseudoephedrine	Stimulant; for lethargy, malaise, diseases of respiratory tract	Sympathomimetic overload: arrhythmias, increased BP; headache, irritability, nausea, vomiting	Synergistic with sympathomimetics, serotonergic agents; avoid with MAOIs	1–2 g/day	Tachyphylaxis and dependence can occur (taken off market)
Ginkgo. L. *Ginkgo biloba*	Flavonoids, ginkgolide A, B	Symptomatic relief of delirium, dementia; improves concentration and memory deficits; possible antidote to SSRI-induced sexual dysfunction	Allergic skin reactions, GI upset, muscle spasms, headache	Anticoagulant: use with caution because of its inhibitory effect on PAF; increased bleeding possible	120–240 mg/day	Studies indicate improved cognition in persons with Alzheimer's disease after 4–5 wks of use, possibly because of increased blood flow
Ginseng. L. *Panax ginseng*	Triterpenes, ginsenosides	Stimulant; for fatigue, elevation of mood, immune system	Insomnia, hypertonia, and edema (called Ginseng abuse syndrome)	Not to be used with sedatives, hypnotic agents, MAOIs, antidiabetic agents, or steroids	1–2 g/day	Several varieties exist; Korean (most highly valued), Chinese, Japanese, American (*Panax quinquefolius*)
Heather, L. *Calluna vulgaris*	Flavonoids, triterpenes	Anxiolytic, hypnotic	Undetermined	Undetermined	Undetermined	Efficacy for claimed uses is not documented
Holy Basil formula. *Ocimum tenuiflorum*	*Ocimum tenuiflorum*, an aromatic plant native to the tropics, part of the Lamiaceae family. Flavonoids	Used to combat stress, also used for common colds, headaches, stomach disorders, inflammation, heart disease	No data exists regarding the long-term effects. May prolong clotting time, increase the risk of bleeding during surgery and lower blood sugar	None	Dosage depends on the formulation type, recommended dose is 2 softgel capsules taken with 8-oz water daily	None

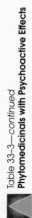

Herb	Constituents	Uses	Adverse effects	Interactions	Dose	Comments
Hops, L. Humulus lupulus	Humulone, lupulone, flavonoids	Sedative, anxiolytic, hypnotic; for mood disturbances, restlessness	Contraindicated in patients with estrogen-dependent tumors (breast, uterine, cervical)	Hyperthermia effects with phenothiazine antipsychotics and with CNS depressants	0.5 g/day	May decrease plasma levels of drugs metabolized by CYP450 system
Horehound, L. Ballota nigra	Diterpenes, tannins	Sedative	Arrhythmias, diarrhea, hypoglycemia, possible spontaneous abortions	May enhance serotonergic drug effects, may augment hypoglycemic effects of drugs	1–4 g/day	May cause abortion
Jambolan, L. Syzygium cumini	Oleic acid, myristic acid, palmitic and linoleic acids, tannins	Anxiolytic, antidepressant	Undetermined	Undetermined	1–2 g/day	In folk medicine, a single dose is 30 seeds (1.9 g) of powder
Kanna, Sceletium tortuosum	Alkaloid, mesembrine	Anxiolytic, mood enhancer, empathogen, COPD treatment	Sedation, vivid dreams, headache	Potentiates cannabis, PDE inhibitor	50–100 mg QID	Insufficient data
Kava kava, L. Piperis methysticum	Kava lactones, kava pyrone	Sedative, hypnotic antispasmodic	Lethargy, impaired cognition, dermatitis with long-term usage, liver toxicity	Synergistic with anxiolytics, alcohol; avoid with levodopa and dopaminergic agents	600–800 mg/day	May be GABAergic; contraindicated in patients with endogenous depression; may increase the danger of suicide
Kratom, Mitragyna speciosa	Alkaloid	Stimulant and depressant	Priapism, testicular enlargement, withdrawal, depression, fatigue, insomnia	Structurally similar to yohimbine	Undetermined	Chewed, extracted into water, tar formulations
Lavender, L. Lavandula angustifolia	Hydroxycoumarin, tannins, caffeic acid	Sedative, hypnotic	Headache, nausea, confusion	Synergistic with other sedatives	3–5 g/day	May cause death in overdose

(continued)

Table 33-3—*continued*
Phytomedicinals with Psychoactive Effects

Name	Ingredients	Use	Adverse Effects[a]	Interactions	Dosage[a]	Comments
Lemon balm, sweet Mary, *L. Melissa officinalis*	Flavonoids, caffeic acid, triterpenes	Hypnotic, anxiolytic, sedative	Undetermined	Potentiates CNS depressant; adverse reaction with thyroid hormone	8-10 g/day	Insufficient data
L-methylfolate	Folate is a B-vitamin found in some foods, needed to form healthy cells, especially red blood cells. L-methylfolate and levomefolate are names for the active form of folic acid.	Adjunctive L-methylfolate is used for major depression, not an antidepressant when used alone. Folate and L-methylfolate are also used to treat folic acid deficiency in pregnancy, to prevent spinal cord birth defects	Gastrointestinal side effects reported	None	15-mg, once a day by mouth with or without food	Considered a "medical food" by the FDA and only available by prescription. Safe to take during pregnancy when used as directed
Mistletoe, *L. Viscum album*	Flavonoids, triterpenes, lectins, polypeptides	Anxiolytic: for mental and physical exhaustion	Berries said to have emetic and laxative effects	Contraindicated in patients with chronic infections (e.g. TB)	10 mg per day	Berries have caused death in children
Mugwort, *L. Artemisia vulgaris*	Sesquiterpene lactones, flavonoids	Sedative, antidepressant, anxiolytic	Anaphylaxis, contact dermatitis, may cause hallucinations	Potentiates anticoagulants	5-15 g/day	May stimulate uterine contractions, can induce abortion

N-acetylcysteine (NAC)	Amino acid	Used as an antidote for acetaminophen overdose, augmentation of SSRIs in the treatment of trichotillomania	Rash, cramps, and angioedema may occur	Activated charcoal, ampicillin, carbamazepine, cloxacillin, oxacillin, nitroglycerin, and penicillin G	1,200–2,400 mg/day	Acts as an antioxidant and a glutamate-modulating agent. When used as an antidote for acetaminophen overdose, the doses 20–40 times higher than those used in OCD trials. It has not been shown to be effective in treating schizophrenia
Nux vomica, L. Strychnos nux vomica, poison nut	Indole alkaloids: strychnine and brucine, polysaccharides	Antidepressant; for migraine, menopausal symptoms	Convulsions, liver damage, death; severely toxic because of strychnine	Undetermined	0.02–0.05 g/day	Symptoms of poisoning can occur after ingestion of one bean; lethal dose is 1–2 g
Oats, L. Avena sativa	Flavonoids, oligo and polysaccharides	Anxiolytic, hypnotic; for stress, insomnia, opium, and tobacco withdrawal	Bowel obstruction or other bowel dysmotility syndromes, flatulence	Undetermined	3 g/day	Oats have sometimes been contaminated with aflatoxin, a fungal toxin linked with some cancers

(continued)

Table 33–3—continued
Phytomedicinals with Psychoactive Effects

Name	Ingredients	Use	Adverse Effects[a]	Interactions	Dosage[a]	Comments
Omega-3 Fatty acid	Comes in three forms, eicosapentaenoic acid (EPA), docosahexaenoic acid (DHA), and alpha-linolenic acid (LNA)	Used as a supplement in the treatment of heart disease, high cholesterol, high blood pressure. May also be helpful in treatment of depression, bipolar disorder, schizophrenia, and ADHD. May reduce the risk of ulcers when used in conjunction with NSAID pain relievers	Can cause gas, bloating, belching, and diarrhea	May increase effectiveness of blood thinners, may increase fasting blood sugar levels when used with diabetes medications such as insulin and metformin.	Doses vary from 1–4 g/day	Can be contaminated with mercury and PCBs
Passion flower, *L. Passiflora incarnata*	Flavonoids, cyanogenic glycosides	Anxiolytic, sedative, hypnotic	Cognitive impairment	Undetermined	4–8 g/day	Overdose causes depression
Phosphatidylserine and Phosphatidylcholine	Phospholipids	Used for Alzheimer's disease, age-related decline in mental function, improving thinking skills in young people, attention-deficit hyperactivity disorder (ADHD), depression, preventing exercise-induced stress, and improving athletic performance	Insomnia and stomach upset	None	100 mg three times daily	None

Polygala	Polygala is a genus of about 500 species of *flowering plants* belonging to the family Polygalaceae, commonly known as milkwort or snakeroot.	Used for insomnia, forgetfulness, mental confusion, palpitation, seizures, anxiety, and listlessness	Contraindicated in patients who have ulcers or gastritis, should not be used long term	None	Dosage of polygala is 1.5–3 g of dried root, 1.5–3 g of a fluid extract or 2.5–7.5 g of a tincture. A polygala tea can also be made, with a maximum of three cups per day.	None
Rehmannia	Iridoid glycosides	Stimulates the release of cortisol. Used in lupus, rheumatoid arthritis (RA), fibromyalgia and multiple sclerosis. May improve asthma and urticaria. Used to treat menopause, hair loss, and impotence	Loose bowel movements, bloating, nausea and abdominal cramps	None	Exact dosage unknown	None
Rhodiola rosea	Potentiator, monoterpene alcohols, flavonoids					

(continued)

Table 33-3—*continued*
Phytomedicinals with Psychoactive Effects

Name	Ingredients	Use	Adverse Effects[a]	Interactions	Dosage[a]	Comments
S-adenosyl methionine (SAMe)	S-adenosyl methionine (SAMe)	Used for arthritis and fibromyalgia, may be effective as an augmentation strategy for SSRI in depression	Gastrointestinal symptoms, anxiety, nightmares, insomnia and worsening of Parkinson's symptoms	Use with SSRIs or SNRIs may result in serotonin syndrome. Interacts with levodopa, meperidine, pentazocine and tramadol	400–1,600 mg/day	A naturally occurring molecule made from the amino acid methionine and ATP; serves as a methyl donor in human cellular metabolism
Scarlet Pimpernel, *L. Anagallis arvensis*	Flavonoids, triterpenes, cucurbitacins, caffeic acids	Antidepressant	Overdose or long-term doses may lead to gastroenteritis and nephritis	Undetermined	1.8 g of powder four times a day	Flowers are poisonous
Skullcap, *L. Scutellaria lateriflora*	Flavonoid, monoterpenes	Anxiolytic, sedative, hypnotic	Cognitive impairment, hepatotoxicity	Disulfiram-like reaction may occur if used with alcohol	1-2 g/day	Little information exists to support the use of this herb in humans
St. John's wort, *L. Hypericum perforatum*	Hypericin, flavonoids, xanthones	Antidepressant, sedative, anxiolytic	Headaches, photosensitivity (may be severe), constipation	Report of manic reaction when used with sertraline (Zoloft); do not combine with SSRIs or MAOIs: possible serotonin syndrome; do not use with alcohol, opioids	100–950 mg/day	Under investigation by the NIH; may act as MAOI or SSRI; 4- to 6-week trial for mild depressive moods; if no apparent improvement, another therapy should be tried
Strawberry leaf, *L. Fragaria vesca*	Flavonoids, tannins	Anxiolytic	Contraindicated with strawberry allergy	Undetermined	1 g/day	Little information exists to support the use of this herb in humans.

Tarragon. L. Artemisia dracunculus	Flavonoids, hydroxycoumarins	Hypnotic, appetite stimulant	Undetermined	Undetermined	Undetermined	Little information exists to support the use of this herb in humans
Valerian. L. Valeriana officinalis	Valepotriates, valerenic acid, caffeic acid	Sedative, muscle relaxant, hypnotic	Cognitive and motor impairment; GI upset, hepatotoxicity; long-term use: contact allergy, headache, restlessness, insomnia, mydriasis, cardiac dysfunction	Avoid concomitant use with alcohol or CNS depressants	1-2 g/day	May be chemically unstable
Wild lettuce, Lactuca Virosa	Flavonoids, coumarins, lactones	Sedative, anesthetic, galactagogue	Tachycardia, tachypnea, visual disturbance, diaphoresis	Undetermined	Undetermined	Bitter taste, added to salad or drinks, active compound closely resembles opium
Winter cherry, Withania somnifera	Alkaloids, steroidal lactones	Sedative, treatment for arthritis, possible anticarcinogenic	Thyrotoxicosis, unfavorable effects on heart and adrenal gland	Undetermined	Undetermined	Smoke inhaled

[a]There are no reliable, consistent, or valid data exist on dosages or adverse effects of most phytomedicinals.

[b]Flavonoids are common to many herbs. They are plant byproducts that act as antioxidants (i.e. agents that prevent the deterioration of material such as DNA via oxidation).

ATP, adenosine triphosphate; BID, twice a day; BP blood pressure; CNS, central nervous system; COPD, chronic obstructive pulmonary disease; GABA, γ-aminobutyric acid; GI, gastrointestinal; MAOI, monoamine oxidase inhibitor; NIH, National Institutes of Health; NSAID, nonsteroidal anti-inflammatory drug; OCD, obsessive-compulsive disorder; PAF, platelet-activating factor; PDE, phosphodiesterase; PMS, premenstrual syndrome; QID, four times a day; SSRI, selective serotonin reuptake inhibitor; TB, tuberculosis; TCA, tricyclic antidepressant; TID, three times a day; UTI, urinary tract infection.

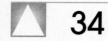

34
Weight Loss Drugs

INTRODUCTION

Obesity is a problem common among persons with mental disorders, either due to poor self-care or as a side effect of psychotropic drug treatment. Not only does obesity adversely affect self-esteem, it can also induce or exacerbate medical conditions such as hypertension, diabetes mellitus, and hyperlipidemia. Effects on body weight and glucose regulation need to be taken into account when selecting medications. Unfortunately, with few exceptions, most psychotropic drugs used to manage mood disorders, anxiety disorders, and psychosis are associated with significant risk of weight gain as a side effect, and are a common cause of treatment refusal or discontinuation. For this and other reasons, it is important for clinicians to be well informed about treatment strategies for mitigating drug-induced weight gain, and obesity in general.

The standard recommendation for weight loss regimens consists of attempting to manage body weight through consistent dietary modifications and regular physical activity. This may be difficult for patients struggling with psychiatric symptoms since their ability to be disciplined in this effort can be compromised by their mental disorder. Also, the physiologic effects of some psychotropic drugs on regulation of satiety and on body metabolism are difficult, if not impossible, to overcome through diet and exercise alone. For these reasons, it may be necessary to use prescription medications to facilitate weight loss.

In this section, drugs used to manage obesity can be categorized in two ways: (1) drugs approved by the FDA as "diet pills"; and (2) drugs with primary indications other than weight loss, but that produce weight loss as a side effect.

DRUGS WITH FDA APPROVAL FOR WEIGHT LOSS

All of the drugs approved by the FDA as weight loss agents are specifically indicated as an adjunct to a reduced calorie diet and increased physical activity for chronic weight management in adult patients with an initial body mass index (BMI) of 30 kg/m^2 or greater (obese), or 27 kg/m^2 or greater (overweight) in the presence of at least one weight-related comorbidity such as hypertension, type 2 diabetes mellitus, or dyslipidemia.

Phentermine

Phentermine hydrochloride is a sympathomimetic amine with pharmacologic activity similar to the amphetamines. It is indicated as a short-term adjunct in a regimen of weight reduction, but in fact, many patients use the drug for extended periods. As with all sympathomimetics, contraindications include advanced arteriosclerosis, cardiovascular disease, moderate to severe hypertension, hyperthyroidism, known hypersensitivity or idiosyncrasy to the sympathomimetic amines, agitated states, and glaucoma.

The drug should be prescribed with caution to patients with a history of drug abuse. Hypertensive crises may result if phentermine is used during or within 14 days following the administration of monoamine oxidase inhibitors (MAOIs). Insulin requirements in diabetes mellitus may be altered in association with the use of phentermine hydrochloride and the concomitant dietary regimen. Phentermine hydrochloride may decrease the hypotensive effect of guanethidine. Phentermine is contraindicated during pregnancy. Studies have not been performed with phentermine hydrochloride to determine the potential for carcinogenesis, mutagenesis, or impairment of fertility.

Phentermine should be taken on an empty stomach, once daily, prior to breakfast. Tablets may be broken or cut in half, but should not be crushed. To avoid disrupting normal sleep patterns, it should be dosed early in the day. If taking more than one dose a day, the last dose should be taken approximately 4 to 6 hours prior to going to bed. The recommended dose of phentermine may be different for different patients. Adults under age 60 taking phentermine using 15- to 37.5-mg capsules should take them once per day before breakfast or 1 to 2 hours after breakfast. Those using 15- to 37.5-mg tablets should take them once per day before breakfast or 1 to 2 hours after breakfast. Instead of taking it once a day, some patients may take 15 to 37.5 mg in divided doses one-half hour before meals. An oral resin formulation is available in 15- and 30-mg capsules, which should be taken once per day before breakfast.

Phentermine/Topiramate Extended Release (Qsymia)

This drug is a combination of phentermine and topiramate (Topamax). It is an extended-release formulation. Both active agents in this formulation are associated with weight loss through separate mechanisms.

Adverse events associated with the use of this drug may include, but are not limited to: parasthesia, dizziness, dysgeusia, insomnia, constipation, dry mouth, kidney stones, metabolic acidosis, and secondary angle closure glaucoma. Use of this drug is associated with a fivefold increased risk of infants with cleft palate and is contraindicated in pregnancy. As a result, it can only be prescribed through certified pharmacies by clinicians who have been certified in the use of this drug.

It is available as a tablet and should be administered once daily in the morning with or without food. Avoid dosing with the drug in the evening due to the possibility of insomnia. The recommended dose is as follows: Start treatment with 3.75 mg/23 mg (phentermine/topiramate extended release) daily for 14 days; after 14 days, increase to the recommended dose to 7.5 mg/46 mg once daily. Evaluate weight loss after 12 weeks of treatment with 7.5 mg/46 mg. If at least 3% of baseline body weight has not been lost on 7.5 mg/46 mg, discontinue the drug or escalate the dose. To escalate the dose, increase to 11.25 mg/69 mg daily for 14 days; followed by dosing 15 mg/92 mg daily. Evaluate weight loss following dose escalation to 15 mg/92 mg after an additional 12 weeks of treatment. If at least 5% of baseline body weight has not been lost on 15 mg/92 mg, discontinue the medication gradually.

Phendimetrazine (Bontril PDM, Adipost, Phendiet, Statobex)

Phendimetrazine is a sympathomimetic amine that is closely related to the amphetamines. It is classified by the DEA as a schedule III controlled substance. It is related chemically and pharmacologically to the amphetamines. Amphetamines and related stimulant drugs have been extensively abused, and the possibility of abuse of phendimetrazine should be kept in mind when evaluating the desirability of including a drug as part of a weight reduction program.

Overall prescribing of this agent is limited. The most commonly used formulation is the 105-mg extended-release capsule, which approximates the action of three 35-mg immediate-release doses taken at 4-hour intervals. The average half-life of elimination when studied under controlled conditions is about 3.7 hours for both the extended-release and immediate-release forms. The absorption half-life of the drug from the immediate-release 35-mg phendimetrazine tablets is appreciably more rapid than the absorption rate of the drug from the extended-release formulation. The major route of elimination is via the kidneys where most of the drug and metabolites are excreted.

Phendimetrazine contraindications are similar to those of phentermine. They include history of cardiovascular disease (e.g., coronary artery disease, stroke, arrhythmias; congestive heart failure, uncontrolled hypertension, pulmonary hypertension); use during or within 14 days following the administration of MAOIs; hyperthyroidism; glaucoma; agitated states; history of drug abuse; pregnancy; nursing; use in combination with other anorectic agents or CNS stimulants and; known hypersensitivity or idiosyncratic reactions to sympathomimetics. Given the lack of systematic research, phendimetrazine should not be used in combination with over-the-counter preparations and herbal products that claim to promote weight loss.

Phendimetrazine tartrate is contraindicated during pregnancy because weight loss offers no potential benefit to a pregnant woman and may result in fetal harm. Studies with phendimetrazine tartrate sustained release have not been performed to evaluate carcinogenic potential, mutagenic potential, or effects on fertility.

Interactions may occur with MAOIs, alcohol, insulin, and oral hypoglycemic agents. Phendimetrazine may decrease the hypotensive effect of adrenergic neuron-blocking drugs. The effectiveness and the safety of phendimetrazine in pediatric patients have not been established. It is not recommended in patients less than 17 years of age.

Adverse reactions reported with phendimetrazine include sweating, flushing, tremor, insomnia, agitation, dizziness, headache, psychosis, and blurred vision. Elevated blood pressure, palpitations, and tachycardia are common. Gastrointestinal side effects include dry mouth, nausea, stomach pain, diarrhea, and constipation. Genitourinary side effects include frequency, dysuria, and changes in libido.

Acute overdose with phendimetrazine may manifest itself by restlessness, confusion, belligerence, hallucinations, and panic states. Fatigue and depression usually follow the central stimulation. Cardiovascular effects include tachycardia, arrhythmias, hypertension or hypotension, and circulatory collapse. Gastrointestinal symptoms include nausea, vomiting, diarrhea, and abdominal cramps. Poisoning may result in convulsions, coma, and death. The management of acute overdose is largely symptomatic. It includes lavage and sedation with a barbiturate. If hypertension is marked, the use of a nitrate or rapid-acting α-receptor–blocking agent should be considered.

Diethylpropion (Tenuate)

Diethylpropion preceded its analog, the antidepressant drug bupropion (Wellbutrin). Diethylpropion comes in two formulations: a 25-mg tablet and a 75-mg extended-release tablet (Tenuate Dospan). It is usually taken three times a day, 1 hour before meals (regular tablets), or once a day in midmorning (extended-release tablets). The extended-release tablets should be swallowed whole, never crushed, chewed, or cut. The maximum daily dose is 75 mg.

Side effects include dry mouth, unpleasant taste, restlessness, anxiety, dizziness, depression, tremors, upset stomach, vomiting, and increased urination. Side effects that warrant medical attention include tachycardia, palpitations, blurred vision, skin rash, itching, difficulty breathing, chest pain, fainting, swelling of the ankles or feet, fever, sore throat, chills, and painful urination. Diethylpropion is pregnancy category B, and has a low-abuse potential. It is listed as a schedule IV drug by the DEA.

Orlistat (Xenical, Alli)

Orlistat interferes with the absorption of dietary fats, causing reduced caloric intake. It works by inhibiting gastric and pancreatic lipases, the enzymes that break down triglycerides in the intestine. When lipase activity is blocked, triglycerides from the diet are not hydrolyzed into absorbable free fatty acids, and are excreted undigested instead. Only trace amounts of orlistat are absorbed systemically; it is almost entirely eliminated through the feces.

The effectiveness of orlistat in promoting weight loss is definite, though modest. When used as part of weight loss program, between 30% and 50% of patients can expect a 5% or greater decrease in body mass. About 20% achieve at least a 10% decrease in body mass. After orlistat is stopped, up to a third of people gain the weight they lose.

Among the benefits of orlistat treatment are a decrease in blood pressure and a reduced risk of developing type 2 diabetes.

The most common subjective side effects of orlistat are gastrointestinal related, and include steatorrhea, flatulence, fecal incontinence, and frequent or urgent bowel movements. To minimize these effects, foods with high fat content should be avoided; a low-fat, reduced calorie diet is advisable. Ironically, orlistat can be used with high-fat content diets to treat constipation that results from treatment with some psychotropic drugs, such as the tricyclic antidepressants. Side effects are most severe when beginning therapy and may decrease in frequency with time. Hepatic and renal injuries are potentially serious side effects of orlistat use. In 2010, new safety information about rare cases of severe liver injury was added to the product label of orlistat. The rate of acute kidney injury is more common among orlistat users than nonusers. It should be used with caution in patients with impaired liver function and renal function, as well as those with an obstructed bile duct and pancreatic disease. Orlistat is contraindicated in malabsorption syndromes, hypersensitivity to orlistat, reduced gallbladder function, and in pregnancy and breastfeeding. Orlistat should not be used during pregnancy.

Absorption of fat-soluble vitamins and other fat-soluble nutrients is inhibited by the use of orlistat. Multivitamin supplements that contain vitamins A, D, E, K, as well as β-carotene should be taken once a day, preferably at bedtime.

Orlistat can reduce plasma levels of the immunosuppressant cyclosporine (Sand-immune), so the two drugs should therefore not be administered concomitantly. Orlistat can also impair absorption of the antiarrhythmic amiodarone (Nexterone).

At the standard prescription dose of 120 mg three times daily before meals, orlistat prevents approximately 30% of dietary fat from being absorbed. Higher doses have not been shown to produce more pronounced effects.

An over-the-counter formulation of orlistat (Alli) is available as 60-mg capsules—half the dosage of prescription orlistat.

Lorcaserin (Belviq)

The exact mechanism of action of lorcaserin is selective activation of 5-HT_{2C} receptors on neurons in the hypothalamus. It promotes weight loss by creating a sense of fullness. In clinical trials, patients taking the drug for 2 years sustained an average weight loss of 12 lb. Belviq should be discontinued if 5% weight loss is not achieved by week 12 of therapy.

Lorcaserin is absorbed from the gastrointestinal tract with peak plasma concentration occurring 1.5 to 2 hours after oral dosing. The absolute bioavailability of lorcaserin has not been determined. Lorcaserin has a plasma half-life of approximately 11 hours; steady state is reached within 3 days after twice-daily dosing, and accumulation is estimated to be approximately 70%. Lorcaserin can be administered with or without food.

Lorcaserin hydrochloride is moderately bound (~70%) to human plasma proteins.

It is extensively metabolized in the liver by multiple enzymatic pathways and the metabolites are excreted in the urine. Lorcaserin and its metabolites are not cleared by hemodialysis. It is not recommended for patients with severe renal impairment (creatinine clearance <30 mL/min) or patients with end-stage renal disease.

The half-life of lorcaserin is prolonged by 59% to 19 hours in patients with moderate hepatic impairment. Lorcaserin exposure (AUC) is approximately 22% and 30% higher in patients with mild and moderate hepatic impairment, respectively. Dose adjustment is not required for patients with mild to moderate hepatic impairment.

No dosage adjustment based on gender is necessary. Gender does not meaningfully affect the pharmacokinetics of lorcaserin. No dosage adjustment is required based on age alone.

Lorcaserin significantly inhibits CYP2D6-mediated metabolism.

Liraglutide Injection (Saxenda)

Saxenda injection 3 mg is a brand of liraglutide indicated as an adjunct to a reduced calorie diet and increased physical activity for chronic weight management in adult patients with an initial BMI of 30 kg/m^2 or greater (obesity) or 27 kg/m^2 or greater (overweight) in the presence of at least one weight-related comorbid condition (e.g., hypertension, type 2 diabetes mellitus, or dyslipidemia).

Saxenda and Victoza both contain the same active ingredient, liraglutide, and therefore should not be used together. Victoza is not indicated for weight loss, but for type 2 diabetes. Saxenda should not be used in combination with any other GLP-1 receptor agonist. Saxenda has not been studied in patients taking insulin. Saxenda and insulin should not be used together. The most common adverse reactions associated with the drug are: nausea, hypoglycemia, diarrhea, constipation, vomiting, headache, decreased appetite, dyspepsia, fatigue, dizziness, abdominal pain, and increased lipase.

The drug may promote thyroid C-cell tumors: If serum calcitonin is measured and found to be elevated, the patient should be further evaluated. Patients with thyroid nodules noted on physical examination or neck imaging should also be further evaluated. Based on spontaneous postmarketing reports, acute pancreatitis, including fatal and nonfatal hemorrhagic or necrotizing pancreatitis, has been observed in patients treated with liraglutide. After initiation of Saxenda, patients should be monitored for signs and symptoms of pancreatitis (including persistent severe abdominal pain, sometimes radiating to the back and which may or may not be accompanied by vomiting). If pancreatitis is suspected, Saxenda should promptly be discontinued and appropriate management should be initiated. If pancreatitis is confirmed, Saxenda should not be restarted. The incidence of acute gallbladder disease is increased in patients treated with Saxenda. Saxenda is contraindicated in pregnancy.

Naltrexone/Bupropion (Contrave)

Contrave is a fixed-dose combination of naltrexone HCl, bupropion HCl 8 mg/90 mg; extended-release tablets. It is indicated as an adjunct to a reduced calorie diet and increased physical activity for chronic weight management in adults with an initial BMI of 30 kg/m^2 or greater (obese) or 27 kg/m^2 or greater (overweight) in the presence of at least one weight-related comorbid condition (e.g., hypertension, type 2 diabetes mellitus, or dyslipidemia). The pill should be swallowed whole and not used with high-fat meals. Dosing should be increased gradually. In those ≥18 years: Week 1: 1 tablet daily in the morning; Week 2: 1 tablet daily in the morning and 1 in the evening; Week 3: 2 tablets in the morning and 1 tablet in the evening; Week 4 and thereafter: 2 tablets in the morning and 2 tablets in the evening. The maximum daily dose is 32 mg/360 mg/day. If after 12 weeks a ≥5% weight loss is not achieved, the drug should be discontinued. With concomitant CYP2B6 inhibitors (e.g., ticlopidine, clopidogrel), moderate or severe renal impairment the maximum dose should be 2 tablets daily (1 tablet each in the morning and evening). With hepatic impairment, 1 tablet in the morning is the maximum dose.

Contrave is not recommended for use during pregnancy. It may harm a fetus. This drug passes into breast milk and is not recommended for use while breastfeeding. Withdrawal symptoms may occur if you suddenly stop taking this medication.

Amphetamine (Evekeo)

Evekeo is an amphetamine, consisting of racemic amphetamine sulfate (i.e., 50% levoamphetamine sulfate and 50% dextroamphetamine sulfate). Amphetamines have long been known to promote weight loss. Curiously, this is the only formulation to have been approved by the FDA for use as a weight loss treatment. Evekeo is available in 5- and 10-mg tablets. Tablets are scored, so they can be split in half. Consult the chapter on psychostimulants for more information on the clinical effects and use of amphetamines.

DRUGS WITHOUT FDA APPROVAL FOR WEIGHT LOSS

Topiramate (Topamax)

Topiramate and the next drug zonisamide are discussed in Chapter 5, but are mentioned here because both agents can have a substantial effect on weight loss.

Topiramate is approved as an antiepileptic drug and for prevention of migraine headaches in adults. The degree of weight loss associated with topiramate may be comparable to the weight loss that other FDA-approved antiobesity drugs induce. Small studies and extensive anecdotal reports indicate that topiramate can help to offset weight gain associated with SSRIs and second-generation antipsychotic drugs. Its impact on body weight may be due to its effects on both appetite suppression and satiety enhancement. These may be the result of a combination of pharmacologic effects including augmenting GABA activity, modulation of voltage-gated ion channels, inhibition of excitatory glutamate receptors, or inhibition of carbonic anhydrase.

The duration and dosage of treatment affect the weight loss benefits of topiramate. Weight loss is higher when the drug is prescribed at doses of 100 to 200 mg/day for more than a month compared with less than a month. In a large study it was shown that compared to those who took placebo, topiramate-treated patients were seven times more likely to lose more than 10% of their body weight. In clinical practice, many patients experience weight loss at a starting dose of 25 mg/day.

The most common side effects of topiramate are paresthesias—typically around the mouth, impaired taste (taste perversion), and psychomotor disturbances, including slowed cognition and reduced physical movements. Impaired concentration and memory impairment, often characterized by word finding and name recall problems, are often reported. Some patients may experience emotional lability and mood changes. Medical side effects include increased risk of kidney stones and acute-angle closure glaucoma. Patients should report any change in visual acuity. Those with a history of kidney stones should be instructed to drink adequate amounts of fluid.

Topiramate is available as 25-, 50- 100-, and 200-mg tablets and as 15-, 25-, and 50-mg capsules.

Zonisamide (Zonegran)

Zonisamide (Zonegran) is a sulfonamide-related drug, similar in many ways to topiramate. Its exact mechanism of action is not known.

Like topiramate, it can cause cognitive problems, but the incidence is lower than that with topiramate.

Zonisamide has been assigned to pregnancy category C. Animal studies have revealed evidence of teratogenicity. Fetal abnormalities or embryo-fetal deaths have been reported in animal tests at zonisamide dosage and maternal plasma levels similar to, or lower than, human therapeutic levels. Therefore, use of this drug in human pregnancy may expose the fetus to significant risks.

The most common side effects include drowsiness, loss of appetite, dizziness, headache, nausea, and agitation/irritability. Zonisamide has also been associated with hypohidrosis. There is between 2% and 4% risk of kidney stones. Other drugs known to provoke stones, such as topiramate or acetazolamide, should not be combined with zonisamide. Serious, but rare, adverse drug reactions include Stevens–Johnson syndrome, toxic epidermal necrolysis, and metabolic acidosis.

Typical dosing for weight loss has not been established. In general, zonisamide is started at 100 mg at night for 2 weeks, and increased by 100 mg daily every 2 weeks to a target dose of 200 to 600 mg/day in 1 or 2 daily doses.

Metformin (Glucophage)

Metformin is a medication for type II diabetes mellitus. Its actions include reduction of hepatic glucose production, reduced intestinal glucose absorption, increased insulin sensitivity, and improved peripheral glucose uptake and regulation. It does not increase insulin secretion.

When used as an adjunct to second-generation antipsychotics, it has consistently been shown to reduce body weight and waist circumference. Metformin probably has the best evidence of therapeutic benefit for the treatment of antipsychotic drug–induced metabolic syndrome. In several studies, metformin has been shown to attenuate or reverse some of the weight gain induced by antipsychotics. The degree of effect on body weight compares favorably with the effect of other treatment options that are approved for weight reduction. The weight loss effect of adjunctive metformin appears to be stronger in drug-naive patients treated with second-generation antipsychotic medications. This effect is most evident for those being treated with clozapine and olanzapine. Based on the existing evidence, if weight gain occurs after second-generation antipsychotic initiation, despite lifestyle intervention, metformin should be considered.

Common side effects include nausea, vomiting, abdominal pain, and loss of appetite. Gastrointestinal side effects can be mitigated by dividing the dose, taking the drug after meals, or using delayed-release formulations.

One serious treatment risk is that of lactic acidosis. This side effect is more common in those with reduced renal function. While very rare (9/100,000 persons/year), it has a 50% mortality rate. Alcohol use along with metformin can increase the risk of acidosis. Renal function monitoring and alcohol avoidance are important.

The weight loss effects of metformin are also evident in chronically ill patients with schizophrenia. Long-term use of metformin appears to be safe and effective.

There is no clearly established dose range for metformin when used as an adjunct for weight loss. In most reports, the usual dose ranged from 500 to 2,000 mg/day. The maximum dose used in treating diabetes is 850 mg three times daily. Patients usually start with a low dose to see how the drug affects them.

Metformin is available in 500-, 850-, and 1,000-mg tablets, all now generic. Metformin SR (slow release) or XR (extended release) is available in 500- and 750-mg strengths. These formulations are intended to reduce gastrointestinal side effects, and to increase patient compliance by reducing pill burden.

Amphetamine

Amphetamine is a psychostimulant approved for the treatment of attention-deficit/hyperactivity disorder and narcolepsy. It has the effect of reducing appetite and has been used off-label for that purpose for many years. Some of the drugs discussed above have amphetamine-like properties which account for their effectiveness. Amphetamines and other psychostimulants are discussed fully in Chapter 29.

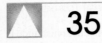 # 35

Medication-Induced Movement Disorders

INTRODUCTION

Medication-induced movement disorders may be associated with the use of psychotropic drugs, most frequently with drugs that block dopamine type 2 (D_2) receptors. Abnormal motor activity may occur with other types of medications as well, including some commonly used drugs that inhibit serotonin reuptake. Sometimes, it can be difficult to determine if abnormal motor movements are an adverse event or a symptom of an underlying disorder. For example, anxiety can resemble akathisia, and alcohol or benzodiazepine withdrawal can cause tremor. The American Psychiatric Association has decided to retain the term *neuroleptic* when discussing side effects associated with drugs used to treat psychosis—the DRAs and second-generation antipsychotics (SGAs). The rationale for continued use of the term is that it was originally used to describe the tendency of these drugs to cause abnormal movements. Based on the specific agent and type of movement disturbance, various strategies are employed to counter these adverse effects.

The most common neuroleptic-related movement disorders are parkinsonism, acute dystonia, and acute akathisia. Neuroleptic malignant syndrome is a life-threatening and often misdiagnosed condition. Neuroleptic-induced tardive dyskinesia is a late-appearing adverse effect of neuroleptic drugs and can be irreversible; recent data, however, indicate that the syndrome, although still serious and potentially disabling, is less pernicious than was previously thought in patients taking DRAs. The newer antipsychotics, the SDAs, block binding to dopamine receptors to a much lesser degree and thereby are presumed to be less likely to produce such movement disorders. Nevertheless, this risk remains and vigilance is still required when these drugs are prescribed.

Table 35–1 lists the selected medications associated with movement disorders and their impact on relevant neuroreceptors.

Neuroleptic-Induced Parkinsonism and Other Medication-Induced Parkinsonism

Diagnosis, Signs, and Symptoms.   Symptoms of neuroleptic-induced parkinsonism and other medication-induced parkinsonism include muscle stiffness (lead pipe rigidity), cogwheel rigidity, shuffling gait, stooped posture, and drooling. The pill-rolling tremor of idiopathic parkinsonism is rare, but a regular, coarse tremor similar to essential tremor may be present. The so-called *rabbit syndrome*, a tremor affecting the lips and perioral muscles, is another parkinsonian effect seen with antipsychotics, although perioral tremor is more likely than other tremors to occur late in the course of treatment.

Table 35-1

Selected Medications Associated With Movement Disorders: Impact on Relevant Neuroreceptors

Type (Subtype)	Name (Brand)	D₂ Blockade	5-HT₂ Blockade	mACh Blockade
Antipsychotics				
Phenothiazine (aliphatic)	Chlorpromazine (Thorazine)	Low	High	High
Phenothiazine (piperidines)	Thioridazine (Mellaril)	Low	Med	High
	Mesoridazine (Serentil)	Low	Med	High
Phenothiazine (piperazines)	Trifluoperazine (Stelazine)	Med	Med	Med
	Fluphenazine (Prolixin)	High	Low	Low
	Perphenazine (Trilafon)	High	Med	Low
Thioxanthenes	Thiothixene (Navane)	High	Med	Low
	Chlorprothixene (Taractan)	Med	High	Med
Dibenzoxazepine	Loxapine (Loxitane)	Med	High	Low
Butyrophenones	Haloperidol (Haldol)	High	Low	Low
	Droperidol (Inapsine)	High	Med	—
Diphenyl-butylpiperidine	Pimozide (Orap)	High	High	Low
Dihydroindolone	Molindone (Moban)	Med	Low	Low
Dibenzodiazepine	Clozapine (Clozaril)	Low	High	High
Benzisoxazole	Risperidone (Risperdal)	High	High	Low
Thienobenzodiazepine	Olanzapine (Zyprexa)	High	High	High
Dibenzothiazepine	Quetiapine (Seroquel)	Low	Low/med	Low
Benzisothiazolinone	Ziprasidone (Geodon)	Low/med	High	Low
Quinolone	Aripiprazole (Abilify)	Med	High	Low
Nonantipsychotic psychotropic	Lithium (Eskalith)	High (as partial agonist)	N/A	N/A
Anticonvulsants		Low	Low	Low
Antidepressants		Low (except amoxapine)	(Varies)	(Varies)
Nonpsychotropics	Prochlorperazine (Compazine)	High	Med	Low
	Metoclopramide (Reglan)	High	High	—

D₂, dopamine type 2; 5-HT₂, 5-hydroxytryptamine type 2; mACh, muscarinic acetylcholine; N/A, not applicable.
Adapted from Janicak PG, Davis JM, Preskorn SH, et al. *Principles and Practice of Psychopharmacotherapy.* 3rd ed. Philadelphia, PA: Lippincott Williams & Wilkins; 2001.

Epidemiology. Parkinsonian adverse effects typically occur within 5 to 90 days of the initiation of treatment. Patients who are elderly and female are at the highest risk for neuroleptic-induced parkinsonism, although the disorder can occur at all ages.

Etiology. Neuroleptic-induced parkinsonism is caused by the blockade of D_2 receptors in the caudate at the termination of the nigrostriatal dopamine neurons. All antipsychotics can cause the symptoms, especially high-potency drugs with low levels of anticholinergic activity, most notably haloperidol (Haldol).

Differential Diagnosis. Included in the differential diagnosis are idiopathic parkinsonism, other organic causes of parkinsonism, and depression, which can also be associated with parkinsonian symptoms. Decreased psychomotor activity and blunted facial expression are symptoms of depression and idiopathic parkinsonism.

Treatment. Parkinsonism can be treated with anticholinergic agents, benztropine (Cogentin), amantadine (Symmetrel), or diphenhydramine (Benadryl) (Table 35–2). Anticholinergics should be withdrawn after 4 to 6 weeks to assess whether tolerance to the parkinsonian effects has developed; about half of patients with neuroleptic-induced parkinsonism require continued treatment. Even after the antipsychotics are withdrawn, parkinsonian symptoms can last up to 2 weeks and even up to 3 months

Table 35–2
Drug Treatments of Extrapyramidal Disorders

Generic Name	Trade Name	Usual Daily Dosage	Indications
Anticholinergics			
Benztropine	Cogentin	PO 0.5–2 mg TID; IM or IV 1–2 mg	Acute dystonia, parkinsonism, akinesia, akathisia
Biperiden	Akineton	PO 2–6 mg TID; IM or IV 2 mg	
Procyclidine	Kemadrin	PO 2.5–5 mg BID–QID	
Trihexyphenidyl	Artane, Tremin	PO 2–5 mg TID	
Orphenadrine	Norflex, Disipal	PO 50–100 mg BID-QID; IV 60 mg	Rabbit syndrome
Antihistamine			
Diphenhydramine	Benadryl	PO 25 mg QID; IM or IV 25 mg	Acute dystonia, parkinsonism, akinesia, rabbit syndrome
Amantadine	Symmetrel	PO 100–200 mg BID	Parkinsonism, akinesia, rabbit syndrome
β-Adrenergic antagonist			
Propranolol	Inderal	PO 20–40 mg TID	Akathisia, tremor
α-Adrenergic antagonist			
Clonidine	Catapres	PO 0.1 mg TID	Akathisia
Benzodiazepines			
Clonazepam	Klonopin	PO 1 mg BID	Akathisia, acute dystonia
Lorazepam	Ativan	PO 1 mg TID	
Buspirone	BuSpar	PO 20–40 mg QID	Tardive dyskinesia
Vitamin E	—	PO 1,200–1,600 IU/day	Tardive dyskinesia

PO, orally; IM, intramuscularly; IV, intravenously; BID, twice a day; TID, three times a day; QID, four times a day.

in elderly patients. With such patients, the clinician may continue the anticholinergic drug after the antipsychotic has been stopped until the parkinsonian symptoms resolve completely.

Neuroleptic Malignant Syndrome

Diagnosis, Signs, and Symptoms. *Neuroleptic malignant syndrome* is a life-threatening complication that can occur anytime during the course of antipsychotic treatment. The motor and behavioral symptoms include muscular rigidity and dystonia, akinesia, mutism, obtundation, and agitation. The autonomic symptoms include hyperthermia, diaphoresis, and increased pulse and BP. Laboratory findings include an increased white blood cell (WBC) count and increased levels of creatinine phosphokinase, liver enzymes, plasma myoglobin, and myoglobinuria, occasionally associated with renal failure.

Epidemiology. About 0.01% to 0.02% of patients treated with antipsychotics develop neuroleptic malignant syndrome. Men are affected more frequently than women, and young patients are affected more commonly than elderly patients. The mortality rate can reach 10% to 20% or even higher when depot antipsychotic medications are involved.

Course and Prognosis. The symptoms usually evolve over 24 to 72 hours, and the untreated syndrome lasts 10 to 14 days. The diagnosis is often missed in the early stages, and the withdrawal or agitation may mistakenly be considered to reflect an exacerbation of the psychosis.

Treatment. In addition to supportive medical treatment, the most commonly used medications for the condition are dantrolene (Dantrium) and bromocriptine (Parlodel), although amantadine (Symmetrel) is sometimes used. Bromocriptine and amantadine pose direct DRA effects and may serve to overcome the antipsychotic-induced dopamine receptor blockade. The lowest effective dosage of the antipsychotic drug should be used to reduce the chance of neuroleptic malignant syndrome. High-potency drugs, such as haloperidol, pose the greatest risk. Antipsychotic drugs with anticholinergic effects seem less likely to cause neuroleptic malignant syndrome. ECT has been used. Table 35–3 summarizes treatments for neuroleptic malignant syndrome.

Medication-Induced Acute Dystonia

Diagnosis, Signs, and Symptoms. *Dystonias* are brief or prolonged contractions of muscles that result in obviously abnormal movements or postures, including oculogyric crises, tongue protrusion, trismus, torticollis, laryngeal–pharyngeal dystonias, and dystonic postures of the limbs and trunk. Other dystonias include blepharospasm and glossopharyngeal dystonia; the latter results in dysarthria, dysphagia, and even difficulty in breathing, which can cause cyanosis. Children are particularly likely to evidence opisthotonos, scoliosis, lordosis, and writhing movements. Dystonia can be painful and frightening and often results in noncompliance with future drug treatment regimens.

Table 35–3
Treatment of Neuroleptic Malignant Syndrome

Intervention	Dosing	Effectiveness
Amantadine	200–400 mg PO/day in divided doses	Beneficial as monotherapy or in combination; decrease in death rate
Bromocriptine	2.5 mg PO BID or TID, may increase to a total of 45 mg/day	Mortality reduced as a single or combined agent
Levodopa/carbidopa	Levodopa 50–100 mg/day IV as continuous infusion	Case reports of dramatic improvement
Electroconvulsive therapy	Reports of good outcome with both unilateral and bilateral treatments; response may occur in as few as three treatments	Effective when medications have failed; may also treat underlying psychiatric disorder
Dantrolene	1 mg/kg/day for 8 days, then continue as PO for 7 additional days	Benefits may occur in minutes or hours as a single agent or in combination
Benzodiazepines	1–2 mg IM as test dose; if effective, switch to PO; consider use if underlying disorder has catatonic symptoms	Has been reported effective when other agents have failed
Supportive measures	IV hydration, cooling blankets, ice packs, ice water enema, oxygenation, antipyretics	Often effective as initial approach early in the episode

PO, orally; BID, twice a day; TID, three times a day; IV, intravenously; IM, intramuscularly.
Adapted from Davis JM, Caroff SN, Mann SC. Treatment of neuroleptic malignant syndrome. *Psychiatr Ann.* 2000;30:325–331.

Epidemiology. The development of acute dystonic symptoms is characterized by their early onset during the course of treatment with neuroleptics. There is a higher incidence of acute dystonia in men, in patients younger than age 30 years, and in patients given high dosages of high-potency medications.

Etiology. Although it is most common with intramuscular (IM) doses of high-potency antipsychotics, dystonia can occur with any antipsychotic. The mechanism of action is thought to be dopaminergic hyperactivity in the basal ganglia that occurs when CNS levels of the antipsychotic drug begin to fall between doses.

Differential Diagnosis. The differential diagnosis includes seizures and tardive dyskinesia.

Course and Prognosis. Dystonia can fluctuate spontaneously and respond to reassurance, so the clinician gets the false impression that the movement is hysterical or completely under conscious control.

Treatment. Prophylaxis with anticholinergics or related drugs usually prevents dystonia, although the risks of prophylactic treatment weigh against that benefit. Treatment with IM anticholinergics or intravenous or IM diphenhydramine (Benadryl) (50 mg) almost always relieves the symptoms. Diazepam (Valium) (10 mg intravenously), amobarbital (Amytal), caffeine sodium benzoate, and hypnosis have also been reported to be effective. Although tolerance for the adverse effects usually develops, it is prudent to change the antipsychotic if the patient is particularly concerned that the reaction may recur.

Medication-Induced Acute Akathisia

Diagnosis, Signs, and Symptoms. *Akathisia* is subjective feelings of restlessness, objective signs of restlessness, or both. Examples include a sense of anxiety, inability to relax, jitteriness, pacing, rocking motions while sitting, and rapid alternation of sitting and standing. Akathisia has been associated with the use of a wide range of psychiatric drugs, including antipsychotics, antidepressants, and sympathomimetics. Once akathisia is recognized and diagnosed, the antipsychotic dose should be reduced to the minimal effective level. Akathisia may be associated with a poor treatment outcome.

Epidemiology. Middle-aged women are at increased risk of akathisia, and the time course is similar to that for neuroleptic-induced parkinsonism.

Treatment. Three basic steps in the treatment of akathisia are reducing medication dosage, attempting treatment with appropriate drugs, and considering changing the neuroleptic. The most efficacious drugs are β-adrenergic receptor antagonists, although anticholinergic drugs, benzodiazepines, and cyproheptadine (Periactin) may benefit some patients. In some cases of akathisia, no treatment seems to be effective.

Tardive Dyskinesia

Diagnosis, Signs, and Symptoms. *Tardive dyskinesia* is a delayed effect of antipsychotics; it rarely occurs until after 6 months of treatment. The disorder consists of abnormal, involuntary, irregular choreoathetoid movements of the muscles of the head, limbs, and trunk. The severity of the movements ranges from minimal—often missed by patients and their families—to grossly incapacitating. Perioral movements are the most common and include darting, twisting, and protruding movements of the tongue; chewing and lateral jaw movements; lip puckering; and facial grimacing. Finger movements and hand clenching are also common. Torticollis, retrocollis, trunk twisting, and pelvic thrusting occur in severe cases. In the most serious cases, patients may have breathing and swallowing irregularities that result in aerophagia, belching, and grunting. Respiratory dyskinesia has also been reported. Dyskinesia is exacerbated by stress and disappears during sleep.

Epidemiology. Tardive dyskinesia develops in about 10% to 20% of patients who are treated for more than a year. About 20% to 40% of patients who require long-term hospitalization have tardive dyskinesia. Women are more likely to be affected than men. Children, patients who are more than 50 years of age, and patients with brain damage or mood disorders are also at high risk.

Course and Prognosis. Between 5% and 40% of all cases of tardive dyskinesia eventually remit, and between 50% and 90% of all mild cases remit. Tardive dyskinesia is less likely to remit in elderly patients than in young patients, however.

Treatment. The three basic approaches to tardive dyskinesia are prevention, diagnosis, and management. Prevention is best achieved by using antipsychotic medications only when clearly indicated and in the lowest effective doses. The atypical antipsychotics are associated with less tardive dyskinesia than the older antipsychotics. Clozapine (Clozaril) is the only antipsychotic to have minimal risk of tardive dyskinesia and can even help improve pre-existing symptoms of tardive dyskinesia. This has been attributed to its low affinity for D_2 receptors and high affinity for 5-hydroxytryptamine (5-HT) receptor antagonism. Patients who are receiving antipsychotics should be examined regularly for the appearance of abnormal movements, preferably with the use of a standardized rating scale. Patients frequently experience an exacerbation of their symptoms when the DRA is withheld or its dose is lowered, whereas substitution of an SDA may limit the abnormal movements without worsening the progression of the dyskinesia.

Once tardive dyskinesia is recognized, the clinician should consider reducing the dose of the antipsychotic or even stopping the medication altogether. Alternatively, the clinician may switch the patient to clozapine or to one of the new SDAs. In patients who cannot continue taking any antipsychotic medication, lithium (Eskalith), carbamazepine (Tegretol), or benzodiazepines may effectively reduce the symptoms of both the movement disorder and the psychosis.

In 2017, the FDA-approved valbenazine (Ingrezza) as the first drug approved to treat adults with tardive dyskinesia. Valbenazine inhibits the vesicular monoamine transporter 2 (VMAT2), which results in reversible reduction of dopamine release. Since tardive dyskinesia is believed to be associated with dopamine hypersensitivity, the reduction in levels of available dopamine in the synaptic cleft alleviate symptoms of the disorder. It is available as a 40-mg capsule. The initial dose is 40 mg once daily. After 1 week, increase the dose to the recommended dose of 80 mg once daily. It can be taken with or without food. The recommended dose for patients with moderate or severe hepatic impairment is 40 mg once daily. Consider dose reduction based on tolerability in known CYP2D6 poor metabolizers. There are no absolute contraindications, but its use should be avoided in patients with congenital or drug-induced long QT syndrome or with abnormal heartbeats associated with a prolonged QT interval. Serious side effects include sleepiness and QT prolongation. Patients taking valbenazine should not drive or operate heavy machinery or do other dangerous activities until it is known how the drug affects them. Valbenazine may interact with monoamine oxidase inhibitors (MAOIs), itraconazole, ketoconazole, clarithromycin, paroxetine, fluoxetine, quinidine, rifampin, carbamazepine, phenytoin, St. John's wort, and digoxin.

Tardive Dystonia and Tardive Akathisia
On occasion, dystonia and akathisia emerge late in the course of treatment. These symptoms may persist for months or years despite drug discontinuation or dose reduction.

Medication-Induced Postural Tremor
Diagnosis, Signs, and Symptoms. *Tremor* is a rhythmic alteration in movement that is usually faster than 1 beat/s. Fine tremor (8 to 12 Hz) is most common.

Epidemiology. Typically, tremors decrease during periods of relaxation and sleep and increase with stress or anxiety.

Table 35-4
Drug-Induced Central Hyperthermic Syndromes[a]

Condition (and Mechanism)	Common Drug Causes	Frequent Symptoms	Possible Treatment[b]	Clinical Course
Hyperthermia (↓ heat dissipation) (↑ heat production)	Atropine, lidocaine, meperidine NSAID toxicity, pheochromocytoma, thyrotoxicosis	Hyperthermia, diaphoresis, malaise	Acetaminophen per rectum (325 mg every 4 hours), diazepam oral or per rectum (5 mg every 8 hours) for febrile seizures	Benign; febrile seizures in children
Malignant hyperthermia (↑ heat production)	NMJ blockers (succinylcholine), halothane	Hyperthermia muscle rigidity, arrhythmias, ischemia, hypotension,[c] rhabdomyolysis; disseminated intravascular coagulation	Dantrolene sodium (1–2 mg/kg/min IV infusion)[d]	Familial; 10% mortality if untreated
Tricyclic overdose (↑ heat production)	Tricyclic antidepressants, cocaine	Hyperthermia, confusion, visual hallucinations, agitation, hyperreflexia, muscle relaxation, anticholinergic effects (dry skin, pupil dilation), arrhythmias	Sodium bicarbonate (1 mEq/kg IV bolus) if arrhythmia is present, physostigmine (1–3 mg IV) with cardiac monitoring	Fatalities have occurred if untreated
Autonomic hyperreflexia (↑ heat production)	CNS stimulants (amphetamines)	Hyperthermia, excitement, hyperreflexia	Trimethaphan (0.3–7 mg/min IV infusion)	Reversible
Lethal catatonia (↓ heat dissipation)	Lead poisoning	Hyperthermia, intense anxiety, destructive behavior, psychosis	Lorazepam (1–2 mg IV every 4 hours), antipsychotics may be contraindicated	High mortality if untreated
Neuroleptic malignant syndrome (mixed; hypothalamic, ↓ heat dissipation, ↑ heat production)	Antipsychotics (neuroleptics), methyldopa, reserpine	Hyperthermia, muscle rigidity, diaphoresis (60%), leukocytosis, delirium, rhabdomyolysis, elevated CPK, autonomic deregulation, extrapyramidal symptoms	Bromocriptine (2–10 mg every 8 hours orally or nasogastric tube), lisuride (0.02–0.1 mg/hr IV infusion), carbidopa-levodopa (Sinemet) (25/100 PO every 8 hours), dantrolene sodium (0.3–1 mg/kg IV every 6 hours)	Rapid onset, 20% mortality if untreated

[a]Boldface indicates features that may be used to distinguish one syndrome from another.
[b]Gastric lavage and supportive measures, including cooling, are required in most cases.
[c]Oxygen consumption increases by 7% for every 1°F increase in body temperature.
[d]Has been associated with idiosyncratic hepatocellular injury, as well as severe hypotension in one case.
NSAID, nonsteroidal anti-inflammatory drug; NMJ, neuromuscular junction; CNS, central nervous system; CPK, creatine phosphokinase; PO, orally; IV, intravenously.
From Theocharides TC, Harris RS, Weckstein D. Neuroleptic malignant-like syndrome due to cyclobenzaprine? *J Clin Psychopharmacol.* 1995;15:79–81, with permission.

Etiology. Whereas all the above diagnoses specifically include an association with a neuroleptic, a range of psychiatric medications can produce tremor—most notably, lithium, stimulants, antidepressants, caffeine, and valproic acid (Depakene).

Treatment. The treatment involves four principles:

1. The lowest possible dose of the psychiatric drug should be taken.
2. Patients should minimize caffeine consumption.
3. The psychiatric drug should be taken at bedtime to minimize the amount of daytime tremor.
4. β-Adrenergic receptor antagonists (e.g., propranolol [Inderal]) can be given to treat drug-induced tremors.

Other Medication-Induced Movement Disorders

Periodic Limb Movement Disorder. *Periodic Limb Movement Disorder (PLMD)*, formerly called nocturnal myoclonus, consists of highly stereotyped, abrupt contractions of certain leg, and occasionally of upper extremity muscles during sleep. Patients lack any subjective awareness of the leg jerks. The condition may be present in about 40% of persons over 65 years of age. The cause is unknown, but it is a rare side effect of SSRIs.

The repetitive movements occur every 20 to 60 seconds, most commonly with extensions of the large toe and flexion of the ankle, the knee, and the hips. Frequent awakenings, unrefreshing sleep, and daytime sleepiness are major symptoms. No treatment for nocturnal myoclonus is universally effective. Treatments that may be useful include benzodiazepines, levodopa (Larodopa), quinine, and, in rare cases, opioids.

Restless Legs Syndrome. In *restless legs syndrome*, persons feel deep sensations of creeping inside the calves whenever sitting or lying down. The dysesthesias are rarely painful but are agonizingly relentless and cause an almost irresistible urge to move the legs; thus, this syndrome interferes with sleep and with falling asleep. It peaks in middle age and occurs in 5% of the population. The cause is unknown, but it is a rare side effect of SSRIs.

Symptoms are relieved by movement and by leg massage. The dopamine receptor agonists, ropinirole (Requip) and pramipexole (Mirapex), are effective in treating this syndrome. Other treatments include the benzodiazepines, levodopa, quinine, opioids, propranolol, valproate, and carbamazepine.

Hyperthermic Syndromes

All the medication-induced movement disorders may be associated with hyperthermia. Table 35–4 summarizes the drugs associated with hyperthermia, possible mechanisms as well their symptoms, treatments, and their clinical course.

Index

Note: Page number followed by f and t indicates figure and table, respectively.

About the Authors

BENJAMIN JAMES SADOCK, M.D., is the Menas S. Gregory Professor of Psychiatry in the Department of Psychiatry at the New York University (NYU) School of Medicine, New York, New York. He is a graduate of Union College, received his M.D. degree from New York Medical College, and completed his internship at Albany Hospital. After finishing his residency at Bellevue Psychiatric Hospital, he entered military service, serving as Acting Chief of Neuropsychiatry at Sheppard Air Force Base, Wichita Falls, Texas. He has held faculty and teaching appointments at Southwestern Medical School and Parkland Hospital in Dallas and at New York Medical College, St. Luke's Hospital, the New York State Psychiatric Institute, and Metropolitan Hospital in New York. Dr. Sadock joined the faculty of the NYU School of Medicine in 1980 and served in various positions: Director of Medical Student Education in Psychiatry, Co-Director of the Residency Training Program in Psychiatry, and Director of Graduate Medical Education, and is currently the Administrative Psychiatrist to the NYU School of Medicine. He is on the staff of Bellevue Hospital and Tisch Hospital and is a Diplomate of the American Board of Psychiatry and Neurology and served as an Associate Examiner for the Board for more than a decade. He is a Distinguished Life Fellow of the American Psychiatric Association, a Fellow of the American College of Physicians, a Fellow of the New York Academy of Medicine, and a member of Alpha Omega Alpha Honor Society. He is active in numerous psychiatric organizations and is founder and president of the NYU-Bellevue Psychiatric Society. Dr. Sadock was a member of the National Committee in Continuing Education in Psychiatry of the American Psychiatric Association; he served on the Ad Hoc Committee on Sex Therapy Clinics of the American Medical Association, was a delegate to the conference on Recertification of the American Board of Medical Specialists, and was a representative of the American Psychiatric Association Task Force on the National Board of Medical Examiners and the American Board of Psychiatry and Neurology. In 1985, he received the Academic Achievement Award from New York Medical College and was appointed Faculty Scholar at NYU School of Medicine in 2000. He is the author or editor of more than 50 books, is a book reviewer for psychiatric journals, and lectures on a broad range of topics in general psychiatry. Dr. Sadock maintains a private practice for diagnostic consultations and psychiatric treatment. He has been married to Virginia Alcott Sadock, M.D., Professor of Psychiatry at NYU School of Medicine, since completing his residency. Dr. Sadock enjoys opera, golf, traveling, and is an enthusiastic fly fisherman.

NORMAN SUSSMAN, M.D., is Professor of Psychiatry at the New York University (NYU) School of Medicine. A graduate of Queens College in New York, Dr. Sussman obtained a master's degree from the NYU Graduate School of Public Administration, where he majored in health care administration. He received his M.D. from New York Medical College and completed his residency in psychiatry at Metropolitan Hospital and Westchester County Medical Center. He joined the faculty at NYU

School of Medicine in 1980 and served both as director of inpatient psychiatry at Tisch Hospital—the University Hospital of NYU Medical Center—and director of residency training in psychiatry. Most recently Dr. Sussman served as Interim Chair of the Department of Psychiatry at the NYU Langone Medical Center. He developed one of the first university-based review courses in general psychiatry and in psychopharmacology and is committed to the continuing education of both psychiatric and nonpsychiatric physicians in the rapidly changing field of psychopharmacology. Dr. Sussman served on the American Psychiatric Association's Task Force for the development of the American Psychiatric Association's *Diagnostic and Statistical Manual of Mental Disorders*, 3rd edition (DSM-III), and helped develop the criteria for Factitious and Somatoform Disorders. He is a Distinguished Fellow of the American Psychiatric Association, and he received that organization's Certificate of Recognition for Excellence in Medical Student Education. Dr. Sussman has been an investigator for over 30 clinical trials involving treatment for anxiety and mood disorders. He writes and lectures extensively on psychopharmacology both in this country and around the world. Dr. Sussman has been a contributing editor and section editor in the area of psychopharmacology through several editions of *Kaplan & Sadock's Comprehensive Textbook of Psychiatry*. He and his wife, Susan, live in Hudson River Valley, New York, and have two children, Rebecca and Zachary. Dr. Sussman paints in his spare time and vacations with family in Bozeman, Montana.

VIRGINIA ALCOTT SADOCK, M.D., joined the faculty of the NYU School of Medicine in 1980, where she is currently the Professor of Psychiatry and Attending Psychiatrist at the Tisch Hospital and Bellevue Hospital. She is the Director of the Program in Human Sexuality at the NYU Medical Center, one of the largest treatment and training programs of its kind in the United States. Dr. Sadock is the author of more than 50 articles and chapters on sexual behavior and was the Developmental Editor of *The Sexual Experience*, one of the first major textbooks on human sexuality, published by Williams & Wilkins. She serves as a referee and book reviewer for several medical journals, including the *American Journal of Psychiatry* and the *Journal of the American Medical Association*. She has long been interested in the role of women in medicine and psychiatry and was a founder of the Committee on Women in Psychiatry of the New York County District Branch of the American Psychiatric Association. She is active in academic matters, and served as an Assistant and Associate Examiner for the American Board of Psychiatry and Neurology for more than 15 years; and was a member of the Test Committee in Psychiatry for both the American Board of Psychiatry and the Psychiatric Knowledge and Self-Assessment Program (PKSAP) of the American Psychiatric Association. She has chaired the Committee on Public Relations of the New York County District Branch of the American Psychiatric Association and has participated in the National Medical Television Network series *Women in Medicine* and the Emmy Award-winning PBS television documentary *Women and Depression*. She hosts a weekly radio program on Sirius-XM called *Sexual Health and Well-Being*. Dr. Sadock has been the Vice-President of the Society of Sex Therapy and Research and a regional council member of the American Association of Sex Education Counselors and Therapists; she is currently the President of the Alumni Association of Sex Therapists of NYU

Langone Medical Center. She lectures extensively in the United States and abroad on sexual dysfunction, relational problems, and depression and anxiety disorders. She is a Distinguished Fellow of the American Psychiatric Association, a Fellow of the New York Academy of Medicine, and a Diplomate of the American Board of Psychiatry and Neurology. Dr. Sadock is a graduate of Bennington College; she received her M.D. degree from New York Medical College, and trained in psychiatry at Metropolitan Hospital. She maintains an active practice that includes individual psychotherapy, couples and marital therapy, sex therapy, psychiatric consultation, and pharmacotherapy. She lives in Manhattan with her husband Dr. Benjamin Sadock. They have two children, James William Sadock, M.D. and Victoria Anne Gregg, M.D., both emergency physicians, and four grandchildren, Emily, Celia, Oliver, and Joel. In her leisure time, Dr. Sadock enjoys theater, film, golf, reading fiction, and traveling.

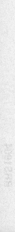